Tina Joyce

W9-CFX-651

Becoming a Clinician

A Primer for Students

Notice

Medicine is an ever-changing science. As new research and clinical experience broaden our knowledge, changes in treatment and drug therapy are required. The editors and the publisher of this work have checked with sources believed to be reliable in their efforts to provide information that is complete and generally in accord with the standards accepted at the time of publication. However, in view of the possibility of human error or changes in medical sciences, neither the authors nor the publisher nor any other party who has been involved in the preparation or publication of this work warrants that the information contained herein is in every respect accurate or complete, and they are not responsible for any errors or omissions or for the results obtained from use of such information. Readers are encouraged to confirm the information contained herein with other sources. For example and in particular, readers are advised to check the product information sheet included in the package of each drug they plan to administer to be certain that the information contained in this book is accurate and that changes have not been made in the recommended dose or in the contraindications for administration. This recommendation is of particular importance in connection with new or infrequently used drugs.

Becoming a Clinician

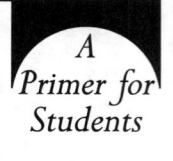

A Primer for Students

Editors

SHIRLEY M. NEITCH, MD

Professor and Chief, Section of Geriatrics
Department of Internal Medicine
Marshall University School of Medicine
Huntington, West Virginia

MAURICE A. MUFSON, MD

Professor and Chairman
Department of Internal Medicine
Marshall University School of Medicine
Huntington, West Virginia

New York St. Louis San Francisco Auckland Bogotá Caracas

Lisbon   London   Madrid   Mexico City   Milan   Montreal

New Delhi   San Juan   Singapore   Sydney   Tokyo   Toronto

McGraw-Hill
Health
Professions
Division

McGraw-Hill

A Division of The McGraw·Hill Companies

Becoming a Clinician: A Primer for Medical Students

Copyright © 1998 by The McGraw-Hill Companies, Inc. All rights reserved. Printed in the United States of America. Except as permitted under the United States Copyright Act of 1976, no part of this publication may be reproduced or distributed in any form or by any means, or stored in a data base or retrieval system, without the prior written permission of the publisher.

1234567890   DOCDOC   998

ISBN 0-07-046515-0

This book was set in Perpetua by Keyword Typesetting Services Ltd
The editors were John Dolan and Peter McCurdy;
the production supervisor was Heather Barry;
the cover designer was Ed Smith
Project management was by Keyword Publishing Services Ltd
R. R. Donnelley & Sons was printer and binder.

This book is printed on acid-free paper.

Visit the McGraw-Hill Health Professions website at
http://www.mghmedical.com

LIBRARY OF CONGRESS CATALOGING-IN-PUBLICATION DATA

Becoming a clinician : a primer for medical students / editors,
    Shirley M. Neitch, Maurice A. Mufson.
        p.   cm.
    Includes bibliographical references and index.
    ISBN 0-07-046515-0
    1. Clinical medicine—Handbooks, manuals, etc.   2. Clinical medicine—Practice.   3. Physician and
patient.   I. Neitch, Shirley M.   II. Mufson, Maurice A.
    [DNLM: 1. Clinical Medicine handbooks.   2. Clinical Medicine case studies.   3. Patient Care
handbooks.   4. Patient Care case studies.
    WB 39 B398 1998]
    RC55.B33   1998
    616—dc21
    DNLM/DLC
    for Library of Congress   98-15024

Contents

v

Preface

The transition from college to medical school represents a substantial challenge. The idea of working with patients in the first year can disconcert the most aggressive medical student. We experienced the same feelings when we were medical students.

We wrote this book as a "handbook" for this transition. Keep it close at hand as a companion during your beginning clinical experiences and use it to answer your clinical questions in the first few years, when you don't know what to ask. It is organized into three sections encompassing the developmental processes of working with patients, understanding their medical complaints, and evaluating their problems.

SECTION I: BECOMING A CLINICIAN

Medicine remains, above all other professions, an honorable and honored career. All of us play a part in maintaining the integrity of the profession, maximizing service to our patients, and ensuring that Medicine continues to reward its practitioners.

Section I surveys the philosophical and ethical foundations of our profession in a pragmatic way. Read it before you meet your first patient. Then, you can reconcile your life experiences and ideological background with your new medical school experiences to mold your identity as a doctor.

SECTION II: PRACTICAL HELP FOR EARLY CLINICAL ENCOUNTERS

Some of you will have the advantage of prior experience in which you formed relationships similar to patient–physician interactions; for example, some medical students trained as nurses or physician assistants. More likely you followed the traditional "high school to college to medical school" route, and therefore you've never experienced anything quite like medical school before! Look to Chapters 3 and 4.

Chapter 3 discusses techniques for interviewing patients and introduces the important concept of therapeutic touch. Your differing family and peer experiences impart a personal comfort level in interacting with other people by voice and touch. If these interpersonal situations are uncomfortable for you, read this chapter closely; it can ease your transition. If, on the other hand, you can handle these interactions, this chapter will identify and emphasize the unique qualities of personal encounters that characterize the special relationship between doctor and patient.

Chapter 4 explains the principles by which you are evaluated. Many of you will be unfamiliar with performance evaluation, as opposed to knowledge testing. This chapter aims to clarify the process.

SECTION III: CLINICAL EVALUATION OF COMMON MEDICAL PROBLEMS

Section III represents the "guts" of this handbook. It describes common clinical situations which you may encounter before your formal classroom instruction provides background information. Students clamor for more patient encounters early in the medical school curriculum. "Show me," we've all asked, "some real patients, so I can understand why the basic-science information is important." Today medical schools respond by introducing clinical experiences in the first year. This creates another dilemma for medical students—how can those very early patient experiences make any sense when you lack the necessary background information?

The chapters in Section III address that question in the following way:

- Each chapter begins with an illustrative case, presented exactly the way patients come to the doctor's clinic or office.

- Each chapter includes definitions of the medical terminology not defined by the text itself.
- The chapters in Section III are organized into three subsections:

  1. The first four chapters encompass the routine or general examinations which patients need at different times in their lives. Often patients who come for prenatal examinations or sports physical examinations don't consider themselves to be patients at all since they are not "sick." Nevertheless, physicians play important roles at these times, whether identifying unexpected problems or alternatively "issuing a clean bill of health."
  2. The next ten chapters discuss common *symptoms* or common *diseases*. Patients come into a medical office to seek care just this way—either they have a symptom which they want to have "checked out" or they need evaluation for a defined disease.
  3. The final three chapters discuss three increasingly recognized, multidisciplinary problems which many patients experience, but which they seldom can explicitly explain. You will be called upon to use certain "detective" skills with patients who have problems because of alcohol abuse, domestic violence, and depression.

- Each clinical chapter discusses the symptom or disease in relatively nontechnical terminology, and in almost exclusively clinical contexts. We have included little pathophysiology and limited emphasis on treatment. Your goal in early clinical encounters should be directed toward one-on-one interactions with your patients, and toward relating "real life" clinical situations to the physiology and pathology as it is taught in the classroom. This concept forms the basis of scientific medicine.
- At the conclusion of each chapter, the case scenario is resolved. You may have a problem-based curriculum in your medical school, and resolving cases will often be your assigned task. These examples give you clues which explain how clinicians seek to solve clinical problems.
- Every clinical chapter includes study questions. Board examinations increasingly emphasize clinically stated questions. We include many of these to help you prepare for this question format.

Finally, as a medical student your challenge is to integrate your scientific knowledge with your patient care skills *to become a clinician*. Medical schools approach this challenge in a new way, by providing patient encounters early and often, through mentoring or other situations in which you meet real patients. The fundamentals of these early encounters are described in this book and its aim is to guide you through them so that you gain confidence and the necessary background for your later clinical years.

Acknowledgments

The editors wish to thank the many excellent clinicians of Marshall University School of Medicine who contributed to this book. We particularly acknowledge the contributions of the coordinators of Marshall's Interdisciplinary Generalist Curriculum Project, Sarah McCarty, M.D., Marie Veitia, Ph.D., and Patricia Kelly, M.D., who have been extremely supportive. We also highlight the contribution of David Carr, Ed.D., of Ohio University, our curriculum and evaluation specialist.

We are grateful to our students; they are indeed the main inspiration for our book, and they have taught us while we taught them. We acknowledge the influence of Roberta Messner, R.N., Ph.D., who is both personally and professionally a sincere inspiration to all who are fortunate enough to know her.

We could not have completed our work without the diligent and cheerful secretarial support of Mrs. Sherry Puckett, who has processed more words than any of us foresaw at the beginning of this project.

And finally, we acknowledge our deepest gratitude to those to whom we dedicate this book:

To: M.S.P., F.R.N., and R.I.N.—my foundation and strength
L.E.K. and S.L.N.—my heart and courage, and
L.T.K.—the wind beneath my wings   S.M.N.

and

To: My loving wife, Deedee, for always being there   M.A.M.

Contributors

The following contributors are located at:

> Marshall University School of Medicine
> Huntington, WV

Editors/Contributors

Maurice A. Mufson, M.D.
Professor and Chairman
Department of Internal Medicine

Shirley M. Neitch, M.D.
Professor and Chief, Section of Geriatrics
Department of Internal Medicine

Contributors

Bruce S. Chertow, M.D.
Professor and Chief, Section of Endocrinology
Department of Internal Medicine

Sachin T. Dave, M.D.
Assistant Professor
Department of Internal Medicine

Renee S. Domanico, M.D.
Assistant Professor
Department of Pediatrics

Henry K. Driscoll, M.D.
Professor of Medicine
Department of Internal Medicine

Lynne J. Goebel, M.D.
Assistant Professor of Medicine
Department of Internal Medicine

Patricia J. Kelly, M.D.
Professor, Adolescent Medicine
Department of Pediatrics

John W. Leidy, Jr., M.D., Ph.D.
Professor of Medicine
Department of Internal Medicine

Sarah A. McCarty, M.D.
Professor of Medicine
Director, Generalist Preclinical Education
Department of Internal Medicine

Diane W. Mufson, M.A.
Instructor
Department of Internal Medicine

Nancy J. Munn, M.D.
Professor of Medicine
Chief, Section of Pulmonary and
    Critical Care
Department of Internal Medicine

Robert C. Nerhood, M.D.
Professor and Chairman
Department of Obstetrics and
    Gynecology

Gretchen E. Oley, M.D.
Professor and Chief, Section of
    General Internal Medicine
Department of Internal Medicine

Thomas C. Rushton, M.D.
Assistant Professor and Chief,
    Section of Infectious Diseases
Department of Internal Medicine

W. Michael Skeens, M.D.
Associate Professor
Department of Internal Medicine

Marc A. Subik, M.D.
Associate Professor and Chief,
    Section of Gastroenterology
Department of Internal Medicine

Marie C. Veitia, Ph.D.
Director of Educational
    Development
Office of Academic Affairs

Ralph W. Webb, M.D.
Professor and Chief, Section of
    Rheumatology
Department of Internal Medicine

Paulette S. Wehner, M.D.
Assistant Professor
Department of Cardiovascular
    Services

Jayson L. Yap, M.D.
Assistant Professor and Chief,
    Section of Neurology
Department of Internal Medicine

Kevin W. Yingling, M.D.
Associate Professor
Internal Medicine Residency
Program Director
Department of Internal Medicine

Additional contributor:

David B. Carr, Ed.D.
Assistant Professor
Coordinator of Physical Education
    and Sports Studies
Ohio University
Athens, OH

Becoming a Clinician

A Primer for Students

Becoming a Clinician

Students in Patient Care—the Honor

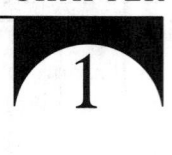

Maurice A. Mufson

INTRODUCTION

Today, more than any time during the past fifty years, first-year medical students work with patients very early in their first year when they know little more about this process than they did when they decided upon a career in medicine. It seems appropriate to coordinate patient care encounters in the first year with the basic science curriculum. The scientific basis of medical care depends in a major part on the knowledge base available in the basic science courses as much as it does on the knowledge base taught in the clinical years. By this approach, first-year medical students learn the importance of working with patients, explore interactions with patients, and develop an appreciation of professionalism and the patient–physician relationship. This early clinical experience can provide a deep-felt appreciation for the many aspects of working with patients and a sense that this requires much skill and dedication by the medical student to succeed at it.

OATHS OF THE PROFESSION OF MEDICINE

Medicine is the noblest profession. It demands the highest standards of devotion to duty. It requires the highest ethics in the care of patients, broad intellect in understanding disease and its treatment, profound empathy in reaching out to all patients, and genuine understanding of the balance that must be maintained between the altruistic and pragmatic facets of the practice of medicine. Unlike almost any other profession, physicians swear oaths to act and practice medicine in a noble manner. The first recorded oath originated during the early Greek

civilization and it is attributed to the Greek physician Hippocrates of Cos (Table 1-1). The Oath of Hippocrates demanded of the ancient physician not only ethical conduct and competence, but also strict obedience and acquiescence to certain limitations of their practice of medicine. As a historical writing, it provides insights into a few of the issues that held importance for physicians of that time, or at least to the Hippocratic school, which are moot today.

The Oath of Hippocrates does not, and could not be expected to, reflect the many issues of importance to physicians of today. Mostly, it is archaic and out of date. Many schools of medicine which administer this oath to its graduating students use a modified version that seems more in accord with contemporary ideas and ideals (one example is shown in Table 1-2).

Table 1-1. Oath of Hippocrates

I swear by Apollo the physician, by Aesculapius, Hygeia and Panacea, and I take to witness all the gods, all the goddesses to keep according to my ability the following Oath:

To consider dear to me as parents him who taught me the art and to live in common with him and, if necessary, to share my goods with him; to look upon his children as my own brothers; to teach them this art if they so desire without fee or written promise; to impart to my sons and the sons of the master who taught me and the disciples who have enrolled themselves and have agreed to the rules of the profession according to the law of medicine, but to none others. I will prescribe regimens for the good of my patients according to my ability and my judgement and never do harm to anyone. To please no one will I prescribe a deadly drug if asked, nor suggest any such counsel. Nor will I give a woman an instrument to procure abortion. But I will preserve the purity of my life and my art. I will not cut for stone, even for patients in whom the disease is manifest. I will leave this operation to be performed by practitioners in the art. In every house where I come, I will enter only for the good of my patients, keeping myself from all intentional ill-doing and all seduction, and especially from the pleasures of love with women or with men, be they free or slaves. All that may come to my knowledge in the exercise of my profession or in daily commerce with men, which ought not to be spread abroad, I will keep secret and will never reveal. If I keep this oath faithfully, may I enjoy my life and practise my art, respected by all men and in all times, but if I swerve from it or violate it, may the reverse be my lot.

Table 1-2. A Modified Oath of Hippocrates

I swear by all I hold most sacred that according to my ability and judgement I will keep this oath and this stipulation: That I will be loyal to the profession of medicine, and just and generous to its members. That I will lead my life and practice my art in uprightness and honor. That into whatsoever home I shall enter, it shall be for the good of the sick and the well to the utmost of my power, and that I will hold myself aloof from wrong and corruption and from tempting to vice. That I will exercise my art solely for the care of my patients and the prevention of disease, and will give no drugs and perform no operation for a criminal purpose and far less suggest such thing. That whatsoever I shall see or hear of the lives of men which is not fitting to be spoken, I will keep inviolably secret. While I continue to keep this oath inviolate may it be granted to me to enjoy life and the practice of the art, respected by all men in all times. But, should I trespass and violate this oath, may the reverse be my lot.

Recently, new oaths have been conceived which attempt to represent more appropriately the contemporary medical issues and provide physicians with an oath consistent with the issues and honor of medicine today (5,6,7). A new oath for physicians encompasses all aspects of contemporary medicine and challenges the physician to live up to medicine as the noblest profession (Table 1-3) (5). Oaths do not need to be restricted to the end of medical school or at graduation. When medical students enter medical schools, they become a part of the profession and the administration of an oath can signal this in a symbolic manner. A new oath for medical students encourages them to honor the profession, their medical education, and the ideals of the profession from the very first day of the start of their career as physicians-to-be (Table 1-4) (6). Lastly, the oath and prayer of Moses Maimonides has been revised in poem form to express the essence of the practice of medicine today (Table 1-5) (7). It touches the issues, as do the longer, more itemized oaths, but more succinctly and lovingly.

Why oaths for medicine at all? Physicians fulfill an especial role in any community because they are entrusted with its health and well being and oaths remind physicians of this responsibility and honor. Starting from medical student days and extending through all the days of your practice, you will be expected to honor the profession and care for the sick

Table 1-3. A New Oath for Physicians (5)

In the name of suffering humanity, with humility, compassion, and dedication to the welfare of the sick according to the best of my ability and judgement, I will keep this oath and stipulations:

I will be honest with my patients in all medical matters. When this honesty reveals bad news, I will deliver it with understanding and sympathy and tact.

I will provide my patients with acceptable alternatives for various forms of diagnosis and medical and surgical treatment, explaining the risks and benefits as best I know them.

I will allow my patients to make the ultimate decision about their own care. In circumstances where my patients are incapable of making decisions, I will accept the decision of family members or loved ones, encouraging them to decide as they believe the patient would have decided.

I will not sit in moral judgement on any patient, but will treat their illness to the best of my ability whatever the circumstances.

I will be empathetic to patients with illnesses caused by substances such as alcohol or drugs, or other forms of self-abuse usually believed to be under voluntary control.

Knowing my own inadequacies and those of medicine generally, I will strive to cure when possible but to comfort always.

I shall perform medical tests only if I believe there is a reasonable chance that the results will improve the outcome.

I will not perform any tests or procedures or surgery solely to make money. I will freely refer my patients to other physicians if I am convinced that they are better able to than I to provide treatment.

I will freely furnish copies of medical records to patients or their families upon request.

I will do unto patients and their families only what I would want done unto me or my family. I will not experiment on patients unless the patients give truly informed consent. I will strive to instruct patients fully so their informed consent is possible.

I will remain a student all my professional life, attempting to learn not only from formal medical sources but from patients as well.

I will attempt to function as a teacher for my patients so that I can care for them more effectively and can apply the lessons they provide to the care of other patients.

I will provide care to all patients seeking it, regardless of sex, race, color, creed, sexual preference, lifestyle, or economic status. In particular, I will volunteer some of my time to providing free care to the poor, the homeless, the disadvantaged, the dispossessed, and the helpless.

Table 1-3. Continued

I will turn away no patient, even though with dreaded contagious diseases.

I will encourage my patients to seek medical opinions other than my own before agreeing to accept my opinion.

I will treat my professional colleagues with respect and honor, but I will not hesitate to testify openly about physicians and medical institutions that are guilty of impatience, malfeasance, cupidity, or fraud.

I will defend with equal fervor colleagues who are unjustly accused of malpractice, malfeasance, cupidity, or fraud.

Table 1-4. An Oath for Entering Medical Students (6)

As I embark upon the study of medicine at this school of medicine, I will:
Respect the patient's right to privacy;
Accept responsibility only for those matters for which I am competent; maintain the trust expected of a physician and never take advantage of the patient–doctor relationship;
Enter into a relationship of mutual respect with my teachers and my colleagues to enhance the learning environment and gain the knowledge, skills, and attitudes of a good physician;
Continue this learning throughout all the days of my life;
Value the knowledge and wisdom of the physicians who have preceded me and endeavour to contribute to this tradition; and
Recognize my weaknesses and strengths and strive to develop those qualities that will earn the respect of my patients, my colleagues, my family, and myself.

without regard for your personal advantage. Oaths remind all of us of the traditions of medicine, of the frailty of your patients, and of your responsibility to the profession. By swearing an oath, you rededicate yourself to the ideals of the profession of medicine. The oath for medical students encourages reflection by you of your responsibilities for educating yourself and to your new profession and reminds you of your commitment to professionalism.

Table 1-5. Only the Human Being: Modification of the Oath and Prayer of Moses Maimonides (7)

Always keep me seeing
In suffering and in strife
Only the human being
And not an "insured life."
Show me to keep apart
From venal attitude
Poison to the healer's heart;
Teach me to know the good.
Permit me to recognize
Unworthy, ill-won gain,
No matter its disguise,
Whatever its name.
Give me the will to dare
To practice with integrity,
To sustain, to love, to care.
Support, oh strengthen me!

PROFESSIONALISM

Professionalism represents the demeanour of physicians in their caring for patients, including: conducting themselves in an ethical and moral manner; investing the patient in their own care and in maintaining their own health; applying the latest advances in the scientific basis of medicine in initiating appropriate and compassionate treatment; and fulfilling the role of a confidant of the patient in the good times and bad.

Project Professionalism of the American Board of Internal Medicine asserts that professionalism in medicine requires the physician to serve the interests of the patient above the interests of the physician (1). Professionalism, it states, aspires to altruism, accountability, excellence, duty, service, honor, integrity, and respect for others. The elements of professionalism required of physicians who seek certification from the American Board of Internal Medicine encompass:

A commitment to the highest standards of excellence in the practice of medicine and in the generation and dissemination of knowledge.
A commitment to sustain the interests and welfare of patients.
A commitment to be responsive to the health needs of society.

This canon defines the dedication of physicians to the practice of medicine in the service of their patients and society. For the medical student, professionalism in medicine begins the first day of medical school. Patients expect their physicians to act professionally and other physicians expect the same.

PATIENT PRESENTATIONS

Consider the following descriptions of two patients and the student physicians attending to them in light of the issues of professionalism and decide whether you would have approached these patients as they did.

CASE 1: A Patient Admitted in Hospital for the First Time and an Insensitive Student Physician

The first patient, Mr. Charles Simon, 68 years old, the owner of a large construction firm in town, was admitted to the inpatient medical service only a few minutes ago after undergoing a very quick assessment and the start of prompt medical care in the emergency room. This episode began about 2 hours ago when, for the first time, he developed oppressive chest pain, which he described as "taking his breath away" and "the worst pain he ever experienced." He told the Attending Physician in the emergency room that he never wants to have such pain again. The Attending Physician told the patient that his pain likely signified serious heart disease requiring medical care in the hospital and subsequently several diagnostic and treatment procedures.

As the patient, Mr. Simon, has not previously suffered any heart disease, he does not know what to expect at this point in his illness. Nether his wife nor any close relatives have had any serious illnesses so that he has not visited a hospital in the past few years. However, he has read in the weekly news magazines and watched on television ample reports of the seriousness of heart disease and of the high number of persons dying from "heart attacks," the result of occlusion of one or more coronary arteries because of arteriosclerosis. Clearly, he is very concerned, anxious, and scared. We can see it in his face—one means of nonverbal communication.

At this time, the third-year medical student—called the Clerk—assigned on the Medicine Clerkship, and next on the list to conduct a full history and physical examination of a new patient, enters the room to examine Mr. Simon. We can observe the medical student without his being aware of us. His name is Mr. Robert Rollins. Custom dictates that on the hospital medical service the medical students are not usually addressed as "Doctor," unless the Attending Physician introduces the medical student to the patient

and indicates that Mr. Rollins can be called "Doctor" for this session. In this case, the Attending Physician does so.

Dr. Rollins greets Mr. Simon. "How are you Charlie? What's up? Not doin' too well today, are you? Well, we'll see to that. What happened?" Dr. Rollins sits on the foot end of the bed and takes out his notepad. Mr. Simon answers by telling Dr. Rollins about his chest pain and his coming to the hospital. He admits, "it was the worst pain I had ever experienced and I thought I was going to die even before I reached the hospital." Dr. Rollins has been entering notes in his pad, without looking at Mr. Simon. Mr. Simon ends his story, and, finally, Dr. Rollins looks at Mr. Simon. "But you didn't die, did you Charlie." "I guess not, doctor, not yet, at any rate. What is your name? Are you really my doctor?" "Of course I'm your doctor; who did you expect? I'm Dr. Rollins. I have just one or two more questions." Mr. Simon answers these questions the best he can. He realizes he is tired, and asks Dr. Rollins whether he can rest with his eyes closed for about 15 minutes before Dr. Rollins examines him. Dr. Rollins insists on starting his examination then, and he prevails on Mr. Simon. He begins his examination; after listening to Mr. Simon's heart, Dr. Rollins chides Mr. Simon, "your heart sounds a little off, but not too bad Charlie, did you know that?" Dr. Rollins finishes his examinations, collects his belongings and starts for the door. "If you need anything, Charlie, call the nurse by ringing the bell next to your bed."

Would you have treated Mr. Simon as Mr. Rollins did? What mannerisms of Mr. Rollins did you like or dislike? If you were in Mr. Simon's place, how would you react to being questioned and examined by Mr. Rollins? Why? By his actions, Mr. Rollins typifies the vexatious student, lacking a professional manner. Patients want understanding, sensitivity, and courtesy by their physicians, and all health care personnel with whom they come in contact in the hospital. After all, they come to the hospital because they are ill and they expect their physician to care for them in a caring manner. Compare Mr. Rollins's handling of Mr. Simon with Ms. Sandra Williams's interactions with Mr. John Peterson in the next case presentation.

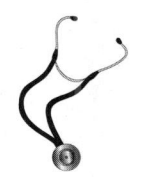

CASE 2: A Patient with Many Admissions in Hospital and a Thoughtful Student Physician

The day has not gone well for the second patient, Mr. John Peterson, 64 years old, employed as an accountant with supervisory responsibilities in a large local firm. Soon after breakfast, he felt a sense of discomfort in the upper part of his abdomen, which he thought was caused by something he

ate that morning. His discomfort did not go away after he drank some milk and he thought that the usually busy morning in the office intensified it. By lunch time the discomfort had become pain in the lower part of his chest, which seemed to radiate down his left arm. Now, his pain mimicked the pain he had a few months ago, and also a few years ago, when he suffered a heart attack. He called 911 and the ambulance came promptly and took him to the hospital. In the emergency room (ER), he felt more comfortable and the senior physician examined him promptly, started the necessary medications, and arranged for him to be moved to the medical service.

He is settled in bed when the third-year Clinical Clerk, Ms. Donna Williams, enters the room, alone. "Good afternoon, Mr. Peterson; I'm Donna Williams, a third-year medical student, and I am assigned as one of your doctors on this service's medical team. How are you feeling? Do you have chest pain now? If you do, I will ask the Resident Physician on the team to order pain medication for you now." Mr. Peterson responds that he does not have chest pain now, apparently the pain medications given to him in the emergency room have been sufficient. "I am pleased to meet you, Ms. Williams. I am feeling better, but I had a terrible scare this morning and I don't know if the next time I have pain I can get to the hospital in time." Ms. Williams stands by the bed and holds Mr. Peterson's hand to feel his pulse. "Your skin feels warm, and its color is good, and your pulse is normal. I'd have to say that you are doing a little better than when you came to the ER. Tell me about your chest pain and how it began this morning." As Ms. Williams listens to Mr. Peterson relate the events leading up to his admission to the hospital, she stands near the bed, in his line of sight, and listens intently to his story, interrupting from time to time to ask a question. Finally, she completes her questioning. "I need to examine you now Mr. Peterson. Do you feel up to it?" Mr. Peterson asks for a minute to rest. Ms. Williams responds, "I will get the few things I need for my examination of you and return in 10 minutes. Will that do?" Mr. Peterson answers that it will be fine. He rests and Ms. Williams leaves for a few minutes.

In this scenario, the medical student, Donna Williams handles the introduction and interview with Mr. Peterson in an entirely satisfactory manner. If you were Mr. Peterson, would you feel comfortable with Ms. Williams as your doctor. Why?

Clearly, the two medical students described in these case presentations used dissimilar approaches to their patients. In the second case presentation, Ms. Donna Williams established a welcoming bond with the patient and she treated the patient as an individual deserving of her attention, interest, and respect. In return, the patient liked her and they worked well together. In all likelihood, they would maintain a strong and

enduring patient–physician relationship. The other student, Mr. Robert Rollins, failed in these respects. He proved insensitive and unprofessional. In all likelihood the patient felt uncomfortable having to deal with Mr. Robert Rollins and would not want someone who acted as Mr. Rollins did to be his physician. These case presentations illustrate the importance of establishing a welcoming and interactive working relationship with the patient, one which establishes a bond between the patient and physician so that the patient and physician trust each other and work together for the patient's benefit—this defines the patient–physician relationship. It cannot be carried forward except in an atmosphere of professionalism.

THE PATIENT–PHYSICIAN RELATIONSHIP

Patients must trust their physicians and physicians must gain their patient's trust because it forms the basis of the patient–physician relationship. The patient–physician relationship requires that the patient and physician trust each other so that at those times when the patient most needs the physician, the physician can act on behalf of the patient (2). It forms the quintessence of the profession of medicine and distinguishes it from all other professions.

The patient–physician relationship begins at the moment of first contact with the patient. The physician must do everything necessary to initiate the relationship in a warm and caring manner, to gain the trust of the patient, and to make it clear that at that time the patient is the most important person in the world to the physician. In the two case presentations, medical students meet patients for the first time in the hospital, when the patient is most vulnerable, and more than at any other time, needs the understanding and friendship of the physician, albeit the medical student. Often, the first time first-year medical students examine patients will be in the doctor's office or a similar ambulatory setting. Usually, the patient arranges the appointment with the physician and their situation doesn't require in-hospital care; they may be well and come for preventive measures. At any rate, the patient may feel under less stress in the physician's office, but the physician must act appropriately to establish and maintain a meaningful patient–physician relationship. Medical students also must fill this role from the start of their education, especially now that patient encounters begin in the first year of medical school. This requires a determined effort on the part of the medical student, now and through their career.

THE MEDICAL STUDENT "WHITE COAT CEREMONY"

Recently, many medical schools began a distinctive welcome for incoming medical students designated as the "White Coat Ceremony" (3). At this ceremony, each of the incoming medical students receives a white coat and the recognition that accompanies their introduction to the faculty and classmates denoting their starting their educational program leading to a Doctor of Medicine. The Dean of the medical school presents the white coat during orientation or at an appropriate opening day exercise when family and friends can attend. The white coat symbolizes the physician.

The white coat also signals to the patient that the person in the white coat represents a physician. When medical students meet patients for the first time, the white coat provides an unspoken message that the wearer is a physician or someone in training to become a physician. Without question, the patient defers to this person in the white coat, whether they are a senior physician, resident physician, or medical student. The patient works with them and confides in them personal information they would otherwise keep secret. The aura of the white coat encompasses both power and responsibility. The medical student must recognize this and respect it. Because medical students represent a physician to the patient, the patient will answer questions of a personal nature that you would feel uncomfortable asking, or never ask, of your closest friend or relative. Medical students must honor this responsibility; your patient wants to trust you because by doing so they can achieve maximum care. The white coat can ease the medical student through the first few difficult questions that must be asked, but afterwards the trust that the medical student establishes carries forward the patient–physician relationship.

APPROACH TO EXAMINING A PATIENT

As a student physician, your first encounters with patients begin in the first year before you take the introductory medicine courses which begin the discussion of disease. This need not represent a barrier to working with patients as a student physician. It does mean that you will need to learn to handle yourself in a professional manner and establish a meaningful patient–physician relationship, albeit a patient–*student physician* relationship. Here are guidelines for your first patient encounter.

Your First Patient Encounter

Your first and subsequent encounters with patients should be enriching experiences, instilling a sense of accomplishment, caring, and empathy. They should improve your ability to deal with patients and add to your knowledge base. However, for this to occur, your faculty teacher must instruct you in advance. You may ask many pertinent questions about your first encounters with patients, usually just outside the room of the patient. Your questions deserve discussion much before that time so that you can more effectively conduct these patient encounters. It's a case of "everything you've always wanted to know about examining your first patient, but were afraid to ask!"

Faculty expect most medical students to exhibit ambivalence about their role as a student "physician" because they are *not* (graduate) physicians. Although you carry the mantle of a physician during the process of learning to examine patients in the first and second years, you will likely remain uncomfortable during this period of your development. Sometimes, it continues during your clerkships in the third and fourth years of medical school, but more often you will adapt to this role by that time.

How to Introduce Yourself to the Patient

Typically, faculty hear medical students expressing their concern by asking "How I am to introduce myself?" "Shall I say that I am Doctor Name?" "By what title should I be called in the patient's presence?" Invariably, they ask, "As I am not a physician, is it correct for me to be addressed as Doctor? Do I deceive the patient if I am called Doctor by them?" The obvious answer is that it is a deception, of sorts. Let's examine the answer to these questions because they can substantially assist you in understanding your role as a surrogate physician during the evolving process of becoming a physician.

Medical students in their first and second years appear to patients as physicians, albeit beginning ones. Surprisingly, many patients know when it is a medical student in the white coat standing at their bedside waiting to examine them. They know this even when you introduce yourself as "Doctor." How do they know? Several reasons account for this. Patients admitted to a teaching hospital usually have been told by a number of people that medical students and resident physicians will examine and treat them. The patient doesn't recognize the student as one of the physicians who examined him or her when they were

admitted and who had the authority and credentials to begin treatment. Medical students usually come to the patient's room with the faculty teacher who introduces them to the patient, or should do so. I always accompany first- and second-year medical students and introduce them to the patient, explaining to the patient "This is student Doctor Name who is working with me today; he or she will talk to you about your complaints and examine you. I will be back later." Then, they alone examine the patient. You should ask the faculty teacher to introduce you to the patient if it appears that the faculty teacher does not intend to do this or did not do it the first time you examined a patient in the course.

How to Avoid Impropriety

A few words of caution and advice—male medical students should examine female patients only when another female medical student, nurse, or nurse's aide, remains in the room throughout the examination, even if it involves only talking to the patient and examining them without any need to unclothe them at all. Although this approach may seem overly cautious, it will, without exception, preclude any misunderstandings about the examination and avoid embarrassment on the part of both the patient and you. Also, it will prevent the threat of law suits. On the other hand, female medical students can examine male patients without another man standing by during the examination. Here, I would caution that some male patients find it titillating to be examined by a female medical student. The faculty teacher needs to be aware of this possibility and if it appears that this is the case, then the female medical student should be assigned another patient immediately or a male student, nurse or aide must remain in the room during the examination. If the possibility of this situation is not immediately apparent to the faculty teacher, but the female student confronts it any time during her examination of the patient, then she needs to leave the room and inform the faculty teacher, who will make the appropriate arrangements.

How to Address Patients

When you examine your first patient alone, you must maintain a professional demeanor at all times. This attitude personifies the physician. *Always call the patient "Mr." or "Miss" or "Mrs." as appropriate*. Formality keeps the relationship on a professional level; *you are not a friend of the patient, but you can be friendly*. Often the patient is older than you and deserves the courtesy usually extended to someone senior to you. I consider it demeaning to the

patient when they address their physician as "Doctor" and then their physician calls the patient by their first name or nickname.

Approach to the Difficult Patient

What do you do when the patient refuses some part of the examination?

What do you do when the patient says "No," for example to questions about certain personal or social information or the patient disallows examination of his or her abdomen or the patient refuses to remove their clothes for an examination of their genitalia? These scenarios represent examples of a patient's unwillingness to cooperate, perhaps because your are a student physician, or perhaps for other reason(s) which the patient chooses not to tell. You should excuse yourself from the room and notify the faculty teacher; anyone assisting you should leave with you also. The faculty teacher will handle the situation—the student must not force the issue either by cajoling or by arguing with the patient. When it can not be settled, end the examination. You can prepare the written history and physical examination for as much of your assignment as you completed, or if too little of the examination was done, the faculty teacher should assign you to a new patient.

What do you do when the patient questions you too much during your examination?

What do you as a first- and second-year student do when the patient you are examining asks about their illness or about the results of their laboratory tests or X-rays or wants to discuss whether or not they should undergo surgery or a biopsy? The patients ask in earnest because they perceive any medical student as knowledgeable, notwithstanding that you are not a graduate physician. One approach is to tell the patient that you are "not their primary doctor and can not discuss their case; however, you will speak with the patient's primary physician and that physician will answer their questions." After this you complete your examination. *Medical students should not reach beyond their expertise at any level of their training.* They risk telling the patient information that the ward team may not want discussed or the wrong information. *Any attempt on your part to answer the patient's questions may interfere with the plans of the ward team.* If the patient continues to ask for answers to their questions, ask the faculty teacher to handle the situation.

The situation differs for third- and fourth-year students assigned as clerks on the hospital ward or the ambulatory center. In their case, they

have some responsibility for care of the patient as a member of the team and they will have had an opportunity to discuss the patient's illness. They may want to answer some of the patient's questions appropriately. However, they also will need help doing so and they should ask the attending physician in charge of the ward team, or the senior resident physician.

What Do You Do When The Patient Becomes Acutely Ill During Your Examination?

What should you do as a first- and second-year medical student when the patient you are examining becomes acutely ill; for example, the patient develops severe chest pain or any condition necessitating urgent medical care? Quickly go to the door of the room and shout down the hallway to the nurses' station for help. Medical students who have been certified in basic cardiac life support (BCLS) should do what they judge as appropriate until the ward team arrives. Those with no certification should get nursing assistance as rapidly as possible.

As part of the curriculum at entry into medical school, most new medical students should be instructed in BCLS; by their fourth year they should qualify in Advanced Cardiac Life Support.

What Do You Do When You Discover a Physical Finding Not Previously Noted by the Attending and Resident Physicians?

Sometimes a first-year or, more likely, a second-year medical student may discover a new physical finding not previously noted by either the Attending or Resident Physician. For example, you may hear a murmur and incidentally inquire of the patient as to whether any one told them about it. If the patient has no knowledge of it, you search the patient's chart and also fail to find a record of the murmur. At this point, what do you do? A good approach is to inform the faculty teacher instructing the class and ask him or her to examine the patient. When they also hear the murmur, they will alert the Attending and Resident Physicians. Even if you are unsure of your observation, in this case a murmur, and you decide not to search the chart, the best approach remains to have the faculty teacher listen to the patient's heart to confirm or deny your findings and to instruct you. Any finding you discover when assigned to examine a patient as part of course work in the first 2 years should be reported to your faculty teacher for verification. Not only does the instructor's verification substantiate your physical diagnosis acumen, but they can explain or clarify your understanding of the finding. Some physical findings are fleeting, such as pleural friction rubs, or changeable, such as murmurs, and deserve confirmation immediately.

ADDITIONAL THOUGHTS ON THE HONOR OF WORKING WITH PATIENTS

Throughout your medical career the experience of working with patients will provide endless satisfaction. Unlike anything else you do as a physician, or any other professional does in their field, caring for patients represents the giving unselfishly of yourself for the welfare of others. It involves more than that single act. It's also being there for your patients and being knowledgeable when they need you the most—when they are sick and the only person they know to turn to is their physician. If you never let them down, you will honor the profession and yourself.

Your education for this unparalleled role of the physician begins immediately in the first year of medical school. Many first-year students fail to grasp this concept, understandably, because of their preoccupation with the task of learning the large body of basic science knowledge which forms the infrastructure of clinical medicine. Nonetheless, early on in medical school, you develop the patterns of behavior which will influence your demeanor with patients for your entire career. You, and every first-year medical student needs to examine their feelings towards patients from their very first encounter and handle these relationships with patients in a professional manner. If you respect patients as individuals who need your help when they suffer illness and you help them through this vulnerable time, they will respect you and trust you. This shared responsibility in the patient–physician relationship will carry you through the good times and the bad and you will enjoy "doctoring" thoroughly for all your years in the practice of medicine (4).

A GLOSSARY OF MEDICAL TERMS

Clerk or Clinical Clerk

Medical students in their third and fourth years are called Clerks by faculty, resident physicians and nursing staff during their clinical assignments on the ward or in the emergency room of a hospital and in the ambulatory care of a hospital or free standing center. Patients call medical students "Doctor". The term clerk originated in England sometime during the middle 1800s to designate medical students assigned as apprentices to the physician-in-charge of the medical care of patients. These clinical assignments are called Clerkships (see Clerkship or Clinical Assignment). First- and second-year medical students are not called clerks.

Clerkship or Clinical Assignment

During the third and fourth years of medical school, medical students learn clinical medicine by serving as Clerks in a structured curriculum (or Clerkship) offered by each of the Clinical Departments. These Clerkships provide the Clerk with the experience of direct patient care at a beginning level. The Clerk is responsible for taking a history and performing a physical examination on a specific number of patients each week, preparing the necessary write-up for review by the senior resident physician and Attending Physician, assisting the Resident Physicians with ordering laboratory studies, and discussing the patient when the Attending Physician and Resident Physicians meet at the bedside to consider the patient's condition and plans for their treatment. Assignment in surgery or one of the surgical specialties also involves participating in surgery as an assistant to the Attending Surgeon and Surgical Residents who perform the operation. In this case, the medical student follows the usual procedures including the necessary careful scrubbing of their hands and forearms and gowning without contaminating their hands or forearms or their gowns with bacteria.

Attending Physician or Attending Surgeon

The terms Attending Physician and Attending Surgeon, usually in common usage abbreviated to Attending, refer to faculty members who are assigned to supervise the clinical instruction of resident physicians and medical students either in the hospital or the ambulatory center and who retain legal responsibility for the medical care of the patients of the medical service to which the resident physicians are assigned.

Resident Physician

A Resident Physician is a graduate physician enrolled in post-medical school education (or training) called a residency program which provides them with the opportunity for meaningful direct patient care responsibilities under the supervision of Attending Physicians or the opportunity to perform operations under the supervision of Attending Surgeons. Each specialty specifies the length of the training period. In the primary care residencies it is 3 years; additional training to become eligible for certification as a subspecialist—a "fellowship"—is 2 to 3 years. In general surgery the training period is 4 or 5 years depending upon

the individual program and in the surgical subspecialties the length of training varies from 2 to 4 years. Residents in their first year may be referred to as junior residents and after that year as senior residents; the resident physician-in-charge is the Chief Resident. In the second and subsequent years of the residency, Resident Physicians usually hold a valid state medical license to practice medicine.

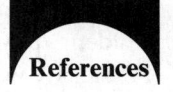

References

1. Project Professionalism. A Report from the American Board of Internal Medicine. Philadelphia, PA, 1995. pp. 5–10.
2. Peabody, F.E.W.: The care of the patient. JAMA 88: 877–882, 1927.
3. Broder, M.I.: The more things change, the more they stay the same. Am. J. Med. 102: 223–226, 1997.
4. Reynold, R. and Stone, J. (Eds): "On Doctoring: Stories, Poems, Essays." Simon and Schuster, New York, NY, 1991.
5. Robin, E.D. and McCauley, R.F.: Cultural lag and the Hippocratic Oath. Lancet 345: 1422–1424, 1995.
6. Newman, A. and Park, I.R.A.: An oath for entering medical students. Academic Medicine 69: 214, 1994.
7. Janis, M.: Only the human being: Modification of the oath and prayer of Moses Maimonides. JAMA 276: 1534; 1996.

Students in Patient Care—the Ethics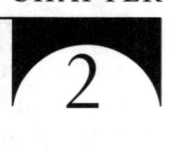

Shirley M. Neitch

INTRODUCTION

Ethics—the discipline dealing with what is good and bad and with one's moral duties and obligations.

To most people, medicine represents the epitome of ethics in action. Though we have always had our detractors, the relationship of ethics to the practice of medicine is clear and strong. Increasingly, medical practitioners and the public focus on ethics in medicine to guide the way toward desirable outcomes and to assure quality of care.

The ethical framework supporting the early years of medical education is far more subtle than medical practice ethics. However, recognizing the ethical principles which underlie your experiences as a medical student will ease the transition to applying ethical precepts to patient-care situations. Toward that end, we discuss some of the ethical issues which you will confront in the medical school classroom, and subsequently introduce the ethics of medical practice.

THE STUDENT'S ETHICAL RELATIONSHIPS

Medical school matriculation creates at least four new relationships for students, whose development over the ensuing years influences much of the physician you will become. We explore the ethical aspects of each of these relationships and we encourage you to reflect on your personal experiences in these contexts.

- Individual and student-to-student
- Student-to-teacher
- Student-to-school
- Student-to-patient.

Individual and Student-to-Student

The depth of the bond which develops among the members of a medical school class cannot be overestimated. Shared experiences, different in most cases from anything you have experienced before, form the basis of lifelong relationships and friendships. Yet these experiences represent more than camaraderie. As medical students are each other's first professional peers, how you interact with your classmates may indicate how you will approach your patients, other physicians, and all health care professionals. The ethics of medicine begins on the first day of medical school.

Fortunately, society mainly highly regards physicians and their role in our culture. Medical students receive automatic respect because they will become physicians. To maintain this public trust, medical students must not only practice ethically, but also remain open to scrutiny by their peers and teachers. An overview of some common ethical problems and suggested ways for medical students to cope with them follows:

Cheating

Remember, medical schools have a lot invested in their students and if you're having problems academically, you *will* be given help.

Cheating is the most obvious example of unethical student behavior. Faculty and medical students would like to believe that in striving to become physicians, students would not cheat. However, this is not the case. In a study at Johns Hopkins University, Dans (1) reported that a vast majority of graduating medical students (90%) believe that cheating makes a less trustworthy physician. Yet cheating occurred; in his study group, the incidence of self-reported cheating reached as high as 24%. Students who cheated rationalized it on the basis that the pressure for grades is so high and the volume of material so enormous.

However, students need to realize that help is available and cheating should not be an answer. Every medical school offers some form of tutoring, counseling, or decelerated curriculum program to assist the struggling student. Because virtually every student can find him or herself in that position at some time, seeking help from these programs is expected.

Developing an ethical interrelationship with fellow medical students requires honesty, confidentiality, and sensitivity. Students *witnessing* cheating must deal with conflicting feelings of disapproval, empathy, and compassion in resolving this problem. *Confidentiality is one of the cornerstones of the practice of medicine and is as important in our interactions with each other as it is with patients. It does not, however, constitute a Code of Silence regarding unethical behaviors.* Sensitive assessment of a situation and reporting to appropriate third parties can be done in a way which will protect confidentiality but still address the breach of ethics.

A practical model for your dealing with cheating by a fellow student that also applies to addressing dishonesty in a fellow practicing physician later in your career follows:

- Approach the offender as cordially as possible, share your concern and get their side of the story.
- If no adequate explanation is forthcoming, report the incident to administrators by following the procedure established by your school (some may have Honor Councils, others may handle such concerns internally in each department).
- If you find it impossible to confront the student, and there is *proof* of cheating, report the problem to administrators. *Serious or repeat offenses cannot go unaddressed!*

Impaired students

Impaired students—students who use illicit drugs, consume excess alcohol, or suffer medical or emotional illnesses—pose ethical dilemmas to themselves and to their fellow students. Recognizing and dealing with the impairment by another student is even more urgent than addressing cheating.

Examples of impairment include: drug or alcohol use, excessive distraction by stress and serious medical or emotional illness.

- First, students are directly involved with patients in their first year, and significant impairment may place patients at risk. Clearly this is unacceptable.
- Secondly, while cheating is a conscious decision, impaired students may not recognize their impairment, much less acknowledge it.

No one wishes to be the first or only person to call attention to impaired behavior among classmates for fear of interpreting the situation wrongly, or for being held responsible for damaging a career. However, you must act first and foremost to protect patients. This requires a

Suspicious actions
include extreme
anxiety or rage
reactions, *unexplainable*
sleepiness, erratic
attendance patterns or
sudden changes in
grades, signs of
depression, weight
loss, or other signs of
physical illness.

compassionate, but honest and thorough investigation, and if needed, a disciplinary process.

A suggested approach for a student who encounters impairment in fellow students is as follows:

- Confide your suspicions to a trusted peer. Unlike cheating, which could well be witnessed by only one person, behaviors indicating impairment have probably been seen by others.
- Whether you then confront the student suspected of being impaired or directly report them to school administrators depends upon the nature of your concern. Certainly if you only suspect physical illness, a direct approach to the fellow student would be warranted.
- If you believe there is a significant possibility of substance abuse or psychiatric illness, a direct approach may be met with denial and a deepening entrenchment of the impairment. In this case report directly to a school official.

Other student behavior

Though less serious than either cheating or student impairment, "laziness" bears mentioning. This unethical behavior pattern is called "slacking off," "lack of conscientiousness," or "just getting by." As most medical students are overachievers, this may seem an unlikely problem, but it is all too familiar to medical educators.

The problem may be rooted in the many stresses on medical students. One of these stresses is that having been accustomed to being at the top of your high school and college classes, suddenly you're in a new peer group where *all* members have similar high academic records. This drives some students to attempt even higher goals and grades. Others adjust well to sometimes being at the "middle of the pack." Unfortunately, some students seem to accept that, if they're no longer "best," mere survival by minimal effort will suffice. Such an attitude irritates faculty, but more importantly, hurts students and ultimately, patients. Common "slacking off" behaviors often relate to future practice of medicine (Table 2-1).

Medicine is inordinately demanding as an academic pursuit and as a "real world" practice. It requires dedication and a sincere commitment to excellence. This is not to say that it must be an all-consuming passion, crowding family or other personal concerns out of your life. A mature and well-rounded individual will undoubtedly be a more effective physician. *Nevertheless, an attitude of intent to learn as much as possible and to put true patient needs ahead of noncritical personal needs is a requirement in a medical*

Remember,
"Perfection is the
goal, but excellence
will be tolerated."

Table 2-1. Relationship of "Lazy" Student Behaviors to Future Practices

Behavior	Implications in future practice
Consistently skipping or being late for lectures or other activities.	Learning to respect your teachers' time now will establish respect for your patients' and staff members' time later.
Consistently choosing less demanding or less closely monitored electives.	"Easy" courses may not adequately equip you to handle infinitely *challenging* patients.
Complaining about and/or manipulating schedules perceived to be unfair.	Your patient's coronary arteries don't care that you worked two weekends last month.
Parroting a resident's work-up rather than doing your own.	"Maybe not today, maybe not tomorrow, but someday . . ." and often, you will be *alone* to do this work. Learn to do it while you can still freely ask questions.
Excess attention to outside activities.	Patients come to your office to see John Doe, *MD*, not John Doe, Olympic swimmer. Pursuit of non-medical passions is not discouraged, but simply must be done on non-school time.

career. Balancing the search for maximum knowledge and effectiveness with acceptance of one's limitations should be the aim of every medical student.

Students-to-Teachers

The association of students with their medical school teachers represents one important relationship which has been recognized for centuries, even honored in the venerable Hippocratic Oath. Hippocrates asked each student to pledge to "hold my teacher . . . equal to my own parents . . ." Professors exert enormous influence on us as sources of information and more importantly as role models.

Students and professors alike have certain obligations to fulfill in making the learning process successful, but this relationship holds the potential for unethical behaviors. Professors may abuse students, deliberately or inadvertently. Students may fail to maximally participate in learning opportunities. We briefly explore both and suggest some guidelines for handling the situations.

Unethical teaching behaviors

"Teachers" include upper level students, resident physicians, faculty, volunteer teaching physicians, and school administrative personnel.

Fifty years ago, it was largely accepted that students would be targets of verbal abuse as part of the teaching technique. It was condoned as a part of the "ritual" of the education of doctors that students endure. They were deliberately humiliated upon demonstrating the slightest lapse of knowledge. Today, blatant forms of verbal abuse and punitive work assignments occur rarely. However, some medical teachers publicly criticize or deride students too quickly, explaining that as "they lived through it, so should their students."

Worse abuses, lacking even the far-fetched disguise of being teaching techniques, are sexual harassment and ethnic prejudice. It is painful, but necessary, to acknowledge that such attitudes still occasionally exist among the educated populace of medical school faculties and administrations.

False accusations of harassment can be extremely damaging to the accused, and later when the truth is discovered, to the accuser. Be sure before you report.

If you experience any of the above behaviors from any medical school teacher, you should respond as follows:

- First, of course, reflect upon the situation to determine if a real infraction has occurred; not every instance of physical touching constitutes sexual harassment, for example.
- If you ascertain that a situation was a real infraction then you should report it through your school's procedure for handling such complaints. Each school has a policy and each will differ somewhat. The Dean's office will be able to assist you.

Unethical student behaviors

Students behave unethically toward their professors when they cheat, when they fail to communicate candidly, when they demand "spoon-feeding" of information, and when they refuse to accept honest evaluations of their performance. Having already addressed cheating, we will briefly discuss the other scenarios and appropriate student responses.

Candor Only through frank and candid interactions with your teachers can you maximally benefit from learning situations. *You will never*

benefit from misrepresenting your level of knowledge. For example, stories abound in medical schools of students who report normal eye exams in patients with prosthetic eyes, or normal gait in amputees, because they omitted the examinations in question but were afraid to admit it. The embarrassment these students experience upon being "found out" far outweighs any temporary chagrin at having to admit "I don't know."

> It will always be uncomfortable (perhaps it should be), to admit a knowledge gap, but it is in no way as problematic as being discovered to be intellectually dishonest.

"Spoon-feeding" As educators and experienced clinicians, medical school teachers understand the necessity of challenging students in situations which they may feel quite inadequate to handle. While the old adage "See one, do one, teach one" surely exaggerates the proper pace of medical education, it does emphasize the sometimes uncomfortable learn-by-doing aspect of clinical medicine. *Certain things in medicine (first and foremost the history and physical examination) simply cannot be learned from the textbook alone.* Teachers, having "been there," know that information can't always be handed to students in neat little textbook bites. The successful student must be willing to venture forth from the safety of old academic work habits and be willing to experience new ways of learning.

Another aspect of medicine which defies teaching by "spoon-feeding" is clinical ambiguity. You may be totally unaccustomed to tolerating, much less acting upon, incomplete or equivocal information. Yet much of clinical medicine demands just such action. Your professors and mentors are *not* shortchanging you by exposing you, early and often, to highly challenging clinical situations. *While it is never acceptable for you as a medical student to independently provide clinical care in such a circumstance (either to be forced to do so or to volunteer), it is important to experience such situations as a protected observer.*

Accepting evaluation Medical students are inordinately grade-conscious. For most students, it has been a long, hard road to secure a place in medical school; one which required not only mastering material but also producing high grades as proof of that mastery. You are also grade conscious because medical school graduation is not the end of the road. High quality residencies, good "board scores," and ultimately, favorable practice positions must be sought. It is no surprise then that medical teachers see a demand for total objectivity in grading, or that you feel anxious or even threatened, in situations where subjective components of evaluation are important.

Chapter 4 will offer more detail about the grading process but these random observations may ease your transition into the world of performance assessment.

- Broad, deep, accurate, and up-to-date "book knowledge" *does not guarantee* excellent performance in clinical settings. Likewise, an academically struggling student may be clinically capable. A different set of skills are being taught and tested, and in the early years of medical school only the rare and gifted student will shine in both the classroom and the clinic.
- A good coach recognizes all aspects of a player's performance and will sometimes assign a starting position to an enthusiastic and doggedly persistent low scorer, ahead of a sometimes brilliant, but erratic "star." Medical students should not be surprised if clinical evaluations sometimes reflect this same approach. *A medical career is work as well as a profession, and it is as important to willingly manage the mundane aspects as it is to dramatically intervene in the crisis.*
- No one evaluation will make or break your grade for a course or a clerkship. If you *do* have a personality conflict with one evaluator which may affect your grade, that person's comments or grades will be counterbalanced by the comments of other evaluators.
- It is trite but true that an honest criticism is meant to help you improve your performance. If your automatic response is to contest any adverse evaluation, you may miss many learning opportunities.

This is not to imply that you passively accept all negative evaluation. Just be willing to take a mature "big picture" look at the evaluation and accept honest criticism.

Student-to-School

Much of what we have discussed about student–teacher relationships applies as well to interactions between students and school administrators. Administrators as well as individual faculty must honor certain obligations, such as maintaining an abuse-free, positive learning environment.

Schools bear the additional responsibility of protecting students from undue external influences. Changing political pressures compete with educational agendas in every medical school, and part of the school's obligation to its students is to shield them from society's unreasonable demands. You should expect your school to provide a solid basic medical education. This in turn will enable you to fulfill your obligation to the school, namely to individually respond to the needs of society-at-large, via your choices of practice styles and settings.

Student-to-Patient

The most ethically complex and multifaceted relationship is that of student to patient. This relationship will be remodeled and refined throughout your career, but a few aspects are especially important for your very earliest contacts with patients.

"Primum non nocere"

This time-honored principle, "First, do no harm," represents the earliest step and sometimes the first obstacle to development of the student-to-patient relationship. A palpable tension, ranging somewhere between anticipation and terror, occurs when you begin examining patients in the clinics and hospitals; much of it stems from a fear of causing harm. You may be more afraid of patients, however, than they need be of you, because medical education is specifically designed to provide supervised experiences and a gradual assumption of responsibility. At first, you will only observe physicians interacting with patients, then move up to performing history and physical examinations, and finally progress to performance of procedures or tests.

Remember:

- You should only do procedures which are indicated for the patient; you will never put a patient at risk for educational purposes.
- Even multiple history and physical examinations are of potential benefit to patients because someone may ask a question no one previously thought to ask.
- Many patients highly appreciate the attention they receive from students, and will be very tolerant; sometimes patients bond very closely with students in a relationship similar to a "true" patient-to-physician relationship.

Confidentiality

The sooner you learn the importance of confidentiality in medicine, the better.

- Never discuss patient information in public—not in elevators, not with your family, not in any setting where unauthorized persons may hear.
- Never release medical information to anyone without permission. Only a competent patient, or the power-of-attorney of an incompetent patient, may authorize you to discuss their case with anyone, even their next of kin. As a medical student, you should always refer requests for medical information to the faculty member whose patient it is.

Professionalism

Of the many aspects of professionalism which will become a part of your patient encounters, none is more important for the beginning medical student to understand than the line between professional and personal relationships. *Never enter a sexual or similarly intimate relationship with a patient. Should you become involved in such an association, you must withdraw from any professional affiliation with the patient.*

There are many more facets to professionalism which will develop through all the years of your career and will enable you to maximally provide the best of care to your patients. (See Chapters 1 and 3.)

Patients' responsibilities

As in each of the relationships we have discussed, the ethics of student-to-patient encounters apply to both parties. Patients have no right to abuse a student in any way.

Report to your supervisor:

- verbal abuse
- gender, racial, or ethical harassment
- physical aggressiveness or violence by a patient

AN INTRODUCTION TO MEDICAL PRACTICE ETHICS

These cases are often heavily laden with the emotions of all parties, and are extremely individual and patient-specific.

All our discussion so far has centered on your personal growth as students becoming clinicians. But what about the larger issues of the ethics of medical decision making? When your patients' medical problems are complicated by ethical issues, providing adequate and appropriate care may become a labyrinthine task. You will surely encounter ethical concerns at every level of patient contact; many may be too complex for even the most experienced clinician to solve alone. Nevertheless, certain general principles provide a guide upon which solid ethical decisions can be made.

Four primary principles underpin medical practice ethics:

- autonomy
- nonmaleficence
- beneficence
- justice.

A number of secondary ethical concerns, for example, confidentiality and truth-telling, are derived from the application of the primary principles, as we illustrate in our discussion and several examples.

Autonomy

Most ethicists regard autonomy as the most important tenet of medical ethics, the one which overrides all others whenever a conflict among principles occurs. *Autonomy is defined as the idea that a competent adult has the right to make his or her own choices in every aspect of life, including medical matters.*

This seems straightforward enough; but consider these few corollaries and complications of the autonomy principle:

- What is it that makes one competent or incompetent? When do we determine that a person no longer has decision making capacity? And *who* decides? Answers to these questions evolve continually, and the legal aspects differ from state to state.
- Judgement does not enter into the competency decision. In other words, patients' decisions are valid, whether you would have made the same decision or not. Granted, some decisions are very hard to accept! But that is the point: competent adults decide for themselves.
- The whole concept of informed consent derives from the autonomy principle. To make reasonable decisions in their own best interests about medical matters, adult patients must understand the consequences of their decisions, and they must be free of coercion.
- It is possible (and highly desirable) to document your autonomous choices for your own care by a Living Will or advance directive. Many ethical dilemmas of physicians in critical medical situations could be avoided if patients prepared these documents in advance of their needing them.

Nonmaleficence

This is another way of saying "Do no harm." Our medical practices must be driven by the principle of nonmaleficence, with the implied understanding that nothing which is potentially harmful may be offered to a patient unless the potential harm is far overridden by the chance for benefit.

- This principle is the reason that research protocols for new drugs and medical procedures are so stringent and carefully monitored.
- Nonmaleficence is not equivalent to nonaggressiveness. Sometimes chances are worth taking.
- The important secondary principle of *confidentiality* is derived from both autonomy and nonmaleficence. An autonomous patient "owns" information about him or herself; improper disclosure of medical information may certainly be a maleficent act, causing enormous, sometimes irreparable harm.

Beneficence

Related to, but somewhat different than nonmaleficence is beneficence, *the idea of supplying a positive benefit, or doing good, for the patient*. It implies an active role for the physician in making things better for patients.

- Benefit has to be defined *in the patient's terms*. Communicate with your patients to clearly understand their goals. You may be surprised to discover they are sometimes very different from yours.
- The "downside" of beneficence is that it may give rise to paternalism. You cannot be your patients' fathers or mothers and therefore cannot make their decisions for them.

Justice

Justice is the principle that *equals should be treated equally*. We would all like a society in which every patient with disease "X" had equal access to sure-fire treatments "Y" and "Z." Several real world problems stand in the way, however:

- Every physician is not equally expert and every community does not have equal facilities.
- Patients' abilities to physically access medical care are extremely variable. This variability is caused by geographic, financial and other factors.
- Financial resources for medical care are finite and in many cases diminishing. If a state's Medicaid (medical assistance for the needy) program has a million dollars to spend, should it be used to provide vaccinations for 50 000 children or bone marrow transplants for five children? A year's nursing home care and

For a fascinating dramatized account of this situation, read George Bernard Shaw's *The Doctor's Dilemma*.

medicines for 20 elderly Alzheimer's patients, or prenatal and obstetrical care for 200 women?

- The dilemmas arising from the justice principle are problems for society as a whole. *A physician should never need to make a resource allocation decision at the bedside.*

CASE ANALYSIS

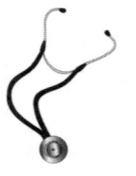

The following brief case analysis illustrates some of the more commonly encountered ethical problems, as well as a framework you can use to work through some of these difficult problems.

Mr. L.C. is a 72-year-old man you have cared for in your office practice for the past 10 years. He has been reasonably healthy except for some well controlled hypertension and mild osteoarthritis. He comes to your office complaining of a cough productive of a small amount of blood-streaked sputum. Your physical exam is negative, but you notice a 7 lb weight loss since his last routine visit about 2 months ago. A chest X-ray shows a small mass in the right lung, and you arrange to have him admitted to the hospital for additional tests, including bronchoscopy.

While he is undergoing bronchoscopy, his wife and daughter approach you in the hallway, and discuss his case. "Whatever you do, doctor, if this is cancer, don't tell Dad," his daughter implores you. "He gets nervous so easily. He won't be able to take it."

What is the ethical concern here and what should your response be? The family believes that information would be harmful and therefore they ask you to apply the "nonmaleficence" principle. That is, it may harm him to hear bad news, so you should withhold the news. However, the autonomy principle overrides other considerations. He is a competent adult with no signs of mental incapacity, and therefore he has the right to know medical information about himself. Is it then entirely his decision to share it with others or not. The only exception to this rule is in the case of certain communicable diseases.

The biopsy results return and Mr. L.C. does have lung cancer. It is "small cell carcinoma," a type known to be fast-growing and quick to spread to other organs. You do tell the patient this information and, with his permission, his wife and daughter also. You also refer the patient to an oncologist, Dr. T.F., who examines him the next day, to discuss treatment options.

Dr. T.F. explains to the patient that he should have scans of his brain and liver, and that his best treatment option would be a multidrug chemotherapy regimen. (While small cell carcinoma is still almost universally fatal, the average life expectancy with treatment has been extended to over a year. Previously, most patients died a few weeks to a few months after diagnosis.) Treatment requires a few days in the hospital about once a month, and side effects would potentially include nausea, vomiting, hair loss, and increased susceptibility to infection. Mr. L.C. considers this information, and the next day he asks you to discharge him because he wants nothing further done. Outside his room, his daughter begs you to make him change his mind. "If it would make him live longer, he just *has* to get treatment." What is the ethical concern, and what might be an appropriate response?

The patient exercised his autonomy, and the family looks to you for beneficence, to do something positive to benefit him. His request overrides theirs. However, because of the gravity of this decision, you may want to have considerably more discussion with Mr. L.C. to clarify the following points: Is he definitely mentally intact? Did he clearly understand the information from Dr. T.F.? Is his decision to forego treatment based on hearsay reports from others about the perils of chemotherapy? Does the decision seem to be consistent with his previous habits and major decisions?

After your discussion, the patient does not immediately agree to further intervention, but does agree to return to your office in one week. He will think seriously about taking treatment, if you will discharge him so he can go home and consider all his options with his family members. You agree with this plan.

SUMMARY

Full development of your personal ethical creeds and standards is a lifetime evolutionary process. We encourage you to build upon the idealism, which you undoubtedly bring with you to medical school, by recognizing the ethical components of your student experience and developing a solid platform for assisting patients with their most difficult decisions.

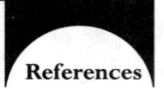

References

1. Dans, P. "Self-Reported Cheating by Students at One Medical School."
    Academic Medicine 71(1): S70–S72; Jan suppl. 1996.

Suggested Reading

Messner, Roberta L. and Lewis, S. J. Increasing Patient Satisfaction. Springer
    Publishing Co., NY, 1996.

Project Professionalism. The American Board of Internal Medicine.
    Philadelphia, PA, 1995.

Reed, J.L. and Hallock, D. "Encouraging Ethical Behavior in Class." The
    Teaching Professor 19(1): 1; Jan. 1996.

Reiser, S.J. "The Ethics of Learning and Teaching Medicine." Academic
    Medicine 69(11): 872–876; 1994.

Thomas, L. The Youngest Science: Notes of a Medicine-Watcher. Viking Press,
    NY, 1983.

Practical Help for Early Clinical Encounters

Interviewing and 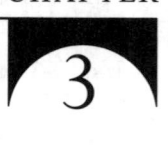 3
Touching Patients

Sarah A. McCarty and Marie C. Veitia

INTRODUCTION

As you begin medical school, you will often hear that communication skills are essential to the development of a therapeutic relationship with your patients. But the reality of the basic science years, with the enormous amount of scientific information that you will be asked to assimilate, may make it hard for you to recognize the significance of developing good communication skills. You will be bombarded with exciting scientific breakthroughs, amazing technological advances, and political upheaval in health care. Ultimately where will you and your patient be amidst all of this growing science and recent political change? The two of you are still sitting in a room together trying to chart an appropriate course of action. How can you know the right course of action if you know little or nothing about your patient other than the name of his disease?

The patient–physician relationship has been described as "a powerful, sometimes mysterious, frequently healing interaction *between human beings*" (1). It is a process that develops collaboratively over time and at its core is effective communication. It is *not* simply good "bedside manner" or being nice to patients. The patient–physician relationship is founded on the "therapeutic core qualities" of respect, genuineness and sympathy described by Carl Rogers (Table 3-1). Throughout this chapter you will learn how your actions in the interview process can make these qualities manifest in your relationships.

The skills and attitudes that create a therapeutic relationship are a critical component of the "art" of medicine. Separating these skills from "science" is not without risk, as both are important to modern medical

> The patient–physician relationship is a healing partnership that is central to the success or failure of patient care.

Table 3-1. Essentials of the Patient–Physician Relationship (2)

Respect	Suspend critical judgment and fully accept the patient
Genuineness	Be yourself in the relationship
Empathy	Accurately understand your patient's feelings and communicate this to them

care. The effective interviewing and communication skills described in this chapter, *when combined with clinical confidence*, can lead to the acquisition of more accurate data, improved diagnostic skills, more comprehensive treatment and an overall improved therapeutic alliance.

How should you, then, go about developing the requisite knowledge, skills, and attitudes to foster such relationships with patients in light of the multiple competing demands of medical school? Practicing the skills discussed in this chapter, will help you develop good communication skills over time, and you will begin to feel more comfortable with patients and your role as a beginning physician.

COMPONENTS OF THE PATIENT–PHYSICIAN ENCOUNTER

When you communicate effectively, your patients will perceive that more time has been spent with them and will be generally more satisfied with their medical care. They will be more likely to adhere to your treatment recommendations and less likely to pursue malpractice claims against you.

The skills involved in interviewing patients are learned by practicing certain behaviors. While keeping in mind the fundamental principles of a therapeutic relationship, it is also important to work toward meeting the goals of the medical interview described in Table 3-2. Building rapport is always the first goal. The medical interview, even in today's technological world, remains key in the development of a differential diagnosis. A differential diagnosis is a list of possible disease processes which may explain the etiology of a patient's complaint. Details in obtaining an appropriate history for the purpose of developing a differential diagnosis are discussed in Chapter 8. Other information gathering

Table 3-2.   Goals of the Medical Interview

Establish *Rapport*
Gather Information
  Develop a *problem list* and *differential diagnoses*
  Understand patients' *fears* and *expectations*
  Assess patients' *adaptation to illness*
  Evaluate patients' *knowledge of disease*

goals are discussed below and illustrated in the following example case. As you read it, ask yourself two questions:

"Why did Mr. Smith seek medical care now?"
"What does he expect me to do for him?"

Mr. Smith is a 54-year-old man who presents with left sided abdominal pain of three years duration.
You begin the interview by asking: "Mr. Smith, can you tell me about your pain?"
"Well doctor it started about three years ago and comes about two or three times a month. It lasts about an hour or so and goes away."
"Does anything you do help your pain?"
"Well, I usually just wait it out and it goes away. Never worried about it much but then my neighbor had some bleeding. Now he is real sick with colon cancer."
"Have you had any bleeding?"
"Well, a little but only when I am constipated. I think it is from my hemorrhoids."

Now, review your interview. *Why did Mr. Smith seek care now?* His neighbor has been recently diagnosed with colon cancer and he probably fears that he too has colon cancer. Recognizing that, you pursue further evaluation to be sure you **meet his expectations**.

"Mr. Smith, I think we need to do further testing. Your pain does not sound severe. However, your bleeding could be because of your hemorrhoids, or it could be from some other cause. I believe we should do some further testing to find out whether it is your hemorrhoids or not."
"Yes, doctor, I agree. I want you to do whatever is necessary to be sure that I do not have cancer. I can live with the pain, but I am worried that I have ignored something I should not."

What did Mr. Smith expect you to do for him?

Mr. Smith *expected* at this visit to be evaluated for colon cancer. Had you not discovered this fear or explored this expectation, you might have appropriately decided that his pain did not need further evaluation, but he *would not have been satisfied* with his visit. Every patient has one of several expectations from a visit which may vary from reassurance, to pain control, to cure for an incurable disease.

The following case illustrates the importance of **understanding your patient's adaptation to their disease** and their knowledge of their disease. As you read this case, ask yourself two further questions:

"How has Mrs. Jones' life been affected by her illness?"
"How well does Mrs. Jones understand her disease and its potential prognosis or complications?"

Differential diagnoses guide the tests you order and the treatments you recommend.

Patient satisfaction ratings are higher when expectations are met.

> Mrs. Jones is a 67-year-old woman who presents for follow-up of her diabetes.
> During your interview, you ask about her medication.
> "Mrs. Jones are you taking your pills for your sugar?"
> "Yes, usually I am."
> "Are you checking your blood sugars?"
> "Oh yes and they are all really good."
> You conclude the interview, "Sounds like you are doing really well. I just need you to go to the lab for a blood test to see how well your sugar has been controlled for the last 3 months."

The blood test you ordered is a glycosylated hemoglobin. In diabetic patients, the goal is a level less than 8. Mrs. Jones' level was 13 which implies very poor control of her diabetes. Are there statements in the interview which if, had you pursued them, would have improved the quality of this interaction?

Review the interview. Now note that Mrs. Jones said that she *usually* takes her pill. This turned out to be a clue which should have been recognized. Then you might have asked:

> "Usually? Are there times that you do not take the pill?"
> She openly and honestly replies, "Yes, at the end of the month I do not."
> "Why?"
> "Because I get paid at the beginning of the month and have very little food at the end of the month. If I take my pills, I get weak and shaky so I just don't take them the last week."

This woman has adapted to her disease by making a choice. She avoids taking her pills when her food supply runs low, a reasonable choice under the circumstances. What can you do? You can explore her knowledge and understanding of her disease. Her statement that her sugars were "good" needed further elaboration, for example:

> "What are your sugars in the morning?"
> "They are less than 200."
> "And the rest of the day?"
> "Oh, I don't know because as long as they are low in the morning, I figure I can eat all I want and in fact if they are less than 140 I always reward myself with a piece of cake. I never check them during the day."

Two hundred is *not* the desired level for a fasting blood sugar and reasonable blood sugars of 140 should not be rewarded with pieces of cake. This patient needs more education and she needs more money. You can refer her to Social Services but recognize that the education deficit is far easier to rectify than the financial problem.

If the clues in the interview are pursued, the physician can help the patient early and more thoroughly. In this case, the physician would have

been able to predict that the patient's diabetes was not controlled, and would better understand some of the limitations this patient had in her own ability to control her disease and in her understanding of it.

Facilitating the Interview

The medical interview is a process that requires purposeful use of techniques that encourage the patient to continue to talk. These skills are summarized in Table 3-3. *Nonverbal communication skills, such as eye contact, body language, and facial expression are essential interview facilitators* that indicate to the patient you are interested and concerned about their illness. You are probably familiar with the need for maintaining personal space, and you know that there are important cultural differences among differing groups in the amount of space needed for comfort. This concept applies to your medical interview as well as to everyday conversation.

The appropriate use of **silence** also encourages continued interaction but, because of our own discomfort, we have greater difficulty using this facilitative technique. Silence is a much discussed, yet difficult to develop, interview skill, and you may perceive moments of silence as awkward and uncomfortable. It is important to recognize that silence is a normal consequence of human interaction which occurs especially when we attempt to convey uncomfortable, complex or emotion-laden material.

> Resist the temptation to jump in, and instead, allow some silence to occur in the interview.

Table 3-3. Facilitating the Interview

Nonverbal skills
Eye contact
Body language
Facial expression
Use of personal space

Verbal skills
Silence
Non-directive open-ended questions
Reflection and clarification
Summarization

Verbal communication tools also include the ability to direct questions in a manner that begins broadly and gradually narrows the focus. **Non-directive, open-ended questions** that require more than yes or no responses are very useful in gathering information. For example, much more information may be gathered by asking your patient to *describe* their abdominal pain, rather than just asking "Do you have abdominal pain?" (to which the entire response may be just "yes"). **Reflection**, a technique by which the interviewer repeats the patient's last few words either verbatim or by paraphrasing encourages continued conversation. Reflection also allows you to clarify information and to demonstrate that you understand what the patient is trying to convey. Simple responses such as "I see" can greatly enhance the interviewing process. Verbal facilitation skills such as reflection and **summarization**—that is, using summary statements at strategic points during the interview—are useful when the interview inevitably begins to slow down or when the interviewer needs to move on to other concerns.

Components of the Medical Interview

The medical encounter has three components:

- The opening
- The information gathering phase
- The summary, which includes patient education.

In the opening, introduce yourself and explore the patient's reasons for the visit. Information gathering to form diagnostic hypotheses, and the physical examination, take place in the middle of the interview. The patient education phase, which completes the interview, is the time when diagnoses and treatment plans are discussed. Your final statements summarize the visit, explore patient understanding and make arrangements for follow-up. During all three components of the encounter, you must *remember the importance of your patient's needs and expectations*.

Opening the interview

Introducing yourself The manner by which you begin the interview is important in establishing rapport with your patient. Introduce yourself and shake your patient's hand. *When you greet the patient, use a title (e.g. Mr., Ms.) in order to demonstrate your respect for them.* Using their name also provides assurance that you are in the right room and have the right

Your very first words to your patient can demonstrate the critical therapeutic quality of respect.

chart. The introduction should also *establish your role in the patient's care. Introduce yourself as a medical student*. By doing so, you create appropriate expectations by your patient.

For example, let us consider this scenario with Mr. Smith who came to be sure he did not have colon cancer.

As it turns out, Mr. Smith did have cancer and is in the hospital recovering from his surgery. The surgeon has told him that other therapy will be needed and that the oncologist will see him today.

In the meantime, you walk in and introduce yourself; you are anxious during your encounter as this is your first interview, and you forget to tell him why you're there. Mr. Smith keeps asking you questions about his treatment plans which you cannot answer and he is clearly becoming upset with you. Finally, out of frustration and fear you say, "Mr. Smith, I am only a first-year medical student and the surgeon told me to talk with you before he came back from his office."

"Why didn't you tell me? I thought you were the oncologist. My doctor did mention a student might be in and I said I was a former teacher and would be glad to talk to you."

In this case, both the student and the patient would have been saved a lot of frustration and even anger if the role of the interviewer had been pre-established.

> Usually your faculty mentor or preceptor will introduce you. If you first meet the patient by yourself, be sure to make it clear that you are a student.

The environment of the interview

Having introduced yourself and established your role in your patient's care, you need to next establish the environment of the interview. Both of you should be as comfortable as possible. If at all possible, sit down (but not on the patient's bed). An ideal interview should be conducted with both of you on the same physical level so you can use appropriate eye contact throughout the interview. There should be no physical barriers between the two of you and you should be seated at a comfortable distance from one another. Be sure to close the examining room door or draw the curtain fully around the bed. Avoid distractions as much as possible. In the hospital setting, televisions need to be turned down (ask before doing so). Once you are both as comfortable as possible, begin your interview.

> You need to create an atmosphere of privacy for the interview because the medical encounter is confidential.

Your opening question is designed to establish the symptoms which motivated the patient to seek medical care. It is referred to as the **chief complaint**. A simple question such as, "Why did you come to see us today?" is an example of an open-ended question that invites the patient to express his or her concerns. One study demonstrated that physicians interrupted their patients, on average, within 18 seconds of their

Allowing your patient to express all their concerns in the beginning of the interview establishes an interview style which is "patient centered" and not "physician centered."

Don't forget to ask the patient, "Do you have any questions for me?"

response to the opening questions. Yet, if left uninterrupted, most patients completed their responses by two and a half minutes following the opening question so, *avoid the temptation to interrupt your patient.* Allowing patients to enumerate their complaints also helps you to organize your interview so that you can explore all of the patient's concerns. The two of you can choose with which problem to begin. The patient's choice of which problem to discuss first may give you insight into the significance of the various concerns in his or her life.

"Oh, by the way . . ."

There is a well-known phenomenon in the medical world known as, "Oh, by the way." You have just spent 45 minutes doing a "full" history and physical examination on an apparently healthy person. You have closed the interview and your hand is on the doorknob as you are about to leave the room. After a brief moment of silence when all seems well, the patient says, "Oh, by the way, I don't have chest pain but at times when I walk I get this pressure in my chest." *It is not unusual for problems of major proportion to be mentioned only at the end of the interview.* Patients need to feel comfortable with you in order to discuss those things which most frighten or embarrass them so the "Oh, by the way" problem is not entirely preventable. However, a few well spent minutes at the beginning of the interview may indeed save such a crisis at the end of the interview. If you interrupt your patient during their answer to the very first question you ask, you are sending the message that you are not really listening to them, and are not interested in all the issues which brought them to you for care. In the worst case, the patient may leave your office having never addressed their real reason for coming.

The information-gathering phase

Once you have opened your interview and established with your patient the issues to be discussed, you move on to the information-gathering portion of your encounter. This includes the traditional medical history as well as the physical examination. These aspects of the patient encounter are further discussed in Chapter 8.

The summary

The end of the physical examination marks the transition to the third and final portion of the interview, the summary, which consists of:

- reviewing the findings
- discussing potential diagnoses
- making plans for further evaluation, treatment, and follow-up.

A critical concept here is that this portion of the interview *must* be a two-way conversation instead of a lecture to the patient. Surveys of patient expectations reveal that *patients expect to be asked about their own ideas regarding treatment*. Failure to do so at this point in the interview may adversely affect several aspects of the patient–physician relationship.

In the outpatient setting the patient should be clothed during the final part of the interview. Leaving your patient wrapped in a paper sheet, which is often tattered and torn after the physical examination, does not create an atmosphere conducive to free discussion. Begin this part of the interview by summarizing your findings. Encourage your patient to add to or correct anything you have said. Discuss your diagnostic and treatment plans and explain why you have made your recommendations. During this exchange, be sure that you ask your patient about their ideas for treatment. *Your goal is to reach a treatment plan that is understood by and agreed upon with your patient in the context of his or her life.*

The medical encounter now comes to final closure. Arrangements for follow-up care are discussed and ways to contact the physician in case of emergency are reviewed. It is appropriate to end the interview with another exchange of pleasantries. This is your opportunity as a student to thank the patient for their time and cooperation. Remember Mr. Smith who became so upset with you earlier in this chapter?

Once you have established your role in his care, he agreed to have you continue with your history and physical examination. He was pleased to have the opportunity to help you learn and enjoyed the time and attention you gave him. Your closing, however, did not include a discussion of the treatment plans because in this case, your role is to be a learner, not health care provider. However, you still summarized and allowed him to correct your story as you understood it. You end your interview with, "Thank you, Mr. Smith, for your time. It has really helped me." Even as a first-year student, you will be surprised how often the response will be, "You're welcome, I really enjoyed it."

The Therapeutic Value of Touch

Students often have difficulty making the transition from interviewing a patient to examining them. We cannot complete a discussion of interviewing and communication skills without addressing the role of touch in overall patient care. The culture of health care has discouraged the therapeutic use of touch, and the scientific model of medicine seems to

Experienced clinicians know that patients expect to be touched by their doctors and may not be quite satisfied until they have been examined.

further diminish its relevance, but patients have a very human need to be touched.

The symbolic dimension of touch, the "laying on of hands," has historically been an important component of the healing process. Many readers will have had the experience of feeling better simply by having gone to the doctor. We may never have the scientific data to understand why or how this happens; however, the current school of thought is that physicians and students should use touch for its symbolic value. Placing your hand on a patient's shoulder while listening to the heart is one example of how the physician can utilize touch to facilitate the patient–physician relationship. *While the physician must clearly exercise sound ethical judgment in all instances of physical contact, he or she should not hesitate to view touch as a valuable skill in nurturing relationships with patients and as a therapeutic intervention in and of itself.*

THE STUDENTS' CONTRIBUTION TO PATIENT CARE

To the medical student, the most distressing problem in communicating with patient is your lack of knowledge, skill, and experience as you approach your first patient encounters. This anxiety about your competence can be overwhelming and can interfere with your ability to recognize and use the skills that you *naturally* bring to the patient–physician interaction (see Table 3-4).

Genuineness will show through your interactions with your patients and will strengthen your relationships to them.

As a medical student, you are often the only person on the health care "team" with the time to interact extensively with a patient. The student–patient interaction may be quite helpful to patient care by revealing new data and clarifying problems. You may enable patients to share feelings in ways that will lead them to consider you as their "doctor". You also have to offer patients the natural **curiosity** and **compassion** that led you to medicine in the first place. While you may not have had

Table 3-4. What Medical Students Can Offer Patients

Time for interaction
Curiosity
Compassion
Observational skills
Sense of responsibility

the benefit of experience to be mindful of the interview at several levels at once (e.g. appearance, words, mannerisms, mood), you do bring certain **observational** skills to the interview. This skill can be better developed with time if you become accustomed to asking yourself questions about the observational process. "What did I notice as I walked into the patient's room?" "What was the patient's facial expression when discussing his neighbor's colon cancer?" Finally, you can bring to the patient interaction a sense of **responsibility**. The overall patient–physician relationship improves when the patient senses that he is cared for and that healing efforts will be made on his behalf.

In short, just remember that you can offer patients a number of skills that greatly offset your inexperience and that you are capable of establishing meaningful, therapeutic relationships with your patients. You can learn to manage anxiety and self-consciousness about your role by recognizing these feelings as normal consequences of learning. Remember that patients are anxious about any new medical encounter. Empathizing with the patient's anxiety about meeting the doctor can help you focus more on the patient and less on your own concerns.

> Approach your interview with confidence in the potential contribution you can make to patients.

PATIENT BEHAVIORS WHICH CHALLENGE EFFECTIVE COMMUNICATION

Some patients exhibit behaviors that are frustrating for the physician. Such individuals are often labeled "problem patients" because they seem manipulative, angry, nonadherent or excessively somatically focused. Remember though that such patients are not always acting deliberately. Rather, weighted down by their fears and anxieties, they are attempting to navigate a confusing health care system in an effort to cope with their illness. It may be useful for you to regard "problem patient behavior" as yet another "symptom"; this may give you some idea as to how this patient interacts with other individuals and may facilitate your understanding the whole person.

> Blaming the patient for "problem" behavior detracts from our ability to examine the situation and ask why the patient is behaving this way.

Two clinical examples of how a patient might challenge communications with their physician deserve special mention. Even experienced clinicians will have problems with these two types of patients: those who are significantly depressed, and patients exhibiting seductive behavior.

- Interacting with a **depressed, tearful patient** can be frightening. Crying patients create anxiety about whether or not they will stop crying and how you should behave in the meantime. Similarly, it is anxiety-provoking to assess **suicidal** ideation or intent; students

Remember that empathy is one of the core properties of the patient–physician relationship.

often worry that their questions will lead patients to harm themselves. As a general guideline for these situations, you need to respond to the patient in a fashion that feels intuitively right for you. For example, simply handing a tissue to a patient sends a message that crying is acceptable in this relationship. You may be sure that your questions will not plant the idea of suicide in the patient's mind. Indeed, the potentially suicidal patient may be quite relieved to see their physician demonstrating interest in their emotional problems.

- Patients who behave seductively when interacting with their physician also present a unique challenge. Professional behavior must be maintained at all times. Under no circumstance is it acceptable for the student or physician to respond sexually to the patient or to pursue a relationship outside the professional realm. Instead, the physician can examine *why* the patient is behaving seductively, while attempting to divert or refocus the patient on the purpose of the interview.

COMMON ERRORS IN THE MEDICAL INTERVIEW

Be curious about your patients and interested in them. Enjoy the interview and see what unexpected things you might learn that no one else on the health care team knows.

As you begin to interview patients, there are some common errors about which you should become aware. These errors, described in Table 3-5, can have significant negative impact upon that atmosphere of open communication you have worked so hard to create.

Overdirecting the interview can occur when you are worried about not getting the "right" information or about taking too long. Because of your own lack of medical knowledge you will not be sure if the information the patient gives you in response to open-ended questions is important or not. In order to "get done" in a reasonable time, you may tend to take control of the interview by asking very direct questions.

Table 3-5. Common Errors in Interviewing

Overdirecting the interview
Leading the patient (verbally or nonverbally)
Making judgmental statements
Asking multiple questions simultaneously
Using medical jargon
Failing to clarify misunderstandings

Leading the patient either verbally or nonverbally is another very common error. Questions should never be asked in the negative form such as, "You don't have chest pain do you?" The implication here is that it must be really bad to have chest pain and the doctor does not want you to have it. The reply will frequently be, "Oh no, I do not." But is it a true response or have you just contributed to your patient's denial of a symptom that they already fear? Shaking your head yes or no as you ask a question is another way you can inappropriately lead the patient. Be sure when you ask a question that it is verbally and nonverbally neutral so the patient is not biased in answering.

The medical interview deals with many sensitive issues. People do not always behave in ways consistent with your own moral, religious, or cultural beliefs. Remember, it is your responsibility to create and maintain an atmosphere in which patients feel free to tell you intimate details of their own lives. Even if you find their behavior totally unacceptable, **never make a judgmental statement**. Such a statement may close the lines of communication forever. Your body language may also make a statement so be aware of your own expression of surprise, shock, or dismay. Even a simple reaction like moving your body away from the patient may signify disapproval.

Ask only one question at a time. Allow the patient time to respond before moving on to the next question. If you ask, "Do you have chest pain, fever, or cough?", to which question is the patient supposed to respond? If the patient is overwhelmed or confused by your questions, they may not ask you to clarify; they may simply say "no." Or if they say, "Yes, I do", does that mean they have one of the symptoms, or all three?

Over the next few years, you will learn a whole new vocabulary. Remember that your patient may not know the meaning of even simple medical terms and abbreviations, so **avoid the use of medical "jargon."** Be careful to use terms your patient understands and always clarify terms your patient uses if you do not understand them.

A great deal of information is exchanged during the medical encounter and this creates enormous opportunity for misunderstandings. **As you end the interview, do not assume that you have both understood each other perfectly**. Observe for nonverbal clues such as frowns or long hesitations in answering questions which may imply that the question is not fully understood. Always ask patients if they have questions, even if they appear to understand.

Reviewing a videotaped interview is useful in pointing out subtle ways you may lead a patient with your body language.

Maintain your professional demeanor.

Avoid misunderstandings by asking only one question at a time.

Will your patients know that "SOB" means "short of breath"?

SUMMARY

The fundamental principles of respect, genuineness, and empathy are central to developing a therapeutic relationship with your patients. You are just beginning to learn the necessary communication skills and these will improve throughout your medical career. We reviewed a number of verbal and nonverbal interviewing techniques to help you as you begin to talk with patients. Remember to keep in mind the multiple goals of the interview. Don't panic if you do not know exactly the right questions to ask as that will come with medical knowledge and experience. *Relax* and enjoy your patient encounters as they are truly the most rewarding aspect of medicine.

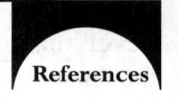

References

1. Cousins, N.: Physician as communicator. JAMA 248: 587, 1982.
2. Rogers, C.R.: The necessary and sufficient conditions of therapeutic personality change. Journal of Consulting Psychology 21: 95–103, 1957.

Suggested Reading

Balint, M.: The doctor, the patient, the illness. Second edition. International Universities Press, NY, 1964.

Beckman, H.B. & Frankel, P.M.: The effect of physician behavior on the collection of data. Annals of IM 101: 692–696, 1984.

Branch, W.T., Levinson, W. & Platt, F.W.: Diagnostic interviewing: make the most of your time. Patient Care, July, 1996.

Harpole, L.H., Orav, J., Hickey, M., Posther, K.E. & Brennan, T.A.: Patient satisfaction in the ambulatory setting: influence of data collection methods and sociodemographic factors. J. Gen. Int. Med. 11: 431–434, 1996.

Hewson, M.G.: Patient education through teaching for conceptual change. J. Gen. Int. Med. 8: 393–398, 1993.

Kravitz, R.L., Callehan, E.J., Azari, R., Antonius, D. & Lewis, C.E.: Assessing patients' expectations in ambulatory medical practice: Does the measurement approach make a difference? J. Gen. Int. Med. 12: 67–72, 1997.

Kravitz, R.L., Cope, D.W., Bhrany, V. & Leake, B.: Internal medicine patients' expectations for care during office visits. J. Gen. Int. Med. 9: 75–81, 1995.

Lane, C. & Davidoff, F.: Patient centered medicine, a professional evaluation. JAMA. 272 (2): 152–1566, 1996.

Lipkin, M.: The medical interview and related skills. In Branch, W.T. (ed.): Office Practice of Medicine, First edition, W.B. Saunders Company, Philadelphia, PA, 1987.

Mangione, S. & Peitzman, S.J.: Physical diagnosis in the 1990s: art or artifact? J. Gen. Int. Med. 11: 490–493, 1996.

Nardone, D.A., Johnson, G.K., Faryna, A., Coulehan, J.L. & Parrino, T.A.: A model for the medical interview: nonverbal, verbal, and cognitive assessments. J. Gen. Int. Med. 7: 437–442, 1992.

Reiser, D.E. & Rosen, D.H.: Medicine as Human Experience. Rockville, MD, Aspen Systems Corporation, 1985.

Thomas, L.: The youngest science: notes of a medicine-watcher. Viking Press, NY, 1983.

White, J., Levinson, W. & Roter, D.: "Oh, by the way . . .": The closing moments of the medical interview. J. Gen. Int. Med. 9: 24–28, 1994.

Assessment  4

David B. Carr and Sarah A. McCarty

INTRODUCTION

Brace yourself! Now that you are a medical student, you must be prepared for an avalanche of information, because you've entered a profession in which the knowledge base literally increases daily. The information you need will be presented to you in novel ways and in multiple venues.

Through: lectures, formal and informal discussions, slides, computer generated technology, and your own reading.
By: dozens of faculty and support personnel each with their own level of expertise and personal teaching style.
In: classrooms, lecture halls, the library, inpatient and outpatient clinics, a variety of hospital settings, hospice, nursing homes, home health agencies, and your own home.

Clearly you and your classmates will be responsible for an awesome amount of information, more than any other students in the history of medicine.

You will be expected to develop a knowledge base in a number of different subject areas. Traditionally, the first 2 years of medical school have been committed to "the basic sciences" such as anatomy, biochemistry, histology, physiology, pharmacology and immunology. You still need to learn these topics in detail. However, the current trend calls for inclusion of more "clinical science" in the first 2 years of medical school. You will be expected to learn communication skills, physical examination skills and clinical problem-solving skills, integrating basic and clinical science early in the curriculum.

While you find ways to come to grips with this information, it is the responsibility of your medical school faculty to determine if you have

learned and developed the appropriate *knowledge, skills and attitudes*. Early evaluation of your clinical skills and attitudes toward patient care becomes crucial.

During your 4 years of medical school, these attributes will be assessed many times. You will be required to take a lot of tests to demonstrate that you have learned well. Expect also to be evaluated by your clinical preceptors in areas such as your level of professionalism and your humanistic qualities. At the conclusion of each course in your curriculum, you will receive a grade indicating that you have achieved a certain level of **knowledge** and **understanding**. In clinical courses this grade also reflects your level of **skill** and **attitudes**. A satisfactory grade allows you to move on to the next phase of the curriculum. An unsatisfactory grade may require remediation.

Each medical school curriculum is unique. While most offer courses with proven content and concepts designed to be delivered at certain comparable points in the program, the curriculum structure and delivery is continually being revised to provide the very latest information through the most effective teaching methods. The goal is to produce the highest possible quality of student learning. *Expectations for you are high!*

> Your student handbook should outline criteria for successful completion of the curriculum, criteria for remediation and even possible dismissal if performance is very poor.

THE ASSESSMENT PROCESS

Medical school curriculums evolved over many years to encompass the salient features of the knowledge that has been developed through research and practice. Assessment of student performance has evolved as well. Now tools can accurately determine if students *demonstrate the intended knowledge*, *understanding*, *and proficiency*. You will be evaluated outside of the classroom setting also. Clinical assessment includes a review of your performance based on observations made in clinical settings. These evaluations include not only mastery of knowledge, but also ability to apply this knowledge effectively. In other words, "How well can you deliver medical care?"

Faculty will assess your knowledge through close observation of you in the process of learning. Multiple monitoring techniques will be utilized throughout each period of your learning to avoid gaps in both *what* is being taught and *how* you come to understand subject matter. Faculty need a continuous flow of accurate information to determine your level of performance.

Summative and Formative Evaluation

An example of formative evaluation is verbal feedback a preceptor may give you during your performance of the heart examination. If you are not listening in the proper areas, they may correct you and show you the appropriate areas in which to listen to the heart.

Summative evaluations include tests and other graded evaluations. While the name may not be familiar to you, most evaluations you have received heretofore are of this type. Good summative assessments must be demonstrably reliable, valid, and free of bias. On the other hand, **formative** evaluation aims to improve the *quality of student learning* by feedback, advice, and hands-on-instruction. It is continuous over time. It is not designed to provide grades. Both techniques are used in medical school to evaluate your knowledge of a number of difficult databases and skills. Faculty must determine your ability to remember, explain, and utilize information that is required of a physician (summative). You will be guided through the learning process by faculty and other nonphysician instructors (formative).

Classroom Assessment

Classroom assessment, usually by written testing, is designed to help the faculty determine what you have learned. It should be learner-centered (you), and teacher-directed (faculty), and thus be a mutually beneficial route to *content* mastery.

Clinical Assessment

Be active in your learning! Ask your clinical preceptors often for feedback so you can improve your performance.

Developing students' understanding is a primary goal of teaching (1). In this case, understanding is defined as the ability to apply facts, concepts, and skills appropriately. Numerous evaluation methods can be used to determine a student's level of understanding. The four most common methods are:

1. Norm-referenced evaluation or comparing students to one another.
2. Criterion-referenced evaluation or evaluation based on absolute, objective performance standards with a focus on mastery of content, standardized tests or outcome.
3. Evaluation based on improvement.
4. Evaluation based on effort.

Norm-referenced and criterion-referenced evaluation are the traditional methods of performance evaluation in medical education. However, concern exists about the adequacy of these conventional

methods, and currently there is a movement embracing **performance assessment** which includes specific task performance, application of knowledge, and presentations of solutions to real medical problems.

This trend accounts for the development of **problem-based learning** which is now part of the curriculum in many medical schools. Problem-based learning involves presenting clinical problems to students, which they attempt to solve. These clinical problems are used, rather than formal lectures, to introduce new knowledge and concepts. Performance assessments seem better suited than traditional tests because they measure "what really counts": whether you can apply your knowledge, skills, and understanding in clinically oriented settings to solve problems.

In order for performance *assessment* to work, the curriculum must include performance-based *instruction* on a regular basis. McTighe (2) described seven strategies of performance-based assessment which demonstrate *how assessment will help you learn*. They form the underpinnings of the curriculum structure. Our discussion aims to help you understand the reasons why you will be challenged with certain performance-based experiences over the next four years.

Performance-based assessment strategies

1. *Establish clear performance targets.* Clear performance targets must be communicated to you in all content areas because attitudes and perceptions toward learning are influenced by the degree to which you understand what is expected of you. Often these performance targets will be presented to you as *goals* and *objectives*. Performance targets help identify curriculum priorities, essential in the assessment process.

2. *Strive for authenticity in product and performances.* Performance tasks should require you to demonstrate your knowledge, skills and attitudes in ways that improve your ability to care for patients. You may be asked to record information or physically perform skills which are necessary in patient care. Your responses should model actual patient care situations. A common method of practical evaluation is the **objective structured clinical examination** (OSCE). Differing formats are available for the OSCE, but the basic format is a multiple station examination using standardized patients. At each station you are asked to perform a specific measurable task in a prescribed period of time (e.g. you may be asked to perform a cardiac examination or interview a patient with a specific complaint, such as chest pain). The evaluator, who

Students who serve on their school's curriculum committee will want to pay particular attention to these teaching and assessment strategies.

watches you, has a preset checklist of performance standards which you are expected to meet.

3. *Publicize criteria and performance standards.* Assessment must be based upon accepted criteria. By sharing the criteria with you, faculty indicate *how* your work will be evaluated. Each of your course syllabuses should outline the criteria for performance, which are essential for summative evaluations. McTighe explains that by highlighting the elements of quality and standards of performance, you will be able to *internalize your responsibility toward your own learning*.

   When you have the opportunity to examine your own work in light of known criteria and performance standards, you will be able to shift your orientation from "What grade did I get?" to "What do I need to do to improve?".

4. *Provide models of excellence. Models* of the various criteria will help you understand how physicians apply basic knowledge to problem-solving situations. These models may be written, can be demonstrations via live performance or videotape, or can be explained by faculty through discussion (often based on physician experience). *You need to see quality models of effective practice in medicine.* You may also be exposed to less than acceptable work and be asked to identify the "bad" characteristics that keep it from being recognized as quality.

   Many schools now have mentoring programs beginning in the first year, which allow you the opportunity to work with a physician/mentor in their office. Seeing your mentor in actual patient care is perhaps the ultimate model.

5. *Teach strategies explicitly.* Professionals in every field seek new ideas, techniques, strategies, and feedback in order to become better at what they do. One effective strategy for the delivery of medical knowledge is to present it in this seven-step sequence:

   (i)   Introduction: what is the knowledge to be learned?;
   (ii) Explanation: purpose and instructional cues;
   (iii) Demonstration: model effective techniques;
   (iv) Participation: guided practice;
   (v)   Solution: share outcomes;
   (vi) Evaluation: how successful was the exercise?;
   (vii) Reflection: effectiveness of the strategies utilized.

   These seven steps enable you to prepare to learn; understand the purpose of learning; understand the sequences leading to mastery; see how the techniques and skills are

performed; spend time practicing those techniques and skills until they are mastered; share in your experiences to broaden understanding and mastery; compare what you have learned with accepted practice; and, think about what you have learned and how you came to know what you know. Though seldom explicitly aware of the process itself, you will repeat this process often, not only while in medical school but throughout your career in medicine.

6. *Use ongoing assessments for feedback and adjustment.* During your medical education, you will be involved in brainstorming by yourself or with others, drafting initial responses to questions or problems, reviewing relevant medical information, receiving feedback from multiple sources, and revising information you collect or construct. You may be asked to submit numerous drafts of written work which will be critiqued and assessed. Performance-based instruction will guide you to improvement throughout your medical school education because, instead of waiting until the end of instruction, you will be participating in the understanding of what you need to know and why you need to know it from the very beginning. *Mastery takes practice.* High levels of mastery and understanding are achieved only as a result of multiple trials, practice with appropriate feedback, adjustments to performance, and repeated practice. Multiple assessments will help in your level of understanding.

> You should approach your entire medical career as an ongoing assessment and adjustment process.

Medical school faculty will involve you in the opportunity for mastery. In the classroom or on the wards there is insufficient time for you to master all of the new skills you need to learn. *Practicing these skills at home is essential.* Neighbors and friends frequently like to have their blood pressures checked. Offer to do it. Many medical students' spouses or even their cats and dogs have had frequent eye examinations.

7. *Document and celebrate progress.* You will be faced with rigorous performance standards and will spend much time improving your levels of knowledge and understanding. *Celebrate incremental achievements.* Collect assessments of successful work done over a period of time and develop a portfolio that documents understanding in a specific medical area. Your successes will be documented by faculty as they help you in your overall development as a physician.

SUMMARY

Faculty have a variety of measurement tools to assess your abilities to think, solve problems, communicate, collaborate, and perform specific physical skills. These assessments will help you develop a sound medical knowledge base, understand practices and strategies, master necessary skills, and reinforce appropriate attitudes toward patient care.

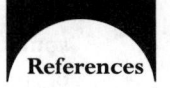

References

1.   Gardiner, H. The unschooled mind. Basic Books, New York, 1991.
2.   McTighe, J. What happens between assessments? Educational Leadership 54, 1: 6–12, 1997.

Suggested Reading

McCombs, B. Processes and skills underlying intrinsic motivation to learn: toward a definition of motivational skills training intervention. Educational Psychologist 19: 197–218, 1984.

Schunk, D. Goal setting and self-efficacy during self-regulated learning. Educational Psychologist 25, 1: 71–86, 1990.

Wiggins, G. Assessing student performance: exploring the limits and purposes of testing. Jossey-Bass, San Francisco, CA, 1993.

Wiggins, G. Practicing what we preach in designing authentic assessments. Educational Leadership 54, 4: 18–25, 1997.

Clinical Evaluation of Common Medical Problems

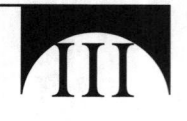

The Prenatal Examination 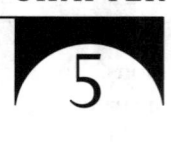 5

Robert C. Nerhood

INTRODUCTION

CASE PRESENTATION

Ms. W.B. and her husband Mr. L.B., both 26 years old, visit your office because they are considering getting pregnant. Married since graduating from college, they have used a variety of birth control measures. Now they are both established in their careers and have decided, "It's time to start a family."

At this preconceptual visit, you do a general examination of Ms. B. and review both of their medical and family histories. You are pleased to be able to tell them that you have identified no significant medical problems.

Seven months later, Ms. W.B. returns to your office. She missed her last menstrual period and last week took a home pregnancy test which was positive.

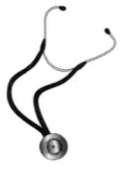

At the turn of the twentieth century, the single most dangerous event that a young woman might face was to become pregnant. In 1900, the maternal mortality rate was 600 to 700 per one hundred thousand live births. This rate decreased to 7.8 per one hundred thousand by 1985. This remarkable reduction in maternal mortality can be attributed to advances in medical care, antibiotics, use of blood products, the control of hypertension and, not insignificantly, the development of an organized, systematic plan of surveillance of a pregnancy. Prenatal care had its origins in England in 1929, as a program of simple biometric measurements. Now it has evolved to include preconceptual counseling, evaluation for pregnancy-related medical conditions, genetic investiga-

Whenever possible,
young women should
undergo examination
and counseling before
becoming pregnant.

tions, fetal assessment, supplementation of diet and vitamins and instruction in neonatal and infant care.

Pregnancy lends itself uniquely to preventive health care because of the well-defined time line and the near universal interest and appeal of the newborn child. The first step, when possible, should be a **preconceptual visit** to provide an opportunity to consider issues of overall health, conditions that might be adversely affected by pregnancy (diabetes/hypertension), immune status (measles/chicken pox/hepatitis B) and the family's genetic history. Then, when the woman becomes pregnant, she and her doctor will already have established a therapeutic relationship which can continue throughout the pregnancy.

Her **prenatal care** will have several important components:

- initial history, physical examination and laboratory assessment
- regular follow-up visits and a flowsheet monitoring the progress of the pregnancy
- special studies to assess specific problems.

A vast array of "prenatal records" are available for documentation of prenatal care. The prenatal form created by the American College of Obstetricians and Gynecologists is probably the most complete and widely used. A portion of this form is reproduced in the appendix at the end of this chapter.

DEFINITIONS

Antenatal, Prenatal: That period in a pregnancy from the time of conception until the onset of labor.

Biparietal Diameter: The biparietal diameter is measured either by abdominal X-ray or more commonly by ultbsound and refers to the greatest transverse diameter of the head which extends from one parietal boss to the other.

Dilation: Dilation is enlargement of the transverse diameter of the cervical opening. In the non-pregnant patient, it is ≤ 5 mm; at complete dilation in labor it is 10 cm.

Eclampsia: Eclampsia is the occurrence of seizures superimposed upon the preeclampsia syndrome.

Effacement: Effacement refers to softening and thinning of the cervix in preparation for dilation.

Engagement: Engagement is the descent of the biparietal diameter of the fetal head into the pelvic inlet.

Estimated date of confinement (EDC): That point in time when labor might be reasonably expected.

Fetal heart tones (FHT): The sound generated by the beating of the fetal heart which may be auscultated over the fundus.

Fundus: The portion of the uterus above the cervix which expands during pregnancy and contains the growing fetus.

Gestation: A pregnancy.

Gravida: The number of times a woman has been pregnant.

HELLP: An acronym which refers to the presence of hemolysis, elevated liver function tests and low platelets superimposed on the preeclampsia syndrome.

Intrapartum: That period of time from the onset of labor until delivery.

LMP: The date of onset of the last menstrual period.

Parity: Completion of a pregnancy beyond what would be considered an abortion. In this country, an abortion is defined as the loss of a pregnancy, *regardless of cause*, of 20 weeks gestation or less or in which the fetus weighs 500 g or less. Note that parity refers to the number of pregnancies, not the number of fetuses. (A multiple gestation is only *one* parity.) Parity is often listed as a series of four numbers (e.g., 2012). These numbers in sequence from left to right refer to the number of term pregnancies, the number of premature pregnancies delivered, the number of abortions and finally, the number of living children.

Postpartum: That period of time beginning with delivery and ending 6 weeks thereafter. The physiologic changes that occur with pregnancy

have resolved at the end of the postpartum period.

Preeclampsia: A syndrome peculiar to pregnancy which is defined by elevated blood pressure, generalized fluid retention and proteinuria.

Quickening: The initial perception of fetal movement by the mother usually occurring at 16 to 18 weeks of pregnancy.

INITIAL HISTORY AND PHYSICAL EXAMINATION

The initial history and physical examination is designed to obtain a comprehensive health history and to establish a baseline of the pregnancy from which follow-up will be established. Ideally, this examination occurs during the first 6 weeks of the pregnancy. The components of the initial examination include general, obstetrical, and family histories, and a physical examination as outlined in Table 5-1.

Initial Laboratory Studies

Pregnant women need more laboratory studies at their initial office visit than almost any other patients. Many conditions which can have an adverse impact on the developing baby can be detected by a comprehensive screening with the following tests.

CBC (complete blood count)
- Iron deficiency anemia is relatively common in pregnancy due to the requirements of the fetus and the common finding of insufficient iron stores in menstruating women.
- Elevated white blood counts will occur in infections.
- Abnormal platelet counts will be important to discover complications.

Rh negative mothers who have Rh positive babies are at risk for isoimmunization and its associated fetal problems.

Blood type and Rh
Some pregnancy complications are associated with unexpected and dangerous bleeding; as transfusion is often required in these circumstances, it is useful to know the maternal blood type. Rh negative mothers who have Rh positive babies are at risk for isoimmunization, a condition in which the mother is exposed to a fetal blood group factor

Table 5-1. Components of the Initial Prenatal Visit

Component	Specific features to be recorded
General medical history	• Any history of hypertension, diabetes, seizure disorder, or bleeding problems • Medication use—prescription or OTC
Obstetrical history	• Past obstetrical experience • Last menstrual period • Regularity of menses • Nausea/vomiting • Breast tenderness • Abnormal bleeding since LMP • Any pelvic pain since LMP
Family history	• Medical illness • Obstetrical history of mother and sisters
Family genetic history	• Both parents
Social history	• Socioeconomic support systems • Nutrition • Emotional factors

Physical examination	• General exam, especially VS and cardio-pulmonary exam
	• Gynecologic exam
	  ▶ Pelvic diameters
	  ▶ Fundal size (Is the fundus the approximate size expected based on time of last menstrual period?)

(Rh antigen) which she (the mother) recognizes as foreign protein and to which she will produce an IgG antibody. This antibody can pass the placenta and cause hemolysis of fetal red blood cells. *Rh isoimmunization is a preventable disorder.*

Blood type antibody screen

Antibody screens are primarily done for determination of the presence of anti-Rh (anti-D) antibodies in Rh negative mothers. Occasionally, unexpected and potentially dangerous rare blood group antibodies are identified (antiKell, Duffy, Kidd, etc.).

STS

A serologic test for syphilis is required by law for public health reasons. Intrauterine syphilis infection is associated with congenital fetal defects that are preventable if treated *in utero*.

Urinalysis and culture

Asymptomatic bacteriuria (the presence of $>100\,000$ colonies of the same species of bacteria in a clean voided specimen of urine from an asymptomatic woman) is common (5 to 12%) in pregnancy and predisposes the patient to urinary tract infections.

Increased rates of urinary tract infections are associated with increased rates of premature labor.

About 25% of pregnant women with untreated, asymptomatic bacteriuria will develop an acute symptomatic urinary tract infection some time during the gestation.

Rubella antibody screen

Rubella infections in pregnancy are dangerous to the developing fetus, and knowledge of the immune status at the onset of a pregnancy is important.

Hepatitis B test

Active hepatitis B is transmissible to the fetus late in pregnancy, and if infection is found, steps can be taken which are very effective in preventing chronic hepatitis in the newborn.

Optional studies

A number of optional but highly recommended tests include:

- HIV status
- Gonorrhea culture
- Chlamydia test (these organisms can cause conjunctival infections in the newborn if there is exposure during labor, and have also been suspected, though not proven, causes of premature labor)
- Hemoglobin electrophoresis in patients of Mediterranean or African origin (sickle cell disease and thalassemia are associated with significant morbidity in the pregnant mother and newborn).

The congenital transmission rate of the HIV virus can be significantly decreased with AZT prophylaxis in the third trimester.

After the initial history and physical examination, you should have a full discussion with the patient including at a minimum:

- The "due date" and whether any confirmatory studies are required.

- A review of significant past medical history, past obstetrical history, family history and/or genetic findings that may affect the pregnancy and any interventions that are indicated.
- A review of general considerations related to pregnancy such as diet, activity, vitamin supplementation, weight gain and the conduct of labor.

Estimated Date of Confinement (EDC)

The determination of the EDC, or "due date," deserves special comments. A human gestation has a duration of 280 days ± 14 (40 weeks/10 lunar months/9 calendar months) and can be calculated by taking the date of the last menstrual period (e.g., 9/10/97) and subtracting 3 months, adding 7 days and 1 year (e.g., 6/17/98). This calculation is quite accurate if the woman is certain of the date of her last menstrual period, and that period was normal with regular cycles. Certain observations during the early part of the pregnancy will support the accuracy of your calculated EDC, including:

> The determination of the EDC is an exceptionally important piece of data with regard to the conduct of a pregnancy and should be determined as early and as accurately as possible.

- appropriate fundal size at first trimester examination
- quickening occurring at about 16–18 weeks
- fundal apex at the umbilicus at 20 weeks
- first auscultation of the fetal heart tones with a fetoscope at 20 weeks.

Any disparity in these observations devalues the accuracy of the calculations and mandates a uterine ultrasound for gestational age.

Ultrasound has evolved as a valuable and safe tool for the evaluation of the fetus and its environment. Standard growth curves based on a number of measurable characteristics (femur length, biparietal diameter, crown–rump length, and abdominal circumference) can accurately determine gestational age in the first and second trimester. As a general rule of thumb, the earlier these determinations are made, the more accurate is the estimated date of confinement (at 6 weeks, the standard error is ± 4 days, at 18 weeks the standard error is ± 10 days). After 24 weeks, the standard error becomes so large that the ultrasound study for gestational age is invalid.

Serial studies for growth, fetal examinations for morphologic abnormalities and placental assessment represent a few of the useful capabilities of ultrasound. The ability of the parents to "see" their baby and identify (sometimes!) the sex of the fetus has made this test a favorite of the patient. However, a controversy continues as to whether

or not an early "dating" ultrasound and a second trimester "morphology" ultrasound should be done as part of standard obstetric care. Most obstetricians and their patients say "yes"; most third party insurance payers say "no."

Follow-up Examinations (Table 5-2)

Following the initial obstetrical consultation, the patient is examined regularly thereafter at 4-week intervals through the 28th week, 2-week intervals through the 36th week and then weekly until delivery. At each of these visits, a number of biometric observations are made, the patient's progress discussed and aspects of prenatal teaching either reviewed or introduced. The standard biometric measurements and their significance include:

Blood pressure It is important to establish a baseline blood pressure early in the pregnancy, to (1) document preexisting hypertension and (2) identify any elevations after the 20th week of gestation which herald the onset of pregnancy-induced hypertension (preeclampsia/eclampsia or transient hypertension of pregnancy). A blood pressure greater than 140/90 is considered significant hypertension during pregnancy.

An elevated blood pressure (140/90 or greater) any time during pregnancy is significant and demands evaluation.

Pregnancy-induced hypertension remains one of the greatest enigmas in medicine and poses a serious threat to the life of the mother and the fetus. This disorder can have a very variable presentation ranging from mild blood pressure increases to fulminant eclampsia (seizures) with multisystem failures; the clinical variability apparently depends upon the location and degree of vasospasm.

Weight In general, weight gain reflects the nutritional status of the pregnant woman and averages 25–40 lb. Lesser gains are acceptable in overweight patients and greater increases are encouraged in underweight patients. One-third of the weight gain occurs in the first one-half of the pregnancy and two-thirds in the second one-half. Weight gain in excess of 2 lb per week in the third trimester may be a sign of fluid retention and the preeclampsia/eclampsia syndrome.

Fundal height A linear measurement of the fundus, from the symphysis pubis to the apex of the uterus, is made each visit. At 12 weeks, the fundal apex should be just at the symphysis, at 16 weeks midway to the umbilicus and at 20 weeks at the umbilicus. From 20 until 38 weeks,

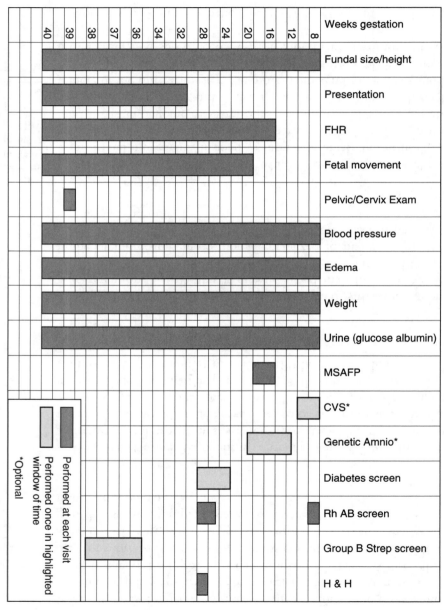

Table 5-2. Follow-up Exams in Uncomplicated Obstetric Patients

Weeks gestation	Performed at each visit / Performed once in highlighted window of time
Fundal size/height	
Presentation	
FHR	
Fetal movement	
Pelvic/Cervix Exam	
Blood pressure	
Edema	
Weight	
Urine (glucose albumin)	
MSAFP	
CVS*	
Genetic Amnio*	
Diabetes screen	
Rh AB screen	
Group B Strep screen	
H & H	

*Optional

MSAFP = maternal serum alpha-fetoprotein; CUS = chorionic villus sampling; Amnio = amniocentesis.

A discordance of ± 3cm from the expected fundal height warrants investigation.

the symphysis–fundal apex measurement should increase about one centimeter per week. After 38 weeks, fundal expansion occurs more laterally and vertical growth becomes less predictable. A discordance of 3 cm or more from expected growth is considered significant. Unusually slow growth suggests fetal growth restriction; greater than expected growth suggests multiple gestation or excessive amniotic fluid accumulation (hydramnios).

Fetal heart tones To confirm continued fetal viability, the presence and rate of fetal heart tones is determined at each visit. Use of Doppler technology allows the fetal heart tones to be determined as early as 10–12 weeks gestation but much variability exists, dependent upon the individual device and the persistence of the observer. Unusually slow (<120 beats per minute) or fast (>180 beats per minute) heart rates warrant more intense scrutiny of fetal health.

Edema Almost all pregnancies are associated with some amount of fluid retention. Usually this is dependent edema which can be ameliorated by intermittent rest periods with the legs elevated and the patient in the lateral recumbent position. Generalized edema (including face and hands as well as feet and ankles) may herald the onset of preeclampsia/eclampsia syndrome.

Any reduction in fetal activity perceived by the mother should be evaluated promptly (within hours).

Fetal movement "Quickening" which is the initial maternal perception of fetal movement, likened to intraabdominal "butterflies", occurs around 16–18 weeks of pregnancy. Thereafter, the increasing activity of the baby is an ongoing reassurance to the mother. The fetus has about a 45-minute sleep cycle and is usually active when awake. Through the middle of the third trimester, the movements tend to be flicks and kicks. As the pregnancy nears its completion and the relative amount of intrauterine free space decreases, the movements are more often rolls and stretches.

Contrary to common belief, babies *do not* quit moving before the onset of labor, and *patients should be counseled to report any notable decrease in fetal activity*. In situations where there is concern for fetal well being, the mother is asked to consciously count fetal movements one or more times each day for a prescribed period of time and report immediately to the obstetrician if the number of movements drops below a specified level.

Fetal position After 28–32 weeks of gestation, the position of the fetus relative to the maternal pelvis can be determined by the application of a series of abdominal palpation maneuvers originally described by Leopold & Sporlin in 1894 (see *Williams Obstetrics*, 20th Edition pp. 180–181, Appleton & Lange, 1997). These maneuvers determine malpresentations (breech/transverse lie) and whether or not engagement has occurred. Engagement indicates full descent of the presenting part (normally the head of the baby) into the inlet of the true pelvis. In general, if engagement occurs you can presume the mother's pelvis is of adequate size for vaginal delivery.

Urine A first-voided urine specimen obtained on the day of each visit is checked for glucose, albumin and ketones. (Glucose is checked to continually screen for diabetes; the presence of albumin is an important sign of the preeclampsia/eclampsia syndrome; and ketones are a nonspecific marker of the state of hydration and nutrition.)

Cervix examinations After the pelvic examination done at the patient's first visit, it is not repeated until 39 weeks' gestation. At that time a gentle digital examination is done to assess cervical dilation and effacement, fetal position and descent (as a very general indicator of the probability of labor). If there are any indicators of premature labor at anytime, digital examination of the cervix is essential, but routine cervical checks from 36 weeks on are uncomfortable and are discouraged.

Other laboratory studies

Maternal serum alpha-fetoprotein An MSAFP should be offered to all patients as a screen for open spinal defects. This blood test is most sensitive when done between 16–18 weeks gestation; an accurate gestational age is essential.

Amniocentesis/chorionic villus sampling All patients should be *offered* genetic evaluation of the pregnancy if familial risk factors exist or if the mother will reach the age of 35 any time during the pregnancy.

Diabetes screen All pregnant women should be screened at least once for diabetes mellitus. The elaboration of placental hormones increases insulin resistance and consequently increases the occurrence of gestational diabetes. The accepted method of screening is for the woman to consume a single loading dose of 50 g of oral glucose, and one

Blood glucose screening, not urine glucose screening, is the standard for evaluation for diabetes mellitus in pregnancy.

hour later have a blood glucose determination. Levels greater than 140 mg/dl should be further evaluated by a full glucose tolerance test.

Rh antibody screen All Rh negative mothers should be retested at 28 weeks for the presence of Rh antibodies. All Rh-antigen negative mothers who are Rh *antibody* negative should be given Rh immune globulin at 28 weeks to prevent Rh sensitization.

Hemoglobin/hematocrit A repeat hemoglobin and hematocrit are usually done at 28 weeks as iron deficiency anemia is very common in pregnancy.

Group B *Streptococcus* screening Group B *Streptococcus* frequently (10–30%) colonizes the lower vagina. This organism occasionally causes postpartum endometritis, and it is also the etiological agent in a rare but dangerous form of neonatal sepsis.

Group B *Streptococcus* has been implicated as an etiologic agent for premature labor. In consequence, screening for the organism is encouraged; the most widely accepted method is culture of the lower one-third of the vagina and perirectal area at or about 36 weeks gestation.

COMMON ISSUES AND COMPLAINTS

Activity

Metabolic demands and the increased weight inevitably increase fatigue and decrease stamina so that most patients will require extra daily rest. Normal employment may be continued until delivery with certain modifications:

- Employment requiring long periods of standing may aggravate dependent edema.
- Employment considered inherently dangerous when balance or dexterity are compromised should be modified or curtailed after 24 weeks.
- Employment involving contact with potential teratogenic substances should be avoided *throughout* pregnancy.

By and large, a pregnant woman can continue her normal activities throughout pregnancy.

Travel

Automobile travel is permissible throughout pregnancy provided that the patient stops, moves about, empties her bladder and drinks some fluids at least every 2 hours, and that she spends no more than 6 hours a day in the car. *Seat belts should be worn but properly positioned* below the abdomen and across the pelvic bone.

Air travel is also permissible in pressurized commercial aircraft. Most airlines require written permission from a physician for air travel after 24–28 weeks gestation.

Any travel after 36 weeks is problematic due to the risk of the patient going into labor while away from home. If such travel is unavoidable, the patient should be provided with a copy of her prenatal record.

Sexual Activity

In general, no restrictions are placed on sexual activity. If significant uterine irritability occurs with orgasm, intercourse *may* be prohibited; if such irritability is caused by the presence of semen, the use of condoms is recommended.

Common Complaints (Table 5-3)

Gastrointestinal problems (nausea/vomiting/heartburn/ hemorrhoids)

Early pregnancy is commonly associated with nausea and vomiting, from the 6th to the 12th weeks. This symptom, almost universally known as **morning sickness**, probably results from the mild physiologic hyperthyroidism which occurs at this time. Pharmacologic intervention is seldom necessary; a myriad of home remedies exists with mixed effects. It seems to be important to never allow the stomach to be empty; consequently, small feedings with bland foods are key. Avoidance of spicy and fried foods helps.

After twelve weeks of gestation, nausea/vomiting usually resolves, and a period of relative gastrointestinal calm persists through 24–28 weeks. After that, **heartburn** (caused by relaxation of the gastroesophageal sphincter) and **constipation** (caused by decreased gastrointestinal motility) become problems. Heartburn is best handled with small, more frequent feedings, avoidance of the supine position and liquid

Table 5-3. Common Complaints

Complaint	Cause	Therapy
Nausea/vomiting (morning sickness) 1st trimester	Physiologic hyper-thyroidism (hypothesized, not proven)	• Small frequent feedings with bland food • Avoid spicy/fried foods
Nausea/heartburn 3rd trimester	Relaxation of gastro-esophageal sphincter	• Small frequent feedings • Avoidance of supine position after eating • Liquid antacids
Constipation	Decreased intestinal motility	• Bulk (fiber) additives, surface active agents
Hemorrhoids	Dilated hemorrhoidal veins due to increased pelvic pressure	• Topical preparations • Avoidance of constipation
Syncope	Venous pooling in legs Delayed response of vascular system to position change	• Change positions slowly • Rest in lateral recumbent position • Avoid sitting, standing or lying flat for extended time
Aches and pains	Increased elasticity of connective tissue Altered body mechanics	• Topical heat • Mild analgesics
Lower quadrant pain, especially on right 2nd trimester	Stretching of the round ligament	• Reassurance

antacids. Constipation is best handled with bulk (fiber) additives or surface active agents.

Hemorrhoids are a common complaint late in pregnancy and in the postpartum period. These dilated hemorrhoidal veins are caused by the increased pelvic pressure of pregnancy. Topical preparations, avoidance of constipation, and time are the best healers. Surgical intervention is to be avoided if at all possible.

Syncope

Pregnant women are predisposed to fainting because of a number of physiologic events. Increased pelvic pressure leads to venous pooling in the legs, delaying the vascular system's response to positional changes. Certain activities such as sitting quietly, standing still, or lying supine, may aggravate these physiologic events sufficiently to reduce cardiac output and allow syncope to occur.

Consequently, patients should be advised to avoid sitting, standing still, or lying flat on their back for extended periods of time and to change positions (sitting or lying to standing) slowly. If she does feel lightheaded, the patient should lie down in the lateral recumbent position immediately, and recovery should occur promptly.

Aches and pains

Progesterone and mechanics are the primary culprits of the aches and pains (low back, pelvis, rib cartilage) of pregnancy. Increased elasticity of the connective tissues predisposes pregnant women to a variety of minor strains and sprains. The mechanical load placed on the pelvis and back, as well as disturbed posture, exacerbate these problems. These aches and pains are seldom more than annoyance, and in general respond to topical heat and mild analgesics. Attention to good posture and flexibility are important preventive measures.

Lower quadrant and groin pains are common in the middle trimester. This discomfort likely results from stretching of the round ligaments as they seek to maintain the position of the fundus as it rises out of the bony pelvis. This pain usually resolves after 24 weeks.

CASE RESOLUTION

Ms. W.B. and her husband Mr. L.B., both 26 years old, visit your office because they're considering getting pregnant. Married since graduating from college, they have used a variety of birth control measures. Now they are both established in their careers and have decided, "It's time to start a family."

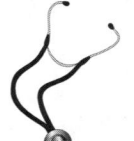

At this preconceptual visit, you do a general examination of Ms. B. and review both of their medical and family histories. You are pleased to be able to counsel and tell them that you have identified no significant problems.

Seven months later, Ms. W.B. returns to your office. She missed her last menstrual period and last week took a home pregnancy test which was positive.

Ms. B. is here for her all-important initial prenatal visit. You perform a complete physical examination and order a full set of laboratory tests as outlined in this chapter.

Ms. B. has a normal examination and laboratory tests. Her blood type is A+, so there will be no concerns about isoimmunization. Both Mr. and Ms. B's grandparents were from the Mediterranean region, so they agreed to have hemoglobin electrophoresis done, and this too is normal.

The EDC is calculated, and gestational age estimated to be about eight weeks. Ms. B. is informed of the routine schedule of follow-up visits. She is a dental hygienist, and you informed her that so long as she used Universal Precautions and very careful radiation protection, she should be able to work until delivery.

The many physiologic changes of pregnancy cause many concerns for pregnant women, especially first-time mothers. Most are very interested in learning all they can about pregnancy, and are grateful for your close attention.

Ms. B. experiences one episode of syncope in the week after her appointment with you, and she has a moderate problem with morning sickness. Your staff are able to reassure her. On her sixth month visit to the office, she is found to have bacteriuria which is successfully treated, and mild ankle edema, about which she is reassured.

At 39 weeks' gestation, Ms. B. goes into labor and after a normal 18-hour labor, she delivers a healthy 6 lb baby boy.

SUMMARY

Prenatal care represents a nearly unique process in health care whereby a physiologic event undergoes intense scrutiny from onset to completion. This scrutiny affords an opportunity not only to identify and forestall untoward outcomes, but also to introduce many aspects of health maintenance and prevention that go beyond the confines of the pregnancy itself. The design of prenatal care will no doubt continue to evolve and change, but the basic concept remains sound and the success unchallenged.

STUDY QUESTIONS*

1. A patient who has been pregnant three times with one miscarriage, one term singleton delivery and one term twin delivery is considered what parity?
    A. 1
    B. 2

---

*For answers, see page 347.

C.   3

D.   4

2. Antibody screens are primarily done for determination of what anti-Rh antibody?

A.   anti-M

B.   null

C.   anti-D

D.   Auntie Mame

3. The congenital transmission rate of the HIV virus can be significantly reduced if the mother is treated with AZT during the third trimester.

True

False

4. The EDC can be determined with fair accuracy:

A.   if the date of the last menstrual period is known and the patient's menstrual cycle is regular with a known interval.

B.   by obtaining a biparietal diameter by ultrasound in the third trimester.

APPENDIX: ACOG FORMS

Patient Addressograph

DATE _____

NAME _____

       LAST   FIRST   MIDDLE

ID # _____ HOSPITAL OF DELIVERY _____

NEWBORN'S PHYSICIAN _____ REFERRED BY _____

FINAL EDD _____   PRIMARY PROVIDER/GROUP _____

BIRTH DATE AGE RACE MARITAL STATUS	ADDRESS:
MONTH DAY YEAR S M W D SEP	
OCCUPATION EDUCATION	ZIP: PHONE: (H) (O)
☐ HOMEMAKER (LAST GRADE COMPLETED)	INSURANCE CARRIER/MEDICAID #
☐ OUTSIDE WORK	
☐ STUDENT Type of Work	
HUSBAND/FATHER OF BABY: PHONE:	EMERGENCY CONTACT: PHONE:

TOTAL PREG	FULL TERM	PREMATURE	AB, INDUCED	AB, SPONTANEOUS	ECTOPICS	MULTIPLE BIRTHS	LIVING

MENSTRUAL HISTORY

LMP ☐ DEFINITE ☐ APPROXIMATE (MONTH KNOWN)   MENSES MONTHLY ☐ YES ☐ NO   FREQUENCY: Q _____ DAYS   MENARCHE _____ (AGE ONSET)
     ☐ UNKNOWN ☐ NORMAL AMOUNT/DURATION   PRIOR MENSES _____ DATE   ON BCP AT CONCEPT. ☐ YES ☐ NO   hCG + ____ / ____ / ____
     ☐ FINAL _____

PAST PREGNANCIES (LAST SIX)

DATE MONTH / YEAR	GA WEEKS	LENGTH OF LABOR	BIRTH WEIGHT	SEX M/F	TYPE DELIVERY	ANES.	PLACE OF DELIVERY	PRETERM LABOR YES / NO	COMMENTS / COMPLICATIONS

PAST MEDICAL HISTORY

	O Neg + Pos.	DETAIL POSITIVE REMARKS INCLUDE DATE & TREATMENT		O Neg + Pos.	DETAIL POSITIVE REMARKS INCLUDE DATE & TREATMENT
1. DIABETES			16. D (Rh) SENSITIZED		
2. HYPERTENSION			17. PULMONARY (TB, ASTHMA)		
3. HEART DISEASE			18. ALLERGIES (DRUGS)		
4. AUTOIMMUNE DISORDER			19. BREAST		
5. KIDNEY DISEASE / UTI			20. GYN SURGERY		
6. NEUROLOGIC/EPILEPSY					
7. PSYCHIATRIC			21. OPERATIONS / HOSPITALIZATIONS (YEAR & REASON)		
8. HEPATITIS / LIVER DISEASE					
9. VARICOSITIES / PHLEBITIS					
10. THYROID DYSFUNCTION			22. ANESTHETIC COMPLICATIONS		
11. TRAUMA/DOMESTIC VIOLENCE			23. HISTORY OF ABNORMAL PAP		
12. HISTORY OF BLOOD TRANSFUS.			24. UTERINE ANOMALY/DES		
	AMT/DAY PREPREG AMT/DAY PREG #YEARS USE		25. INFERTILITY		
13. TOBACCO			26. RELEVANT FAMILY HISTORY		
14. ALCOHOL					
15. STREET DRUGS			27. OTHER		

COMMENTS: _____

The American College of Obstetricians and Gynecologists, 409 12th Street, SW, PO Box 96920, Washington, DC 20090-6920   Copyright © 1997 (Version 4)

ACOG ANTEPARTUM RECORD (FORM A)

Patient Addressograph

SYMPTOMS SINCE LMP

GENETIC SCREENING/TERATOLOGY COUNSELING
INCLUDES PATIENT, BABY'S FATHER, OR ANYONE IN EITHER FAMILY WITH:

	YES	NO			YES	NO
1. PATIENT'S AGE ≥ 35 YEARS				12. MENTAL RETARDATION/AUTISM		
2. THALASSEMIA (ITALIAN, GREEK, MEDITERRANEAN, OR ASIAN BACKGROUND): MCV < 80				IF YES, WAS PERSON TESTED FOR FRAGILE X?		
3. NEURAL TUBE DEFECT (MENINGOMYELOCELE, SPINA BIFIDA, OR ANENCEPHALY)				13. OTHER INHERITED GENETIC OR CHROMOSOMAL DISORDER		
4. CONGENITAL HEART DEFECT				14. MATERNAL METABOLIC DISORDER (EG. INSULIN-DEPENDENT DIABETES, PKU)		
5. DOWN SYNDROME				15. PATIENT OR BABY'S FATHER HAD A CHILD WITH BIRTH DEFECTS NOT LISTED ABOVE		
6. TAY-SACHS (EG, JEWISH, CAJUN, FRENCH CANADIAN)						
7. SICKLE CELL DISEASE OR TRAIT (AFRICAN)				16. RECURRENT PREGNANCY LOSS, OR A STILLBIRTH		
8. HEMOPHILIA				17. MEDICATIONS/STREET DRUGS/ALCOHOL SINCE LAST MENSTRUAL PERIOD		
9. MUSCULAR DYSTROPHY						
10. CYSTIC FIBROSIS				IF YES, AGENT(S):		
11. HUNTINGTON CHOREA				18. ANY OTHER		

COMMENTS/COUNSELING: _____
_____
_____

INFECTION HISTORY	YES	NO			YES	NO
1. HIGH RISK HEPATITIS B/IMMUNIZED?				4. RASH OR VIRAL ILLNESS SINCE LAST MENSTRUAL PERIOD		
2. LIVE WITH SOMEONE WITH TB OR EXPOSED TO TB				5. HISTORY OF STD, GC, CHLAMYDIA, HPV, SYPHILIS		
3. PATIENT OR PARTNER HAS HISTORY OF GENITAL HERPES				6. OTHER (SEE COMMENTS)		

COMMENTS: _____
_____
_____ INTERVIEWER'S SIGNATURE _____

INITIAL PHYSICAL EXAMINATION

DATE ____ / ____ / ____   PREPREGNANCY WEIGHT _____   HEIGHT _____   BP_____

1. HEENT	☐ NORMAL	☐ ABNORMAL	12. VULVA	☐ NORMAL	☐ CONDYLOMA	☐ LESIONS	
2. FUNDI	☐ NORMAL	☐ ABNORMAL	13. VAGINA	☐ NORMAL	☐ INFLAMMATION	☐ DISCHARGE	
3. TEETH	☐ NORMAL	☐ ABNORMAL	14. CERVIX	☐ NORMAL	☐ INFLAMMATION	☐ LESIONS	
4. THYROID	☐ NORMAL	☐ ABNORMAL	15. UTERUS SIZE	_____ WEEKS		☐ FIBROIDS	
5. BREASTS	☐ NORMAL	☐ ABNORMAL	16. ADNEXA	☐ NORMAL	☐ MASS		
6. LUNGS	☐ NORMAL	☐ ABNORMAL	17. RECTUM	☐ NORMAL	☐ ABNORMAL		
7. HEART	☐ NORMAL	☐ ABNORMAL	18. DIAGONAL CONJUGATE	☐ REACHED	☐ NO	_____ CM	
8. ABDOMEN	☐ NORMAL	☐ ABNORMAL	19. SPINES	☐ AVERAGE	☐ PROMINENT	☐ BLUNT	
9. EXTREMITIES	☐ NORMAL	☐ ABNORMAL	20. SACRUM	☐ CONCAVE	☐ STRAIGHT	☐ ANTERIOR	
10. SKIN	☐ NORMAL	☐ ABNORMAL	21. SUBPUBIC ARCH	☐ NORMAL	☐ WIDE	☐ NARROW	
11. LYMPH NODES	☐ NORMAL	☐ ABNORMAL	22. GYNECOID PELVIC TYPE	☐ YES	☐ NO		

COMMENTS (Number and explain abnormals): _____
_____ EXAM BY _____

ACOG ANTEPARTUM RECORD (FORM B)

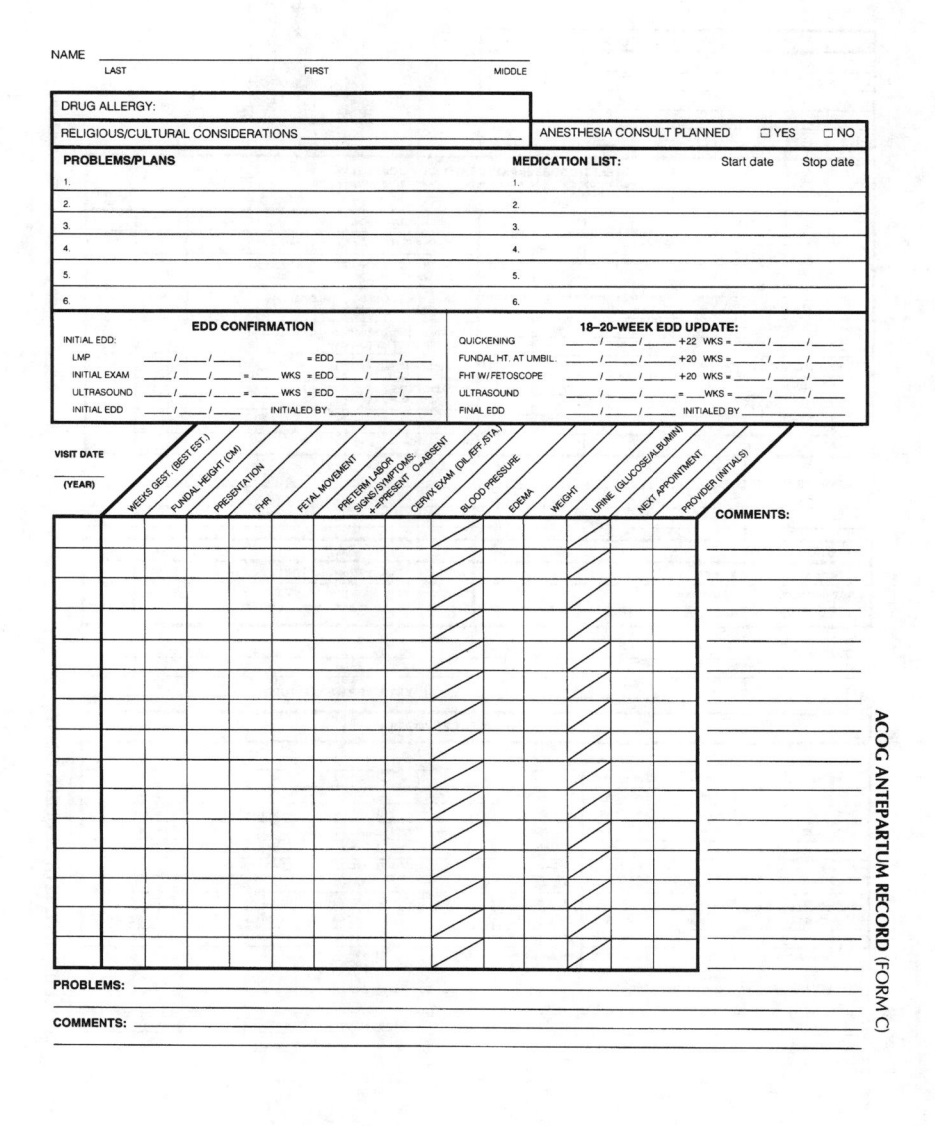

Patient Addressograph

NAME _____
          LAST   FIRST   MIDDLE

DRUG ALLERGY:

RELIGIOUS/CULTURAL CONSIDERATIONS _____   **ANESTHESIA CONSULT PLANNED**   ☐ YES   ☐ NO

PROBLEMS/PLANS   **MEDICATION LIST:**   Start date   Stop date

1.   1.
2.   2.
3.   3.
4.   4.
5.   5.
6.   6.

EDD CONFIRMATION

INITIAL EDD:

LMP   ___/___/___   = EDD ___/___/___
INITIAL EXAM   ___/___/___ = ___ WKS = EDD ___/___/___
ULTRASOUND   ___/___/___ = ___ WKS = EDD ___/___/___
INITIAL EDD   ___/___/___   INITIALED BY _____

18–20-WEEK EDD UPDATE:

QUICKENING   ___/___/___ +22 WKS = ___/___/___
FUNDAL HT. AT UMBIL. ___/___/___ +20 WKS = ___/___/___
FHT W/FETOSCOPE   ___/___/___ +20 WKS = ___/___/___
ULTRASOUND   ___/___/___ = ___WKS = ___/___/___
FINAL EDD   ___/___/___   INITIALED BY _____

VISIT DATE / (YEAR) | WEEKS GEST (BEST EST.) | FUNDAL HEIGHT (CM) | PRESENTATION | FHR | FETAL MOVEMENT | PRETERM LABOR SIGNS/SYMPTOMS; +=PRESENT O=ABSENT | CERVIX EXAM (DIL-EFF-STA.) | BLOOD PRESSURE | EDEMA | WEIGHT | URINE (GLUCOSE/ALBUMIN) | NEXT APPOINTMENT | PROVIDER (INITIALS) | COMMENTS:

PROBLEMS: _____

COMMENTS: _____

ACOG ANTEPARTUM RECORD (FORM C)

LABORATORY AND EDUCATION

Patient Addressograph

INITIAL LABS	DATE	RESULT	REVIEWED
BLOOD TYPE	/ /	A B AB O	
D (Rh) TYPE	/ /		
ANTIBODY SCREEN	/ /		
HCT/HGB	/ /	_____ % _____ g/dL	
PAP TEST	/ /	NORMAL / ABNORMAL / _____	
RUBELLA	/ /		
VDRL	/ /		
URINE CULTURE/SCREEN	/ /		
HBsAg	/ /		
HIV COUNSELING/TESTING	/ /	☐ POS. ☐ NEG. ☐ DECLINED	

COMMENTS/ADDITIONAL LABS

OPTIONAL LABS	DATE	RESULT	
HGB ELECTROPHORESIS	/ /	AA AS SS AC SC AF ↑A$_2$	
PPD	/ /		
CHLAMYDIA	/ /		
GC	/ /		
TAY–SACHS	/ /		
OTHER			

8–18-WEEK LABS (WHEN INDICATED/ELECTED)	DATE	RESULT	
ULTRASOUND	/ /		
MSAFP/MULTIPLE MARKERS	/ /		
AMNIO/CVS	/ /		
KARYOTYPE	/ /	46, XX OR 46, XY / OTHER____	
AMNIOTIC FLUID (AFP)	/ /	NORMAL____ ABNORMAL____	

24–28-WEEK LABS (WHEN INDICATED)	DATE	RESULT	
HCT/HGB	/ /	_____ % _____ g/dL	
DIABETES SCREEN	/ /	1 HOUR_____	
GTT (IF SCREEN ABNORMAL)	/ /	____FBS ____1 HOUR	
		____2 HOUR ____3 HOUR	
D (Rh) ANTIBODY SCREEN	/ /		
D IMMUNE GLOBULIN (RhIG) GIVEN (28 WKS)	/ /	SIGNATURE _____	

32–36-WEEK LABS (WHEN INDICATED)	DATE	RESULT	
HCT/HGB (RECOMMENDED)	/ /	_____ % _____ g/dL	
ULTRASOUND	/ /		
VDRL	/ /		
GC	/ /		
CHLAMYDIA	/ /		
GROUP B STREP (35–37 WKS)	/ /		

PLANS/EDUCATION (COUNSELED ☐)

☐ ANESTHESIA PLANS _____
☐ TOXOPLASMOSIS PRECAUTIONS (CATS/RAW MEAT) _____
☐ CHILDBIRTH CLASSES _____
☐ PHYSICAL/SEXUAL ACTIVITY _____
☐ LABOR SIGNS _____
☐ NUTRITION COUNSELING _____
☐ BREAST OR BOTTLE FEEDING _____
☐ NEWBORN CAR SEAT _____
☐ POSTPARTUM BIRTH CONTROL _____
☐ ENVIRONMENTAL/WORK HAZARDS _____

☐ TUBAL STERILIZATION _____
☐ VBAC COUNSELING _____
☐ CIRCUMCISION _____
☐ TRAVEL _____
☐ LIFESTYLE, TOBACCO, ALCOHOL _____

REQUESTS _____
_____

TUBAL STERILIZATION   DATE   INITIALS
CONSENT SIGNED   ____ / ____ / ____   _____

AA128   12345/10987

PROVIDER SIGNATURE (AS REQUIRED) _____

ACOG ANTEPARTUM RECORD (FORM D)

The Well Baby Examination  6

Renee S. Domanico

INTRODUCTION

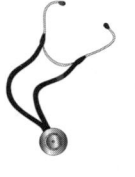

CASE PRESENTATION

A first-time mother and her 2-day-old female infant will be discharged home today. The pregnancy and labor were uncomplicated. The initial newborn examination was normal and her course to this point has been uneventful. The mother is breastfeeding.

When you come into their room, Mom is excited about going home and full of questions. "I hope someone can help me because I feel like I do not know enough. How will I know if I am bathing her correctly? When do we come back to be rechecked? What should I look for?"

The newborn examination is the first and one of the most important complete medical examinations a person will ever have. No other examination offers such a high yield in discovering and intervening in potential abnormalities. Three percent of newborns have at least one major congenital anomaly; more will have complications such as birth trauma, infection, or a problem caused by a maternal medical condition. The initial examination occurs in the first 24 hours of life. With minimal variation, it is repeated at intervals during the first year of life and is referred to as the well baby examination.

The three goals of the well baby examination are:

1. early detection of medical problems
2. facilitation of normal adaptation to extrauterine life
3. protection of newborns from complications to which they are susceptible.

You obtain most information through observation of the newborn's general appearance, behavior, and responses. Additionally, you must assess parental bonding and other psychosocial issues which can significantly influence infant outcomes. This chapter surveys the components of complete newborn and infant examinations and introduces concepts of "anticipatory guidance" which are critically important in pediatrics.

DEFINITIONS

Apgar scores: evaluation of a newborn's physical status by assigning numerical values (0 to 2) to each of five factors: heart rate, respiratory effort, muscle tone, response to stimuli, and skin color (maximum score is 10).

Café-au-lait spots: light brown, sharply defined, usually oval skin lesions.

Circumcision: an operation to remove part or all of the foreskin from the penis.

Erythema toxicum: transient erythematous eruption overlying hair follicles in newborns.

Jaundice: yellowish staining of the skin or other tissue.

Lanugo: very fine, soft embryonic hair.

Meconium: first stool-like material excreted by newborn or by fetus just before delivery.

Postmature: an infant born after 42 weeks' gestation.

Premature: an infant born before 37 weeks' gestation.

Primitive reflexes: any of several involuntary muscle reactions to different stimuli seen normally in newborns.

Pustular melanosis: transient patchy dark brown or black skin eruption in newborns.

HISTORY

The history of the newborn infant is essentially the maternal prenatal history. Any condition or complication of the mother can influence the developing fetus. Table 6.1 summarizes the important historical information.

For well baby visits after the newborn visit, the history must also include the baby's sleeping and eating patterns, state of health since last

Table 6-1. Important Historical Information for the Infant Examination

Maternal History

Age
Number of pregnancies and live births
Blood type and antibodies
Blood product transfusions
Chronic maternal illness
   Hypertension/preeclampsia
   Diabetes
   Renal disease
   Cardiac disease
   Bleeding disorders
Acute maternal illness
   Viral and bacterial infections
   Exposure to infection
   Sexually transmitted diseases

History of this pregnancy
   Bleeding
   Injuries
   Preterm labor
   Amniotic fluid problems
   Fetal testing results
      Ultrasound
      Amniocentesis
      Fetal lung maturity
      α-fetoprotein

Complications of Previous Pregnancies

Abortions/miscarriages
Prematurity
Postmaturity
Malformations

Respiratory distress syndrome
Chromosomal abnormalities
Pathologic jaundice
Group B *Streptococcus*
   infections

Drug Exposure

Prenatal vitamins
Iron
Prescription medicines, especially:
   Insulin
   Anticonvulsants

Illicit drugs
Alcohol
Tobacco

Labor and Delivery (This Pregnancy)

Onset of labor and its duration
Time from rupture of membranes to
   delivery
Abnormality of amniotic fluid
   Meconium-staining
   Blood
   Foul smell
Fetal monitoring information
Type of anesthesia
Presentation of fetus

Method of delivery
Maternal fever
Maternal oxygenation and
   perfusion
Initial neonatal assessment
Apgar scores
Resuscitation required, if any
Placental inspection

visit, and progress of development. Family history and social history have increasing importance in following a baby as it develops.

PHYSICAL EXAMINATION

The sequence of the newborn and well baby examination differs from the adult examination. Since infants are not necessarily cooperative patients, you must *first examine organ systems that require a quiet patient*, then progress to more disruptive maneuvers. Much of your information about the baby comes from close observation, so ideally, the baby should be naked except for a diaper. Always note their overall color, tone, and responsiveness prior to beginning the detailed organ system examination and then proceed to complete as much of the comprehensive examination as possible.

Cardiorespiratory Examination

The baby's color is the best single indicator of heart and/or lung abnormalities. A baby should be pink centrally, i.e., around its head and trunk. If the baby becomes too cool during the examination, the hands and feet may appear bluish, a condition called "acrocyanosis." However, a "dusky" appearance *centrally* is an indication of true cyanosis, i.e., inadequate oxygenation. It may represent either cardiac or pulmonary malfunction.

Usually, the *heart examination* is the first part of a well baby examination when the baby is quiet. If not, you can attempt to quiet the baby by offering a pacifier or a pinkie or holding the baby. If unsuccessful, you should defer the cardiac examination until the baby is quiet.

- Inspect the chest for the *point of maximum impulse* (PMI) and for the presence of a hyperdynamic precordium.
- Palpate for a heave or thrill, for the strength and symmetry of distal pulses.
- Lastly, listen to the heart (auscultate) starting with the **rate** (*which is normally 120–160*) and **rhythm**. Then auscultate the heart sounds carefully to note normal or abnormal S_1 and S_2, possible gallops or clicks, and murmurs. The presence of a murmur in a newborn is less meaningful than at any other time in life. The murmur of a closing ductus arteriosus can be very loud, but very benign. On the other hand, significant cardiac anomalies can be

Assessing normal heart sounds in babies is challenging! However, you should take time to learn this skill since serious congenital heart diseases often produce abnormal sounds.

present without a murmur. A gallop or click is an abnormal finding, suggesting cardiac disease.

Start your lung examination by inspecting the chest.

- *The normal respiratory rate is 30–60 breaths per minute.* Most infants with pulmonary abnormalities are tachypneic. Grunting, which is forced expiration against a closed epiglottis, increases end-expiratory pressures to help the infant keep alveoli open.
- Any increased effort of respiration, including the presence of *nasal flaring, subcostal* and *intercostal retractions*, serves as an important clue to pulmonary problems.
- The respiratory pattern is also important. All infants are periodic breathers which means they alternate periods of regular respirations with short respiratory pauses. This pattern of breathing gradually disappears as the baby ages.
- Apnea is always abnormal.
- Complete your lung examination by auscultating the symmetry of breath sounds, the quality of air exchange and noting the presence of rhonchi or rales.

> Apnea is defined as a respiratory pause sustained for greater than 20 seconds, or associated with development of cyanosis.

Abdominal Examination

Observation is vitally important in the abdominal examination.

- A scaphoid or concave appearing abdomen occurs when air does not enter the intestinal lumen, as in proximal obstruction, or when the intestines are not in the abdominal cavity, as in diaphragmatic hernia. A distended abdomen occurs when air and/or liquid is trapped in the intestine by distal obstruction, such as colonic atresia, meconium plugs or imperforate anus.
- In a newborn, inspect the umbilical cord for the normal appearance of *two arteries and one vein*. Examine the umbilicus of older infants for any erythema, indicative of infection, or any protrusion indicating an umbilical hernia.
- Auscultate the abdomen for the presence and character of bowel sounds. Bowel obstruction may cause high-pitched "tinkling" bowel sounds.
- Gently palpate the abdomen to assess the size of the liver, spleen, kidneys, bladder and the presence of masses.

> Ten percent of neonates with single umbilical artery will also have other gastrointestinal or genitourinary anomalies.

Genitourinary Examination

- Inspection of the external genitalia does not always reveal the actual genetic gender of a newborn. Care should be taken not to assign gender at birth when any ambiguity exists.
- On inspection of the genitalia of a girl, commonly a white or bloody discharge is present from maternal estrogen effects. In a breech presentation, genitalia of a newborn girl may be bruised or swollen. Examine baby girls beyond the newborn period for abnormal discharge, rash, tears or other signs of trauma.
- Examine the penis for size and position of the urethral opening. Palpate the testes to assess whether they have descended into the scrotal sac and are of normal size. Genitalia of a newborn boy may be bruised and swollen also from breech presentation. An older male infant should be examined for descended testes and for abnormal rash, discharge, or signs of trauma.

Musculoskeletal Examination

Inspect the extremities for deformities, asymmetry, and the proper number of fingers and toes. Examine the spine for abnormal curvature, tufts of hair, dimples or sinus tracts. Palpate the clavicles for fracture.

On every well baby visit until at least 1 year of age, examine the hips to assess for possible dislocation.

> Asess for possible hip dislocation with Ortohani's and Barlow's tests of abduction and adduction with posterior pressure.

Skin Examination

Normal newborn skin has uniformly pink undertones and various, often subtle, overtones based upon the child's racial/genetic makeup. **Normal variants** which might be mistaken for abnormalities include:

- dark-pigmented spots, termed Mongolian spots, on the back and sacral region
- nevus flavus on the eyelids ("angel kisses") and at the nape of the neck ("stork bite")
- lanugo
- a mottled appearance, which can be a normal finding in an infant examined in a cold room, providing other signs of infection are absent

- Up to three small (<1 × 1 cm) *café au lait* spots also can be normal.
- "Normal" rashes include the transient findings of erythema toxicum and pustular melanosis in newborns and neonatal acne in young infants.
- Importantly, duskiness, pallor, jaundice and petechiae are *abnormal*.

Head, Eyes, Ears, Nose, Throat (HEENT) Examination

The skull sutures of a normal newborn are not fused to allow for reduction of the head size during normal vaginal birth. Therefore, frequent *normal* findings include molding, overriding sutures, and caput succedaneum, which is edema of the presenting part of the skull. Abnormal findings include cephalohematoma and subgaleal hemorrhage. You should palpate the anterior and posterior fontanelles ("soft spots" at the juncture of the unfused sutures) for size and consistency.

Examine the eyes for size and symmetry, and inspect the integrity of the iris, the color of the sclerae and conjunctivae, the size and symmetry of the cornea. Assess the size and reactivity of the pupils and with your ophthalmoscope, check for the presence of a red retinal reflex.

Examine the ears for size, position, patency of canals, and with your otoscope, the appearance of the tympanic membranes.

The nose is examined for shape, patency, and the presence of any discharge. Inspect the mouth for color and moistness of mucus membranes, an intact palate, the size and color of the tonsils, and the presence of teeth. Assess the neck for any masses, lymphadenopathy, sinus tracts and for mobility.

The posterior fontanelle closes by 2–3 months of age and the anterior fontanelle by 18–24 months.

Absence of a red reflex may indicate cataracts or retinoblastoma.

Neurologic Examination

Most features of the neurologic evaluation are done as part of the general examination. Assessment is made of overall tone, state of behavior (irritable, sleepy, somnolent), symmetry and spontaneity of movement, the quality of the cry, and gross observation of cranial nerves.

- Elicit the deep tendon reflexes with the neurological hammer.
- Check for *primitive reflexes*, including the root, grasp, suck, Moro, and tonic neck reflex. Their presence at birth and disappearance later follows a consistent developmental pattern during the first

Ask your preceptor to demonstrate these reflexes in an infant.

year of life. The abnormal absence or persistence of these reflexes indicates neurologic abnormality.

ANTICIPATORY GUIDANCE

Feeding

The single most important parent education issue during a baby's visit to your office is feeding. Currently, parents have two choices; breastfeeding or commercial formulas. Both provide adequate nutrition.

Breastfeeding, the preferred choice of medical professionals, provides balanced nutritional value and it also assures transfer of immunoglobulins, aiding a baby's immune response to infection. Naturally, it is free, readily available, the correct temperature, and well-tolerated. *However, it is not fool-proof, especially in a first-time breastfeeding mother.* You must closely follow the mother–baby unit over the first few weeks to assess whether the supply of milk is adequate to meet the nutritional needs of the infant and to address possible complications such as jaundice, mastitis, and engorgement.

Commercial formula is available to families who for personal or medical reasons choose not to breastfeed. Quantitating intake is easier with formula so you need not follow these babies quite so closely initially, especially if they are feeding well. Because **iron** is not as bioavailable in cow's milk-based formula, it is routinely supplied in higher quantities in formula. If bottled or well water is used to mix formula, **fluoride** supplementation should be given starting at 6 months of age.

Solid food should not be introduced until after 4 months of age and then only about two new foods per week so as to be able to detect possible food allergies.

If adequate intake is present, a baby will have at least six wet diapers per day. However, stooling patterns are variable. Most breastfed infants have three or four yellow, loose stools a day. Formula-fed infants usually produce more formed, darker stools, usually two or three a day, or as infrequently as once or twice per week.

> Mothers are instructed to breastfeed every two to three hours and alternate the breast that is first offered. Babies usually nurse for ten to twenty minutes at each breast.

> Formula-fed babies usually eat 2 to 3 ounces every 3 to 4 hours and increase the volume over time.

Sleeping

Sleeping habits are a common concern of parents. Newborns average 18–20 hours of sleep daily for the first 2 months, awakening only to eat

and have their diaper changed. Gradually they increase their duration of awake time and condense their sleep time over the next few months. Most infants sleep at least 6 consecutive hours at night by 4 months of age.

All infants except those with specific medical conditions (gastroesophageal reflux, Pierre–Robin syndrome) should *sleep on their side or back*. Remove pillows, excessive bedding, and toys from the bed to reduce the risk of sudden infant death syndrome.

Crying

Some methods of alleviating a colicky infant's distress include rocking, swinging, or riding in the car, but crying usually resumes when these comfort measures are stopped.

Almost all parents think their infants cry excessively. Most infants peak in the frequency of crying between three weeks and three months. Crying in the absence of medical abnormality is normal behavior and represents an infant's method of communicating its needs and disposition.

Some infants manifest intense episodes of crying without medical abnormality. These crying spells usually occur in the early evening and last 2–3 hours; this is typical **colic**. Usually it begins at about 1 month of age and resolves by 4 months. Though frightening and frustrating to parents, it is benign, and probably from an immature intestinal system prone to cramping.

Routine Care Issues

Whether or not to **circumcise** the newborn boy, a highly debated topic, is a personal choice of families, with guidance given that the male infant should resemble the father or male care-giver. Care of a circumcised penis consists of Vaseline gauze wrapping until healing ensues in 3–4 days, and normal washing thereafter. Phimosis, or difficulty in retracting the foreskin, is normal in the uncircumcised infant and parents should be cautioned *not* to force it back. The foreskin will gradually stretch and be retractable by 3 to 4 years of age and the boy should be helped to wash until he is able to do so for himself.

The **umbilical cord** usually falls off by 2–3 weeks of age. The stump should be kept clean and dry until that time and cleansed once or twice daily with rubbing alcohol to aid in drying.

Tub baths usually are not advised until the umbilical cord falls off. Mild, dilute soap should be used to wash the baby, and warm water only

to wash the face. Contrary to what some grandmothers may say, infants do not need a bath daily.

Visitors should not be excessive, to limit potential exposure to infection, but a baby does not need to be restricted to the home for any given time period. Anyone handling the baby must wash their hands!

Infants are seen for follow-up 1–2 weeks after hospital discharge, depending on whether they are breast or bottle feeding or have other problems that may warrant close follow-up.

The health care provider must assess the *quality of the maternal–infant interaction* and address potential problems with bonding. If you detect severe depression or neglect, intervention and possible separation may be necessary. In that case the assistance of members of the extended family, or rarely social service agencies will be needed.

Growth

Growth is an important indicator of health and adequate nutrition. Standardized growth curves can be used to serially plot weight, length, and head circumference over the first 2 years of life. Thereafter, weight and height are plotted at least yearly.

Most infants lose about 10% of their birth weight during the first week of life. Over the next 4 months, they gain on average about an ounce (or 30 g) of weight daily. They should re-achieve their birth weight by the end of the second week, double their birth weight by about 4 months and triple their birth weight by 1 year.

> Insufficient caloric intake, whether from improper nutrition or medical abnormality is first manifest as inadequate weight gain or even weight loss. If a condition continues without intervention over a period of time, length will be affected. The last parameter to be affected is head circumference.

Development

Evaluate infants at each well baby examination for normal progression of development. Infants obtain a sequential series of milestones as they grow and develop, building on past achievements. Neurologic, as well as other medical abnormalities, may cause delays in development.

Monitor infants in four areas: gross motor, fine motor, language, and personal–social skills. Abnormalities in one domain may lead to delays in others. However, success in any one domain does not assure normal development overall.

Cognitive development is difficult to assess in infancy, but is best predicted by language development.

Denver Developmental Assessment is a screening tool used by health care professionals to evaluate for potential abnormalities and provide early intervention if a problem is detected.

Screening and Immunizations

A panel of blood tests performed in the newborn period provides clues to early diagnosis of some inborn errors of metabolism. Most state health departments mandate screening for three: hypothyroidism, galactosemia, and phenylketonuria. The screens provide early detection and early treatment prior to the development of irreversible neurologic damage.

A required series of childhood immunizations provides protection against many communicable and potentially life-threatening infectious illnesses. The immunizations should be administered on the approved schedule (Table 6.2).

- **DPT** or diphtheria, pertussis, and tetanus vaccine is given at 2, 4, 6, and 15–18 months and again at 5 years.
- **HiB** or *Haemophilus influenzae* B vaccine is given at 2, 4, 6, and 12–15 months.
- **HBV** or hepatitis B vaccine is initiated at birth and completed by 6 months. It is recommended also for adolescents if they did not receive it as infants.

Table 6-2. Schedule of Vaccinations

	DPT	HiB	HBV	MMR	Polio
Birth			X		
2 months	X	X	X		X(IPV)
4 months	X	X			X(IPV)
6 months	X	X			
12 months		[X]		X	[X
15 months	[X]				(OPV)
18 months					]
5 years	X			X	X(OPV)
Adolescence			X if not given during infancy		

X=give at this time   IPV=inactivated polio vaccine
[X]=give once during this window of time   OPV=oral polio vaccine

- **MMR** or measles, mumps, and rubella vaccine is given at 1 and 5 years.
- Polio vaccination recommendations have changed very recently. The currently preferred schedule is for **IPV** (inactivated polio vaccine) to be given by injection at 2 and 4 months. Oral polio vaccine (**OPV**) may then be used to complete the immunization at 12–18 months and again at 5 years. IPV should be given for *all* doses if the patient or members of the household are immuno-compromised.

There are many elective vaccines available depending on risk factors of the child, including varicella, pneumococcus, and influenza vaccines. Other vaccines are available for travelers to endemic areas of selected infectious diseases.

COMMON PROBLEMS

Many concerns and problems should be discussed with parents during well baby examinations. The three most common include:

- Jaundice
- "Spitting up"
- Constipation.

Jaundice

Jaundice is the build-up of the yellow pigment bilirubin in the skin of newborns. *Almost all infants develop some degree of normal physiologic jaundice.* Physiologic jaundice occurs because the liver enzyme responsible for conjugation of bilirubin to a more excretable form is still immature. Typically, jaundice peaks on the third day of life at a bilirubin level of about 10 mg/dl and resolves completely by a week. Commonly breastfeeding complicates this condition by enhancing the enterohepatic recirculation of bilirubin. Pathologic jaundice occurs from a number of potentially serious causes. It can be differentiated from physiologic jaundice by the timing of onset, severity, and duration.

"Spitting Up"

Spitting up is a common occurrence in infants and a cause for great concern in parents. Although it can be a sign of metabolic disease, infection, or other medical conditions, in most instances it is only an annoyance. Spitting up usually consists of 5–10 ml of milk vomited shortly after feedings, though it may seem like considerably more to worried parents. Parents should be encouraged by the adequate growth of their infants and reassured that the infant will eventually outgrow this.

- **Bilious emesis** (i.e. vomiting of bile-containing material) is always pathologic and should warrant immediate investigation.
- **Gastroesophageal reflux,** a more pronounced form of spitting, is usually benign. It may be of significant volume; however, most babies consume in excess of their needs. Counsel parents to use frequent, small feedings, and frequent burping, and proper positioning. Occasionally, more intervention may be needed.

Constipation

Constipation represents another area of substantial concern for parents. Our society seems to be fixated on our children's stooling patterns. In most instances, parental education on the normal variation in stooling patterns of infants alleviates their concerns.

In some instances, infants do have hard, infrequent and difficult stooling. They should be examined for abnormalities such as Hirschsprung disease or spina bifida occulta, which may not have been detected at birth. In the absence of these disorders, advise parents to offer small amounts of water or dilute juice during the day to increase the infant's free water intake. *However, the use of honey, molasses, or chronic use of glycerin suppositories should be prohibited.*

Honey and molasses may contain botulism spores and cause infant botulism in infants less than 12 months old.

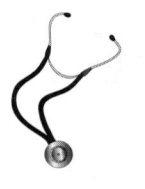

CASE DISCUSSION

A first-time mother and her 2-day-old female infant will be discharged home today. The pregnancy and labor were uncomplicated. The delivery was by NSVD with epidural anesthesia at 39 weeks gestation. The baby received Apgar scores of 9 at 1 minute and 9 at 5 minutes. Her birth weight was 3.0 kg (25%), length was 49 cm (50%), and head circumference was 33 cm (50%). The initial newborn examination was normal and her course to this

point has been uneventful. Today the baby weighs 2.85 kg. The mother is breastfeeding.

When you come into their room, Mom is excited about going home and full of questions. "I hope someone can help me because I feel like I do not know enough. How will I know if I am bathing her correctly? When do we come back to be rechecked? What should I look for?"

This first-time mother will need emotional support, guidance and encouragement for at least the next 18 years! Currently, she will need advice and encouragement on breastfeeding and such problems as sore nipples, breast engorgement, lack of sleep, and disruption to the family unit. Care instructions include establishing routines of eating and sleeping, keeping her daughter warm, clean, and dry.

Follow-up should be in about a week to check the infant's weight and overall state of health, and to reassure the parents of their adequacy in their new roles. The mother should watch for difficulty with feeding, frequency of urination and stooling, jaundice and signs and symptoms of infection including poor feeding, lethargy, irritability, and fever. This may seem overwhelming to new parents who have little prior experience with babies. Frequent communication and reassurance by phone can help new parents through the difficult first months and establish a solid doctor–patient–parent relationship.

SUMMARY

Examining and caring for well babies is the joy of pediatrics. Aiding parents in their task of raising happy, healthy children attracts most health-care providers to pediatrics. Parental education and guidance starts from birth, and can provide an immense measure of satisfaction for parents and doctors alike.

STUDY QUESTIONS*

1. A first-time mother and father bring their 2-week-old infant to your office for a routine well-baby examination. In response to their questions, you offer them all the following advice *except*:
    A. It is normal for the umbilical cord stump to still be attached. They should continue to keep it cleansed with rubbing alcohol.
    B. They should be bathing the baby in a tub once or twice daily.
    C. The baby should be on her side or back to sleep.
    D. It is normal for the baby to sleep 18 hours or more per day.

*For answers, see page 347.

2. All the following are true of breastfeeding *except*:
   A. It aids in the baby's development of normal immune responses.
   B. It provides the most balanced nuritional value for the baby.
   C. Being a natural process it is easy for all mothers to accomplish.
   D. Mastitis is a potential complication.

3. Which of the following sets of vital signs is normal for infants?
   A. Irregular heart rate of approximately 120 beats per minute, regular breathing pattern at a rate of 18 breaths per minute.
   B. Regular heart rate of 200 per minute, periodic breathing pattern of 30 per minute.
   C. Irregular heart rate of approximately 80 per minute, regular breathing pattern at a rate of 30 per minute.
   D. Regular heart rate of 140 per minute, periodic breathing pattern of 40 per minute.

4. Vaccines which should be initiated before age one year include all of the following *except*:
   A. MMR (measles, mumps, rubella)
   A. HiB (*Haemophilus influenzae* B)
   B. IPV (inactivated polio vaccine)
   C. DPT (diphtheria, pertussis, and tetanus)

5. Which of the following "complaints" from the mother of a 2-month-old infant should be of the most concern to you?
   A. The baby, who is formula fed, is having only one stool per day.
   B. The baby cries for nearly 3 hours every evening without being wet or hungry.
   C. The baby spits up one or two teaspoonfuls of its formula after at least three feedings every day.
   D. The baby vomited yellow-green bile-like material twice today.

Suggested Reading

Kendig, J.W. "Care of the Normal Newborn," in Pediatrics in Review 13:38; American Academy of Pediatrics, July 1992.

Oski, F., *et al.*, eds. "Principles and Practices of Pediatrics", 2nd edn, J.B. Lippincott, Philadelphia, 1994.

Taucsch, H.W., R. Ballard & M.E. Avery, eds. "Diseases of the Newborn," 6th edn, W.B. Saunders, Philadelphia, 1991.

The Adolescent  Patient and the Sports Physical

Patricia J. Kelly

INTRODUCTION

CASE PRESENTATION

A 16-year-old boy comes to the office for his school mandated sports physical. He is an avid year round soccer player participating in school-based competition and club soccer. In preparation for his visit, you review his office chart. He has been your patient since moving to the area at age 10 years when you conducted an initial comprehensive history and physical examination.

At the beginning of the interview, the patient tells you he needs a sports physical because he missed the one offered in the physical education department. The previous 2 years he had his physical examination at school; these were done by several different doctors and nurses each doing a small part of the examination. He is eager to have you complete the Pre-Participation Evaluation (PPE) form so he can begin practice with the team today.

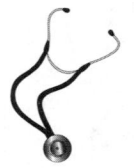

Many adolescent patients, and their parents, regard the sports physical as their only necessary annual medical visit. As both the parent and the patient often are in a hurry to get on with the business of sports participation, they may fail to express any of their concerns to the doctor. However, your job is to fully evaluate the patient for sports participation and your role as the primary care physician includes the added responsibility of addressing medical and psychosocial issues related to the patient's well being. In this chapter we focus on the Pre-Participation Evaluation (PPE) and demonstrate how it provides an excellent opportunity for the physician to address significant adolescent issues.

DEFINITIONS

Acclimatization:
adaptation to environmental conditions such as temperature, humidity and altitude.

Anticipatory guidance:
patient/family counseling which includes information, advice, and suggestions about expected health-related life occurrences, health maintenance, and preventative plans.

Body mass index (BMI):
weight in kilograms divided by the height in meters squared. A BMI of greater than 85th percentile for age and gender is considered *obesity*.

Concussion:
any alteration in mental status induced by trauma (see Table 7.4).

Contusion:
bleeding and damage in the soft tissues, resulting from a direct blow injury.

Dynamic demands:
volume demands on the cardiovascular system created by *isotonic* exercise.

Guidelines for Adolescent Preventative Services (GAPS):
set of recommendations published in 1992 by the American Medical Association providing guidelines for screening and evaluating common causes of adolescent morbidity and mortality (see Table 7.7).

Heat Illnesses:
heat exhaustion and heat stroke.
(a) Heat exhaustion—muscle weakness, dizziness, irritability, hypotension, and tachycardia caused by water depletion.
(b) Heat stroke—a medical emergency which occurs when the body temperature rises above 41 °C; symptoms include confusion, delirium, coma and possible death (a potential 50% mortality rate).

Hepatitis B:
viral infection of the liver contracted from infected blood or body fluids.

Hypertrophic cardiomyopathy (HCM):
primary disease of the myocardium characterized by hypertrophied nondilated left ventricle and septum.

Leukocyte esterase: enzyme produced by neutrophils in the urine; indicates urinary tract infection.

Myocarditis: inflammation of the myocardium (heart muscle) with resultant impairment of cardiac function.

Static demands: *pressure* demands on the cardiovascular system created by *isometic* exercise.

Sexual maturity ratings (SMR) or Tanner Stages:
five stages of visible physical changes associated with pubertal development (see Table 7.8).

Urethritis: inflammatory process involving the urethra, commonly caused by *Chlamydia trachomatis* or *Neisseria gonorrhea,* both sexually transmitted infections.

PRE-PARTICIPATION EVALUATION

An annual physical examination is required for school-based sports participation. The Pre-Participation Evaluation (PPE) may be a **focused** sports related evaluation or it may be **expanded** to provide a comprehensive health review. Objectives of the PPE are to identify medical conditions that may

- interfere with the ability to participate
- be made worse by participation
- increase the risk of injury or death

The American Academy of Pediatrics has published a recommendation guide to assist doctors and parents in deciding whether an athlete with a particular medical condition should participate in competitive sports (selected portions of the guide are summarized in Table 7.1.) *In only two conditions is participation forbidden—carditis (inflammation of the heart) and fever.* All other conditions would allow at least consideration of participation, with the final decision based upon safety features of the sport (see Tables 7.2 and 7.3) and the severity of the medical condition at the time of participation.

The American Academy of Pediatrics does not recommend participation in boxing.

Table 7-1. Medical Conditions and Sports Participation (1)

Condition	Recommendations
Cardiovascular Diseases Hypertension	With significant essential hypertension—avoid weight and power lifting, body building, and strength training. With secondary hypertension (hypertension caused by a previously identified disease), or *severe* essential hypertension—individual evaluation.
Congenital heart disease	With mild disease—participate fully. With moderate or severe disease or after surgery—individual evaluation.
Dysrhythmia	Some dysrhythmias are dangerous in certain sports—individual evaluation.
Mitral valve prolapse	With **symptoms** or evidence of **mitral regurgitation on physical examination**—individual evaluation. All others may participate fully.
Heart murmur	If the murmur is judged "innocent" (no heart disease), full participation is permitted. Otherwise—individual evaluation.
Cerebral Palsy	Individual evaluation.
Diabetes Mellitus	All sports can be played with proper attention to diet, hydration, and insulin therapy. Particular attention is needed for activities lasting 30 minutes or more.
Eyes E.g., functionally one-eyed athlete, detached retina, previous eye surgery or serious eye injury	Significant disability if the better eye is seriously injured. Eye guards, approved by the American Society for Testing Materials (ASTM) may allow participation in most sports, but this must be judged on an individual basis. (*A functionally one-eyed athlete has a best corrected visual acuity of <20/40 in the worse eye.*)
Fever	Fever increases cardiopulmonary effort, reduces maximum exercise capacity, makes heat illness more likely, and increases orthostatic hypotension during exercise. NO SPORTS.
HIV Infection	Minimal risk to others; all sports may be played depending on athlete's state of health.*

Table 7-1.   Continued

Condition	Recommendations
Neurologic	Athlete needs individual assessment for
Convulsive disorder well controlled	collision/contact or limited contact sports, and also for noncontact sports if there are deficits in judgment or cognition.
Convulsive disorder poorly controlled	Individual assessment for collision/contact or limited contact sports. Avoid the following noncontact sports: archery, riflery, swimming, weight or power lifting, strength training, or sports involving heights.
Respiratory	
Asthma	With proper medication and education, only athletes with the most severe asthma will have to modify their participation.
Acute upper respiratory infection	Upper respiratory obstruction may affect pulmonary function—individual assessment for all but mild disease.

*In all athletes, skin lesions should be properly covered, and athletic personnel should use Universal Precautions when handling blood, body fluids, or equipment with visible blood.

Place and Time of the PPE

If you see adolescent patients in your practice, you will at times be asked to do Pre-Participation Evaluations. The PPE *alone* is not a substitute for a comprehensive annual health review. However, because adolescents do not visit their doctors as regularly as younger children, the PPE may afford your only opportunity to address adolescent health issues.

Unfortunately, many adolescents do not have a personal physician to do their PPE's. Therefore, **multiple station screenings** are frequently performed in the school to provide affordable access to medical evaluation for all participants. In this type of PPE, each one of a group of health-care providers is assigned a station with a specific purpose. For example there may be stations for height and weight, vital signs, vision testing, cardiac examination, musculoskeletal examination and male genitalia examination. At the final station, the providers review the findings

> Multiple station screening PPEs also provide an opportunity for medical personnel to interact with the coaching staff.

Table 7-2.   Classification of Sports By Contact (1)

Contact/Collision	Limited contact	Non-contact
Basketball	Baseball	Archery
Boxing*	Bicycling	Badminton
Diving	Cheerleading	Body building
Field hockey	Canoeing/kayaking	Bowling
Football	(White water)	Canoeing/kayaking
Flag	Fencing	(Flat water)
Tackle	Field	Crew/rowing
Ice hockey	High jump	Curling
Lacrosse	Pole vault	Dancing
Martial arts	Field hockey	Field
Rodeo	Gymnastics	Discus
Rugby	Handball	Javelin
Ski jumping	Horseback riding	Shot put
Soccer	Racquetball	Golf
Team handball	Skating	Orienteering
Water polo	Ice	Power lifting
Wrestling	Incline	Race walking
	Roller	Riflery
	Skiing	Rope jumping
	Cross-country	Running
	Downhill	Sailing
	Water	Scuba diving
	Softball	Strength training
	Squash	Swimming
	Ultimate frisbee	Table tennis
	Volleyball	Tennis
	Windsurfing/surfing	Track
		Weight lifting

*Participation not recommended ever for any adolescent.

of the PPE and determine clearance for participation. Confidentiality is a significant challenge with this method of conducting the PPE; however, detection of musculoskeletal abnormalities is maximized.

Ideally, the PPE should occur 4 to 6 weeks prior to participation to permit further evaluation of problems or rehabilitation of recent or unresolved injuries.

Table 7-3.   Classification of Sports by Strenuousness (1)

High to moderate dynamic and static demands	High to moderate dynamic and low static demands	High to moderate static and low dynamic demands	Low intensity (low dynamic and low static demands)
Boxing*	Badminton	Archery	Bowling
Crew/rowing	Baseball	Auto racing	Cricket
Cross-country skiing	Basketball	Diving	Curling
	Field hockey	Equestrian	Golf
Cycling	Lacrosse	Field events (jumping)	Riflery
Downhill skiing	Orienteering		
Fencing	Ping-pong	Field events (throwing)	
Football	Race walking		
Ice hockey	Racquetball	Gymnastics	
Rugby	Soccer	Karate or judo	
Running (sprint)	Squash	Motorcycling	
Speed skating	Swimming	Rodeoing	
Water polo	Tennis	Sailing	
Wrestling	Volleyball	Ski jumping	
		Water skiing	
		Weight lifting	

*Participation not recommended ever for any adolescent.

Sports-Related Anticipatory Guidance

You should also use the PPE to provide sports-related anticipatory guidance, to promote safe and effective participation. Sports participation carries with it an inherent risk of injuries, of which 25–35% may be significant. You need to be familiar with injury risks of the particular sport(s) prior to granting requested clearance, so you can advise appropriately about safety equipment and injury prevention measures. Of special concern are:

- musculoskeletal injuries
- concussion
- eye and dental injuries
- heat illness and sun protection.

Overall, musculoskeletal injuries are the most common, the result of both acute trauma and overuse. *The best predictor of risk for new injury is a recent or non-rehabilitated injury.* You need to emphasize to adolescent athletes, parents, and coaches the paramount importance of conditioning and of allowing resolution of serious injuries.

Concussion, defined as any alteration in mental status induced by trauma, is most often associated with contact/collision sports. *A physician—for example the team doctor—must evaluate the athlete after each concussive event before returning the player to participation* (see Table 7-4). Premature resumption of activity increases the risk of "second impact syndrome" and lethal brain swelling.

Eye and **dental injuries** are more common in some sports than in others. Table 7-5 lists some sports in which eye protectors, mouth guards or helmets and face shields are recommended.

Functionally one-eyed athletes (best *corrected* vision in one eye of less than 20/40) require very careful individual evaluation and counseling. An injury to their better eye may have significant consequences.

Hot and humid weather increases the risk of **heat illness** which is most likely to occur in the first 2 weeks of sports participation. But even acclimated and conditioned athletes may be affected. *Careful acclimatization, avoidance of midday heat and humidity, and scheduled breaks for drinks are essential.* Obesity, dehydration, fever, chronic illness, certain medications, and mental handicaps increase the risk of heat illness. Advise athletes of the need for sun protection by use of protective clothing and sunblocks.

> The soccer maneuver of "heading the ball" is currently a subject of concern and controversy. Does it cause mild brain injuries which could result in cumulative neurological deficits as has been described in boxing?

> Wrestlers should never be allowed to withhold fluids to make a given weight bracket. This will increase their risk for heat illness.

Soccer

Soccer has experienced a phenomenal increase in participation by US youth. Although it's much safer than American Football, musculoskeletal and concussive injuries do occur. Adolescent soccer players undergo more frequent and more severe injuries than adult players, especially knee injuries (see Table 7-6).

Eye injuries related to soccer are relatively frequent, about one per one thousand participants per season. Anticipate heat-related illness in hot summer and early fall weather conditions. The increasing aggressiveness and intensity of soccer play may change the epidemiology and risk for injury.

Table 7-4.   Summary of Recommendations for Management of Concussion in Sports (2)

Grade of concussion	Definition	Management
Grade 1	Transient confusion, no loss of consciousness, and duration of mental status abnormalities of <15 minutes.	Remove athlete from sports activity, examine immediately and at 5-minute intervals, and allow to return to the activity that day only if symptoms resolve within 15 minutes. Any athlete who incurs a second Grade 1 concussion on the same day should be removed from sports activity until asymptomatic for 1 week.
Grade 2	Transient confusion, no loss of consciousness, and a duration of mental status abnormalities of ≥15 minutes.	Remove athlete from sports activity and examine frequently to assess the evolution of symptoms. The athlete should return to sports activity only after asymptomatic for 1 full week. Any athlete who incurs a Grade 2 concussion subsequent to a Grade 1 concussion on the same day should be removed from sports activity until asymptomatic for 2 weeks.
Grade 3	Any loss of consciousness, for any amount of time	Remove athlete from sports activity for 1 full week. If unconscious or if abnormal neurologic signs are present at the time of initial evaluation on the field, transport the athlete by ambulance to the nearest hospital emergency department. An athlete who suffers a second Grade 3 concussion should be removed from sports activity until asymptomatic for 1 month. Any athlete with an abnormality on CT or MRI should be removed from sports activities for the season and discouraged from future return to participation in contact sports.

Table 7-5.   Special Protective Equipment For Selected Sports Activities

Eye protectors	Mouth guards	Helmet with face shield
Basketball	Basketball	Ice hockey
Football	Football	Football
Field hockey	Field hockey	Baseball catcher
Ice hockey	Ice hockey	**Helmet**
Soccer	Wrestling	Cycling
Racquet sports	Rugby	Skiing
Horseback riding	Lacrosse	Baseball
Cycling	Weight lifting	Wrestling
Baseball	Shot put	
Skiing	Discus	

Table 7-6.   Soccer Related Injuries (3)

Type	Location	Knee injuries
59% Contusions	68% Lower extremity	69% Contusions
33% Sprains/strains	15% Upper extremity	21% Sprains
6% Fractures	10% Face/neck	3% Ligament
2% Concussion	7% Trunk	4% Meniscus
		2% Fractures

EXPANDING THE PPE INTO THE ADOLESCENT HISTORY AND PHYSICAL EXAMINATION

The **focused** PPE does not address a number of health-related issues that significantly influence the well being of adolescents, including unacceptable high rates of motor vehicle accidents, homicide, suicide, depression, drug and alcohol abuse, teen pregnancy, sexually transmitted diseases (STDs), and eating disorders. Participation in organized sports does *not* protect the adolescent from high risk behaviors.

Given the reticence of adolescents to see their doctor, the primary care physician may choose to **expand** the school mandated PPE. You can incorporate an annual review of social and behavioral risk into the standard PPE to provide a broader health assessment.

Forms may be obtained from the AMA regarding the Guidelines for Adolescent Preventive Services (GAPS) (Table 7-7), or you may choose to incorporate the suggestions into your practice without specific forms. In either case, the guidelines serve as an excellent model for a comprehensive adolescent health assessment.

Table 7-7.   Preventive Medicine Services for Adolescents (Ages 11–21) (4)

Interval	Recommended service
Yearly	• Guidance regarding: development, diet, physical activity, healthy lifestyles, and injury prevention • Screening for and counseling about: eating disorders, sexual activity, alochol/drug use, tobacco use, domestic violence, school performance, depression, risk for suicide • Physical assessment for: BP, body mass index • If sexually active: Test for gonorrhea, *Chlamydia*, syphilis, and human papillomavirus • If sexually active or >18 years old: Pap smear
Episodically	• Parent health guidance: once during early adolescence (11–14 years) and once during middle adolescence (15–17 years) • Complete physical examination: once during early (11–14 years), mid (15–17 years) and late (18–21 years) adolescence
Once	• Cholesterol: If family history is positive, or once after age 19 • Tuberculosis screening: If history positive for exposure or if in high risk situation (e.g., homeless shelter) • HIV test: If high risk, with pre- and post-test counseling

Modified from AMA Guidelines for Adolescent Preventative Services (4)

Developing the History of Present Illness

An accurate pre-participation history will disclose most medical conditions that affect sports performance. Written questionnaires completed by the adolescent athlete prior to the physical examination facilitate data gathering but should not be used to replace your interview. Whatever the format you use, your initial and interim history for sports participation should include questions to identify:

1. Underlying health problems and chronic conditions
2. Previous musculoskeletal injuries
3. Previous concussions
4. Medications
   - Some medications may increase the risk of heat related illness.
   - Reviewing medications taken by the athlete may reveal illnesses not otherwise mentioned.
5. Risk for cardiac sudden death. Although you will ask relevant questions, you must recognize that *when you do a PPE your chances to identify a risk for sudden cardiac death with athletes is very low*.
6. Tetanus immunization status. A tetanus booster should be given at the time of school entry (age 5), at middle school entry (age 11), and every 10 years thereafter.
7. Menstrual history. The menstrual history (especially disruption of a regular pattern) may provide clues to the presence of eating disorders or undiagnosed chronic conditions. Irregularity or absence of menstruation may be due to vigorous and substantial exercise. You will have to carefully distinguish the causes of menstrual irregularity so as not to miss an important diagnosis.

Eliciting a history from an adolescent may be challenging. The following hints may be helpful:

- Shake hands
- Identify yourself
- Initially focus on the purpose of the examination
- Establish limits of confidentiality
- LISTEN
- Let the adolescent know what to expect
- Approach the psychosocial part of the interview by moving from less personal to more personal questions
- While it may be tempting to take an informal, "buddies" approach to adolescents, it is unwise to do so, as they expect you to be an

---

Unfortunately the PPE seldom identifies hypertrophic cardiomyopathy (HCM) the most common cause of sudden death. HCM, with a systolic murmur that increases in intensity with standing and decreases in intensity with squatting, is rarely discovered by routine auscultation.

authority figure and someone they can entrust with private information. You should *not*, for example, "dress down."

The Physical Examination

Physical examination may create significant anxiety for many adolescent patients, especially younger ones who are not yet comfortable with pubertal changes. Respect the adolescent's modesty! Explain why you are performing specific parts of the examination. e.g., the palpation component of the cardiovascular examination, and the genital examination.

Especially important portions of the physical examination include:

- Vital signs

    Temperature: Presence of **fever** proscribes participation while it is present.

    Blood pressure: **Hypertension** will need to be followed up with diagnostic tests.

    Pulse: Tachycardia may reflect anxiety, or it may be the result of medications or medical conditions. Importantly it also may be a subtle signal of substance abuse. On the other hand, well conditioned athletes usually have bradycardia; however, in the presence of other clinical clues, such as underweight, it may be a sign of **anorexia nervosa**.
- Height, weight, BMI and general appearance: Identify **obesity** and **eating disorders**. (Body habitus suggestive of Marfan's syndrome may be detected. This is associated with **congenital heart disease** and aortic rupture.)
- **Vision**: Measure visual acuity of each eye separately.
- **Mouth and teeth**: Look for oral ulcerations and decreased tooth enamel which may be signs of an eating disorder.
- **Cardiovascular**: Most **heart murmurs** detected in adolescents are benign (or "functional") murmurs. Occasionally a patient with previously unrecognized **congenital heart disease** may be detected by careful examination of the heart.
- **Abdomen**: Look for an enlarged **liver** or **spleen**.
- **Male genitalia**: Look for an atrophied or absent **testicle**.
- **The skin**: Examine the skin lesions suggestive of potentially contagious infection: boils, scabbed or oozing sores.
- **SMR** (sexual maturity rating): (Table 7-8) An advanced SMR is associated with an increase in musculoskeletal injuries.

> Features of Marfan's syndrome include tall stature, long digits, flexible joints and myopia.

Table 7-8. Secondary Sex Characteristics Tanner Stages (mean age ± SD) (5)

Breast Development

Stage I	Preadolescent; elevation of papilla only
Stage II	Breast bud; elevation of breast and papilla as small mound; enlargement of areolar diameter (11.1 ± 1.1)
Stage III	Further enlargement and elevation of breast and areola; no separation of their contours (12.1 ± 1.1)
Stage IV	Projection of areola and papilla to form secondary mound above level of breast (13.1 ± 1.1)
Stage V	Mature stage; projection of papilla only due to recession of areola to general contour of breast (15.3 ± 1.7)

Note: Stages IV and V may not be distinct in some patients.

Genital Development (male)

Stage I	Preadolescent; testes, scrotum, and penis about same size and proportion as in early childhood.
Stage II	Enlargement of scrotum and testes; skin of scrotum reddens and changes in texture; little or no enlargement of penis (11.6 ± 1.1)
Stage III	Enlargement of penis, first mainly in length; further growth of testes and scrotum (12.8 ± 1.0)
Stage IV	Increased size of penis with growth in breadth and development of glans; further enlargement of testes and scrotum and increased darkening of scrotal skin (13.8 ± 1.0)
Stage V	Genitalia adult in size and shape (14.9 ± 1.1)

Pubic Hair (male and female)

Stage I	Preadolescent; vellus over pubes no further developed than that over abdominal wall, i.e., no pubic hair
Stage II	Sparse growth of long, slightly pigmented down hair, straight or only slightly curled, chiefly at base of penis or along labia. (Male: 13.4 ± 1.1, Female: 11.7 ± 1.2)
Stage III	Considerably darker, coarser and more curled; hair spreads sparsely over junction of pubes. (Male: 13.9 ± 1.0, Female: 12.4 ± 1.1)
Stage IV	Hair resembles adult in type; distribution still considerably smaller than in adult. No spread to medial surface of thighs. (Male: 14.4 ± 1.1, Female: 12.9 ± 1.1)
Stage V	Adult in quantity and type with distribution of the horizontal pattern. (Male: 15.2 ± 1.1, Female: 14.4 ± 1.2)
Stage VI	Spread up linea alba: "male escutcheon"

- **Musculoskeletal examination**: The 14-step examination also known as the "2-minute" examination is an efficient screen to detect asymmetrical or limited range of motion, strength and muscle mass. Perform a more thorough individual evaluation of the shoulder, knee or ankle if there is a history of previous injury. The 14-step examination is illustrated below (Figure 7-1).

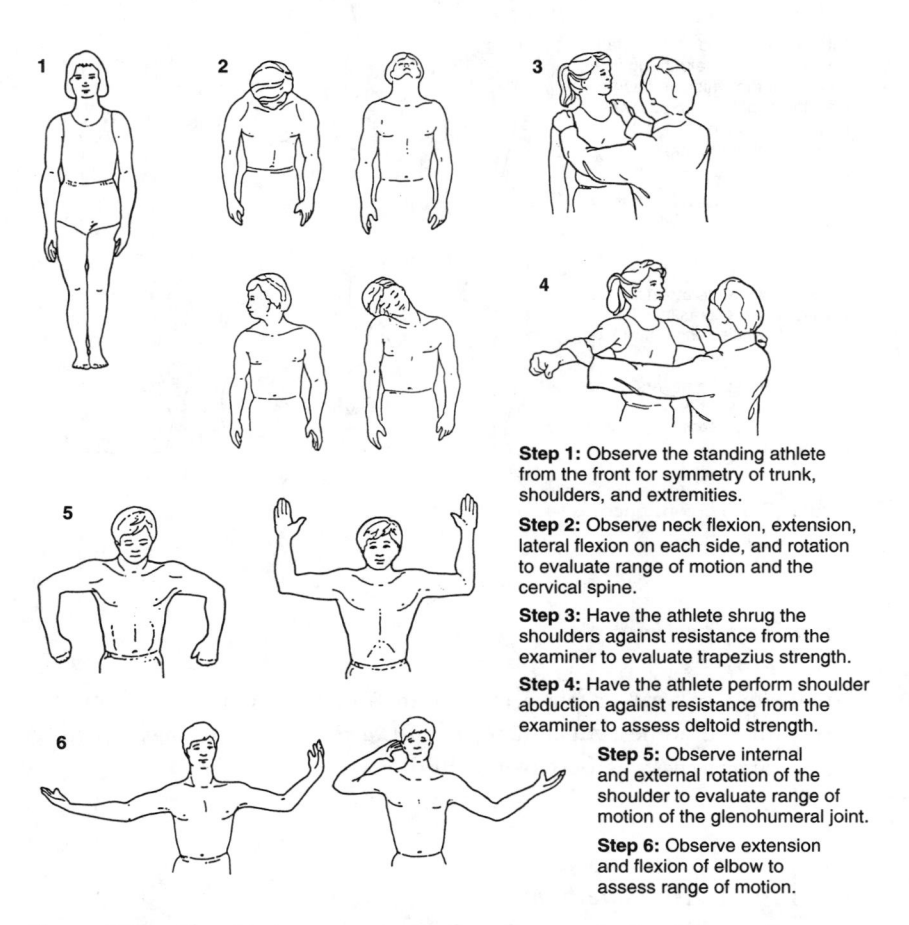

Step 1: Observe the standing athlete from the front for symmetry of trunk, shoulders, and extremities.

Step 2: Observe neck flexion, extension, lateral flexion on each side, and rotation to evaluate range of motion and the cervical spine.

Step 3: Have the athlete shrug the shoulders against resistance from the examiner to evaluate trapezius strength.

Step 4: Have the athlete perform shoulder abduction against resistance from the examiner to assess deltoid strength.

Step 5: Observe internal and external rotation of the shoulder to evaluate range of motion of the glenohumeral joint.

Step 6: Observe extension and flexion of elbow to assess range of motion.

Figure 7-1. The 14-step screening orthopedic examination. (From *Contemporary Pediatrics* 14(3): 196–197, as adapted from D. M. Smith et al., *Pre-Participation Physical Evaluation*, 2nd edn., McGraw-Hill, New York, 1997. Reprinted by permission of the publishers and of the artist, Suzanne Edmonds.)

Step 7: Observe pronation and supination of the forearm to evaluate elbow and wrist range of motion.

Step 8: Have the athlete clench the fist, then spread the fingers to assess range of motion in the hand and fingers.

Step 9: Observe the standing athlete from the rear for symmetry of trunk, shoulders, and extremities.

Step 10: Have the athlete stand with the knees straight and bend backward from the waist. Discomfort with extension of the lumbar spine may be associated with spondylolysis and spondylolisthesis.

Step 11: Have the athlete stand with the knees straight and flex forward at the waist, first away from the examiner, to assess for scoliosis, spine range of motion, and hamstring flexibility.

Step 12: Have the athlete stand facing the examiner with quadriceps flexed to observe symmetry of leg musculature.

Step 13: Have the athlete duck walk four steps to assess hip, knee, and ankle range of motion, strength, and balance.

Step 14: Have the athlete stand on the toes, then the heels to evaluate calf strength, symmetry, and balance.

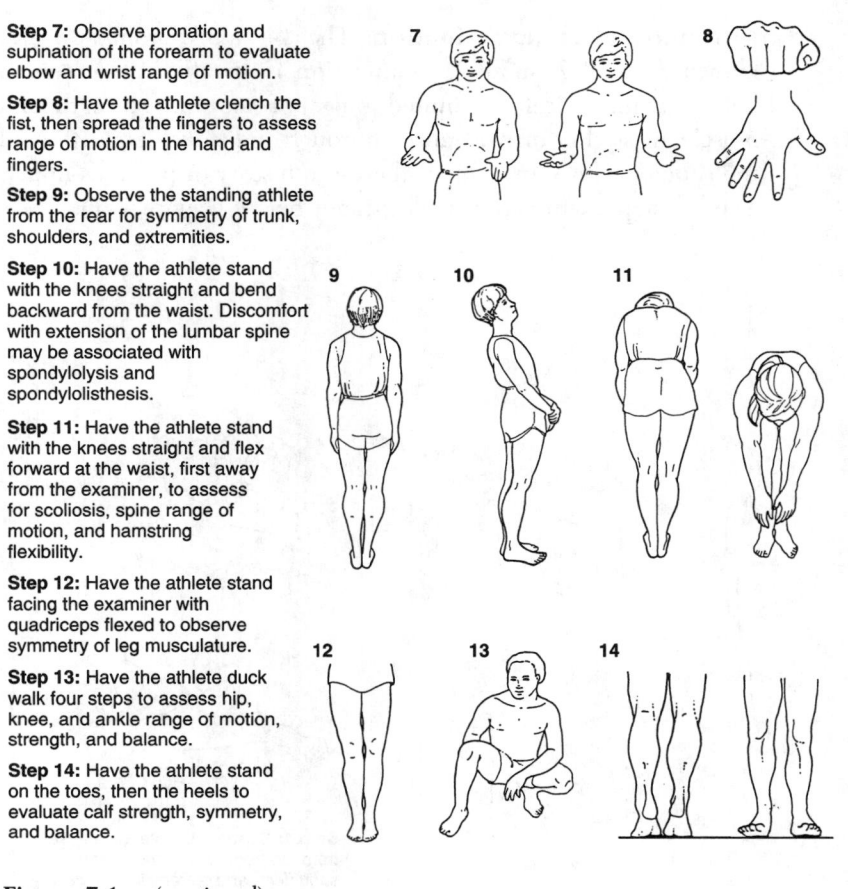

Figure 7-1. (continued)

Ancillary Testing

Unless the history or physical examination raise concerns about the health of the adolescent athlete, *routine laboratory tests or imaging studies are not recommended* as part of the PPE.

Putting It All Together

The following discussion demonstrates resolution of the case presented at the beginning of the chapter by using these basic medical decision making principles:

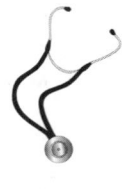

Knowledge of:	medical conditions
	sports-related injuries
	spectrum of adolescent health-related issues
Plus:	History and physical examination; ancillary testing if needed
Leads to:	Participation recommendations
	Treatment of any problems identified
	Anticipatory guidance

A 16-year-old comes to the office for his school-mandated sports physical. He is an avid year round soccer player participating in school-based competition and club soccer. In preparation for his visit, you review his office chart. He has been your patient since moving to the area at age 10 years when you conducted an initial comprehensive history and physical examination. At age 11, you treated him for pharyngitis. There are copies of soccer camp physicals at ages 12 and 13. He was last seen 1 year ago with an extensive contact rash thought to be poison ivy.

The immunization record indicates that his last tetanus vaccination was at age 5. He received his MMR #2 (Measles, Mumps, and Rubella) at the time of his 12-year-old soccer camp physical.

This 16-year-old soccer player has his drivers license and drove to your office for his PPE without his parents, who gave consent for the examination. He completed a sports history questionnaire in your office.

At the beginning of the interview, the patient tells you he needs a sports physical because he missed the one offered in the physical education department. The previous 2 years he had his physical examination at school; they were done by several different doctors and nurses each doing a small part of the examination. He is eager to have you complete the Pre-Participation Evaluation (PPE) form so he can begin practice with the team today.

At this point, organize your historical information. The sports history form discloses no areas of concern. However, review of your office chart indicates that the patient has not had a comprehensive health review since age 10. The patient's main concern is recommendation for sports participation.

You greeted your patient and reviewed with him the reason for his visit. You begin to elicit further history. He is a junior in high school, a member of the school's National Honor Society and he hopes to attend college and major in engineering. He has never had any musculoskeletal injuries or head injuries in soccer or other sports activities. He plans to play baseball in the spring.

Although your patient is anxious to complete the PPE so he can begin practice today, you explain your recommendation that a comprehensive health review be completed today in addition to the PPE. You show him

a confidential history form (such as that from the Guidelines for Adolescent Preventive Services or GAPS) and explain the limits of confidentiality. Although the length of the visit will be longer, the patient agrees to it. You acknowledge his cooperation.

After the patient completes the GAPS form, you will proceed with the physical examination. While the patient undresses, review the GAPS history in your office. Return to the examining room and let the patient know what to expect. Then do the physical examination.

The patient's physical examination, including a 14-step musculoskeletal screen and focused examination of the knee, is normal. You teach him testicular self-examination with an explanation of its importance. After he gets dressed, you return and review the GAPS form and the physical examination.

The GAPS questionnaire discloses that the patient is sexually active and uses condoms. His condom usage has been "frequent," but not "always." After further questioning, you learn that he has experienced a very mild amount of dysuria the past two mornings and is concerned about sexually transmitted disease.

Clearly your patient is at risk for a sexually transmitted disease, and you order a urinalysis to screen for urethritis. You discuss encouraging his girlfriend to seek medical care. Advisability of a tetanus booster and hepatitis B vaccine is discussed with the patient and by telephone with his parents.

Written consent for the tetanus booster and hepatitis B vaccine is obtained from the patient and his parents; the tetanus booster and the first dose of hepatitis B vaccine are given. The urine was positive for leukocyte esterase. A confidential urethral screen was positive for *Chlamydia* and the gonorrhea culture was negative.

The patient receives confidential treatment for *Chlamydia*. His girlfriend has received medical care that addressed her sexual activity and provided treatment for *Chlamydia*.

SUMMARY

Adolescent health care can be a challenge for all concerned, but it also can be a source of great satisfaction. The sports physical, so often needed by adolescents, is an excellent forum through which you may provide a full range of comprehensive services.

STUDY QUESTIONS*

1. Which of the following is true regarding the "functionally one-eyed" athlete?
   A. Athletes in this category have visual acuity in the "bad eye" which is worse than 20/100.
   B. Soccer is one of the safest sports for these athletes.
   C. ASTM approved eye guards will allow these athletes to participate in most sports.
   D. No significant disability would arise from an injury to the better eye.

2. Which of the following is true regarding adolescents and their relationship to the health care system?
   A. Participation in organized sports significantly lessens an adolescent's likelihood of having several problems such as depression, drug and alcohol use, STDs, and eating disorders.
   B. Adolescents see physicians less often and less regularly than young children.
   C. You will have more success in handling adolescent patients if you dress as they do and act as their "buddy."
   D. Adolescents coming in for sports physicals usually freely report all their medical problems and concerns.

3. A 13-year-old boy comes to your office for a Pre-Participation Evaluation so that he can play basketball on his middle school team. He has no previous medical problems and no complaints, and he denies sexual activity. His examination shows he has an I/VI systolic murmur which his mother says has been present all his life; he has scattered facial lesions which are oozing a yellowish clear crusting material (which you diagnose as impetigo); he has a sexual maturity rating of Tanner Stage III. Your recommendations include all the following *except*:
   A. He should not play or practice until his impetigo either resolves with antibiotic treatment or all open sores can be covered.
   B. His heart murmur needs no further evaluation.
   C. His sexual maturity rating is age appropriate and places him at no higher than usual risk of musculoskeletal injury.
   D. He should be tested for STD's before he begins practicing with the team.

4. Heat illnesses are a significant risk in hot weather. Which of the following is true regarding heat illness?
   A. Acclimated and conditioned athletes may suffer heat illness.

*For answers, see page 347.

B. Heat illness most often occurs after the first two weeks of participation.

C. Scheduling practice at midday is the best way to acclimate athletes to heat.

D. Heat stroke is serious but never lethal to young athletes.

5. Which group of clinical findings is most highly suggestive of anorexia nervosa?
    A. Underweight, tachycardia, and hypertension.
    B. Underweight, tachycardia, and fever blisters.
    C. Underweight, mouth ulcers and an enlarged spleen.
    D. Underweight, decreased tooth enamel and bradycardia.

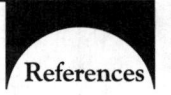

References

1. American Academy of Pediatrics Committee on Sports Medicine and Fitness "Medical Conditions Affecting Sports Participation." Pediatrics 94(5): 757–760; 1994.

2. American Academy of Neurology, Quality Standards Subcommittee, "Summary of Recommendations for Management of Concussion in Sports." JAMA, April 16: 1190; 1997.

3. Roaas, N.S. Soccer Injuries in Adolescents. Am J Sports Med 6: 358–361; 1978.

4. American Medical Association Guideline for Adolescent Preventative Services, Recommendations Monograph. JAMA, 2: 1995.

5. Marshall, W.A. and Tanner, J.M. Archives Dis. Childhood 44: 291; 1969.

Suggested Reading

American Academy of Family Physicians, et al. Preparticipation Physical Examination, 2nd edn. McGraw-Hill, New York, 1997.

Neinstein, L.S. (ed) Adolescent Health Care: A Practical Guide, 3rd edn. Urban and Schwartzenberg, Inc., Baltimore.

The General Medical Examination of an Adult Patient: "The H&P"

Sarah A. McCarty

INTRODUCTION

Your encounters with patients in ambulatory care settings will be interesting and quite variable. They may be very brief contacts where only one specific problem is addressed, or much longer encounters where more information is sought. The traditional history and physical examination (often abbreviated as the "H&P") is an encounter which may take a considerable amount of time. For the H&P you will be trying to gather information about your patient's previous medical problems, current medical problems, and risk factors for future medical problems. The follow-up visit may be much shorter, and has as its goal an *efficient* evaluation of chronic or newly identified problems. The goal of this chapter is to enable you to approach each medical encounter in a way that allows you to make the most of each learning opportunity.

THE INITIAL VISIT

Ms. Kitty Carr is a 65-year-old woman who presents to the office "to establish care." You note that on the schedule for the morning she has been allotted a 60 minute appointment. Your preceptor asks you to go into the room and, "Do a history and physical examination."

Your first response, when you are given any task by your preceptor should be to clarify the preceptor's expectations. If you are not sure what your preceptor means, do not be afraid to ask in order to clarify the instructions. Having done this, you enter Ms. Carr's room with the intention of doing a full H&P (also known as obtaining the database.)

119

What does the full history consist of? It is divided into several sections each of which will be discussed below. In this chapter we will not discuss *every* question which may be asked in the medical interview, but rather give you an overview and suggest an approach to patient evaluation. Your physical examination textbook should be used in conjunction with this chapter.

Now is the time to apply the communication skills discussed in Chapter 3. Before asking the patient any questions, introduce yourself, offer your hand, and then sit down and begin the interview.

Identifying Data

The first part of the history is referred to as the identifying data. It is the **demographic** information on your patient, consisting of information such as name, age, occupation and community in which the patient lives. It is seldom necessary for you to *personally* ask all these questions, as most patient registration forms both in the hospital and in offices will include this information. Review these forms before entering the room. Establishing rapport, a main goal of the interview, will be facilitated by your asking first about a patient's home town or job; this may give an opportunity to chat pleasantly for a few minutes before getting on to the rest of the interview and can help to put both of you at ease. On the other hand, asking the patient's age at the outset is usually not a good idea!

Chief Complaint

The next section of the interview is known as the chief complaint. This is the reason the patient is seeking care and the duration of the problem.

You might begin your structured portion of the interview by asking, "I see that this is your first visit to our office. Are there any problems that you would like to discuss today?"
Ms. Carr responds, "Well, I have been having some chest pain for the last few weeks."

This flows nicely into the next section of the interview, the history of present illness.

History of Present Illness (HPI)

The HPI is a *description of the chief complaint*. (It may actually include a full description of *other* major medical problems in which case it is then the history of medical illness*es*.) A well done history of present illness is essential in the development of a **differential diagnosis**. You want to know not only what is causing the pain, but also what she *thinks* is causing the pain. You want to know how this pain is affecting her life and what she expects you to do about it. A good way to begin to explore all of these issues is with an open-ended question. "How would you describe your pain?"

As a beginning student you may struggle most with the history of present illness. This is because you lack the medical knowledge to be able to formulate a differential diagnosis as you interview the patient and then to ask the appropriate questions. *Do not panic* if you do not know what to ask. Tables 8-1 and 8-2 list a variety of complaints and some characteristics of them that need to be established by your questioning. If you can think of nothing else, ask your patient *what they think* is the cause of the symptom.

Another helpful hint in approaching the history of present illness is to read about the complaint and jot down a few key questions before you

> The differential diagnosis is the list of possible explanations for your patient's problem. Your history and physical is designed to collect the information you need to consider all possible diseases which could explain the patient's problem, then to narrow down the list to the most likely diagnosis.

Table 8-1. Symptoms Commonly Reported by Patients

Pain
    Chest pain
    Abdominal pain
    Headache
    Muscle and joint pains
    Back pain
    Pain on urination
    Pain when swallowing
Shortness of breath
Nausea and/or vomiting
Diarrhea and/or constipation
Fever
Weight and/or appetite changes
Weakness and/or dizziness
Cough
Itching

Table 8-2. Characteristics of Common Symptoms

Time and circumstances of onset
Location*
Radiation*
Quality*
Severity
Frequency
Duration
Associated symptoms
Relieving factors
Exacerbating factors
Treatment tried

* These characteristics are relevant primarily to a complaint of pain.

enter the room. This is of course, possible only if you know the complaint before you go into the room; usually in your early clinical experiences, you *will* be told beforehand the gist of your patient's problems.

Ms. Carr describes her pain as a pressure like pain in her midepigastric area which is always accompanied by shortness of breath. It radiates to the left arm and occurs only when she mows her lawn or mops her floor. It is severe enough to stop her activity but goes away in just a few minutes with rest. She has used no medications for it. She came in to be seen because she cannot mow her lawn and she cannot afford to pay someone to do it. Otherwise, she would not be here. She would like to have the pain taken care of so she can get her lawn mowed sometime this summer. She is afraid that her heart is causing the pain but cannot afford a lot of tests.

You feel comfortable that you have enough information about her chest pain. You now move on to the next section of the interview.

Past Medical History (PMH)

The past medical history, as the title implies, explores **previous medical illnesses** and **surgeries**. It also deals with **prevention issues** such as immunization history and the use of seat belts. A full **medication history**, including **over the counter (OTC) drugs,** should be obtained. **Allergies** are usually asked about in this portion of the history. As a student you may become frustrated as each attending physician

has a somewhat variable list of what they feel should be included in the past medical history. It is reasonable to ask your preceptor what they routinely include in the past medical history.

Ms. Carr reports, "I am lucky because I have been healthy all my life." She has never been hospitalized and has had no surgeries. Her only medication is calcium; she takes 1000 mg a day since menopause at age 56. She is allergic to penicillin which causes a diffuse rash. She has never been pregnant. She has no history of physical abuse, no blood transfusions and wears her seat belt regularly. She has not had a tetanus shot in the last ten years and has never had a pneumonia shot.

The Family History

Now obtain the next portion of the history, the family history. The purpose of the family history is to *identify genetic-based diseases which your patient is at increased risk of developing*. A good way to approach this is to do a family tree and ask about the age and health of each sibling, parent and grandparent. Be sure that you ask both about living siblings and about any who have died. If you ask just, "How many brothers or sisters do you have?" you may only hear about those who are still living. You may want to ask "How many brothers and sisters did you have in all?"

Ms. Carr reports that she is an only child. She knows nothing about her grandparents except that "they died fairly young." Her mother died at 80 of advanced Alzheimer's disease and her father died at 52 from a heart attack.

The Social History

You continue on with the social history. The goal of the social history is to gain an *understanding of your patient's lifestyle*. This helps you to evaluate the impact a disease may have on the patient, as well as the patient's ability to cope with the disease both financially and emotionally. As in much of the history you are also looking for *potential* problems. Your preceptors may vary in what they include in the social history and again it is appropriate to ask them what information they routinely include here.

Habits such as alcohol ingestion and smoking are included here if they have not been discussed in the past medical history. You should also ask about other habits such as **diet, sleep** and **exercise**. A **job history** is obtained to evaluate potential environmental exposures and additionally to get information about financial stability. It is important to determine insurance coverage, but you usually can find this information on

Remember that medical care is very expensive and not everyone can afford tests and medications.

the patient's registration form. Your patient's **home** and their **family unit** are also discussed here in order to help you determine their support system. It is very important, now more than ever, because of acquired immune deficiency syndrome (AIDS), to discuss **sexual activity**. You might mistakenly make assumptions about a patient's risk of sexually transmitted disease based on information such as their age or their general appearance. However, you will not know unless you ask; if you fail to obtain accurate data, your patient will suffer.

Ms. Carr lives in a three-bedroom ranch home with Otto her German Shepherd dog. Her husband died three years ago after a heart attack. He was in intensive care for 2 weeks before his death and she vowed she would never go through anything like that. She has not dated since his death but goes out to dinner or movies with her best friend Judy. She retired 1 year ago after 40 years of teaching high school history. Currently she volunteers as a foster grandparent. Until the last few weeks, she walked a mile every day. She eats no red meat and never fries her food. She has a small garden in the summer and eats its harvest all year as she cans her food. She smokes one pack of cigarettes a day and does not drink alcohol. She does drink five cups of coffee a day. She sleeps 7 hours a night and has no problems getting to sleep.

The Review of Systems (ROS)

Now you begin the last section of the interview: the review of systems. The review of systems consists of a series of questions about each of the organ systems in the body such as the eyes, the heart or the skin. *Your goal is to discover other medical problems that your patients have not told you about or have not themselves recognized as problems.* You may struggle with the review of systems when you first begin taking histories because of the sheer number of questions to be asked. As you learn more about diseases, this task becomes much easier. Ask questions directly and if the response is negative, move on to the next question. Positive responses require further exploration to determine their significance.

Ms. Carr's weight has been stable over the last few years. She has occasional constipation without accompanying abdominal pain or rectal bleeding, for which she takes milk of magnesia about once a month. She has no history of abnormal Pap smears but has not had one since she "went through the change." She has never had a mammogram but does do self breast exams every month. The remainder of the review of systems is negative.

The Physical Examination

Physical examination skills will be taught to you employing a variety of formats over the next 1 or 2 years. There are very specific skills involved in performing the physical examination which may take years to fully develop. Generally the physical examination is taught one organ system at a time. When your preceptor plans to discuss a specific organ system, for example, the heart examination, read that chapter in your textbook and jot down any questions you may have. Your preceptor will show you how to do the examination, answer your questions and allow you an opportunity to practice with him or her present. But that is not enough. *Just as it takes years of practice to perfect your golf game or your tennis game, it takes years of practice to perfect your physical examination.* Practice on your friends, your family or on your fellow students. If you are struggling with a particular aspect of the examination ask your preceptor to review it with you.

Inspection, a very important part of the physical examination, is just observing the area of the body being examined or the person as a whole. Your patient's general appearance, how they walk, and how they talk are all part of the physical examination. Inspection is a skill you can work on almost constantly. When you are in crowds look at the people around you. Do they look happy or sad? Do they look healthy; if not ask yourself what it is about their appearance that makes you think they are not well. In the next few years you will be surprised how your power of observation will improve.

You are now ready for the physical examination. You appropriately step out of the room so that Ms. Carr can undress.

Ms. Carr is a healthy appearing 65-year-old woman. She appears to be in no distress. Her blood pressure is normal at 124/80 and her pulse is 72 beats per minute and regular. Her head and neck examination is normal. She has no jugular venous distention and her carotid artery pulses are normal. Her lungs are clear. Her heart examination is normal. She has no swelling of her legs and her peripheral pulses are intact.

Presenting Your Patient

Now discuss with your preceptor the information you have just gathered. This is known as **presenting the patient.** Explain to Ms. Carr that you are going to talk to your preceptor about her and ask her to remain in the room. You explain that your preceptor may want to verify

Remember, if you are a male student, you need to have a chaperon with you when you return to the room to perform the physical examination. Under some circumstances, female students may need chaperons to examine male patients. Always check with your preceptor.

Your patient presentation should be well organized and contain *pertinent* information; it does *not* need to include every single item you have learned about Ms. Carr.

some of the physical findings and ask her to wait to dress until after your preceptor has examined her.

As a beginning student you may have difficulty presenting patients because you do not know what is important and what is not. Most preceptors understand this and will help you sort out the important information. Because every preceptor prefers a slightly different style of presentation, this may cause you some frustration. Be flexible and once again ask your preceptor how they prefer their presentations to be done. Throughout this chapter Ms. Carr has been presented to you about as most preceptors would want her case presented to them, with the exception of the physical examination. More specific information on the heart examination would likely be requested, but was excluded from this chapter, as our goal is to present an overview to you, rather than to serve as a comprehensive physical examination text.

Problem Formulation

Formulation or analysis of your patient's case has three components:

- *Problem list.* The problem list is just that, a full list of all of the patient's problems, both past and present, and may include major risk factors for future problems such as a family history of coronary artery disease.
- *Assessment.* The assessment includes an evaluation of the stability of the problem and the differential diagnosis.
- *Plan.* The plan includes your plans for diagnostic evaluations such as the tests you will order, and the treatment you will initiate. Plans for patient education are also important.

After your presentation, your preceptor discusses your differential diagnosis and plans for diagnostic evaluation and treatment. Chest pain is Ms. Carr's primary problem. You feel strongly that her pain indicates heart problems but she is not having any pain now and has it only with a lot of exertion. She seems stable and you decide to treat her as an outpatient, but you want to do further studies to evaluate her pain. You are not sure which study would be best and you and your preceptor explore the possibilities. After some discussion you decide to order a dobutamine echocardiogram (a test in which the medication dobutamine is used to increase the workload of the heart, and then an ultrasound is done of the heart; abnormal movements of the heart suggest poor blood supply to that area). In the interim you decide to prescribe an aspirin every day and start her on a medication to control her pain such as metoprolol (a drug which blocks the beta receptors of the sympathetic nervous system used in coronary artery disease). You also feel she needs to stop smoking and plan to address that as well.

Health Care Maintenance

As an intimate part of the initial visit, prevention of disease or looking for early treatable disease is addressed. This is known as health care maintenance.

You decide Ms. Carr should be given cards to test her stool for blood as a screen for colon cancer. She should undergo sigmoidoscopy (a sigmoidoscopy consists of inserting a fiberoptic scope into the rectum and into the sigmoid colon in order to view the walls and look for tumors or other abnormalities) but you and your preceptor decide that her chest pain should be stabilized before pursuing sigmoidoscopy. You also recommend pneumonia and tetanus immunizations. You have done her Pap smear today and her breast examination and plan to order a mammogram. In postmenopausal women prevention of osteoporosis is an important issue. You note that she does exercise and take calcium but plan to discuss estrogen replacement therapy which is important in prevention of osteoporosis and coronary artery disease. You discuss the need to obtain baseline laboratory information including a cholesterol determination.

> A screening test is one that is designed to detect a disease before symptoms occur.

Patient Education

You and your preceptor now return to Ms. Carr's examining room. Introduce your preceptor to Ms. Carr (unless they are already acquainted). Your preceptor checks the major points of the history with Ms. Carr, then does at least a partial examination to verify your findings. Here, practice styles may differ. Your preceptor may begin the final portion of the interview now or may step out of the room to allow Ms Carr to re-dress before beginning this discussion. It is preferable to conduct the closing interview with your patient clothed, but under some circumstances this may be too time consuming. At least be sure she has a sheet which covers her well for this part of the interview.

Your preceptor steps out briefly to allow Ms. Carr to dress; at this time the preceptor reassures you that the history you obtained is accurate and your physical findings are correct. Preceptors may use this few minutes to correct you if you have made any major errors in your history and physical and to revise the plan if this is necessary after seeing the patient. This is not needed today and you return together to discuss the plan with Ms. Carr.

You tell Ms. Carr that you believe her chest pain is coming from poor blood supply to her heart. She nods her head and says, "I thought so, but this is not angina is it?" You explain that you do indeed think that this is

angina. "Oh," she replies, "That can be bad. I could have a heart attack like my husband." "Yes, you could and that is what we would like to avoid," is your response. You begin to discuss the test you would like to do but she interrupts you. "I told you no tests. I do not want to end up like my husband. He had a lot of tests and died anyway. I just want to be able to do the things I need to do, like mow my lawn. Can't you just give me medication and see how I do?" Your preceptor steps in and re-explains to her about the possibility of a heart attack and possible death. "I know all that but I don't want any tests." Together you decide to treat her with the medications previously discussed and give her some sublingual nitroglycerin to take if she has pain. You explain that mowing her lawn could be dangerous for her. She understands and agrees that if she has pain that is not relieved with three nitroglycerin, she will call 911.

You now discuss health care maintenance issues with Ms. Carr.

You discuss a pneumonia shot and a tetanus shot. You explain the reasons they are important. She asks whether her insurance will pay for them and you explain that they will pay for the pneumonia shot only. She agrees to this but refuses the tetanus shot. She agrees to the mammogram as she knows it is important and she has been thinking for a while that she should have one because breast cancer is so very common. She reluctantly agrees to collect stool samples for blood after you explain the reason but quickly adds she knows a lot of people who have "the light put up their rectums and I am not doing that." She has been reading about estrogen replacement therapy and knows it is important in preventing heart disease but at this point is not interested in anything that might restart menstrual bleeding. She asks you to let her think about this. Smoking cessation is now discussed. She realizes it is a bad habit and "might kill her". She is planning to quit and will try if you think it is important. You tell her you think it is essential and give her literature on smoking cessation. She is agreeable to laboratory work as she has been wondering about her cholesterol and has not had any blood work in many years.

Closing the Interview

You covered all the issues you want to discuss. Now ask her if she has any questions and if she is comfortable with the plan.

She does not have any questions and feels she understands and agrees with the plan. To be sure, ask her to review her new medications which she does without a problem. She knows the proper use of her sublingual nitroglycerin and agrees to call 911 for unrelieved chest pain.

You explain you want to see her back in the office in 6 weeks and to call if any problems arise. You confirm that she has the office number and

remind her that it rings into the answering service after hours. Your preceptor or a partner is on-call 24 hours a day should she have problems.

You once again offer your hand and say, "Well Ms. Carr, I was pleased to meet you and I hope you will feel better. I will hopefully be here when you return in 6 weeks. If not, thank you for allowing me to talk to you today." Ms. Carr takes your hand and responds, "I thank you for your time and attention. I too hope I will see you in 6 weeks."

Documentation

After Ms. Carr leaves, your preceptor may ask you to "write up" the visit. This refers to preparing a written (or dictated) document detailing the medical interview, the physical examination and the final assessment and plans (see Table 8-3). When you are just beginning this may take several hours and can be frustrating as you frequently do not know what to include in the history of present illness or review of systems. As your medical knowledge increases it will become easier but at this time just try your best. Your preceptor should review your write-up and point out key points in the history. *Like the skills of the physical examination, perfecting your written histories and physical examinations will take a lot of time and patience.* Take advantage of every opportunity. And once again if you have a question, do not hesitate to ask your preceptor. Their role is to help guide you through this sometimes difficult transition to the world of medical practice.

THE FOLLOW-UP VISIT

Ms. Carr returns in 6 weeks for her follow-up visit. You note that she is scheduled for just 15 minutes. The purpose of this visit is to assess her response to treatment for her chest pain and to re-discuss any health maintenance items that remain unsettled from the last visit. A repeat of the full history and physical examination is unnecessary and inappropriate. The questions and examination at the follow-up visit should be problem focused. Once again your preceptor sends you into the room by yourself.

"Hello Ms. Carr, good to see you again. How is your chest pain doing?" Ms. Carr responds that her pain is better, but (although she knows she shouldn't) she has tried on several occasions to mow her lawn. She is still unable to do so. She is taking her medicine regularly and thinks it might make her tired. She has not needed any nitroglycerin and is afraid to try it because she heard it gives you "an awful headache." In the interim a very

Table 8-3. Example of Documentation of Symptom Inquiry (HPI of Ms. Carr's Chest Pain)

Time and circumstances of onset
    ". . . when I mow my lawn or mop my floor"
Location
    ". . . right at the lower part of my breastbone or high up in my stomach" (midepigastric)
Radiation
    ". . . goes to my left arm"
Quality
    ". . . a pressure-like pain"
Severity
    ". . . to have to stop mopping"
Frequency
    ". . . every time I mow my lawn or mop my floor"
Duration
    ". . . goes away when I rest a few minutes"

good friend had a heart attack and was treated by a cardiologist in town. She had angioplasty (opening up of a coronary artery during catheterization) and is doing great. Ms. Carr has decided she would like to see this cardiologist for further evaluation. You ask about smoking. She replies that her last cigarette was the day you saw her and she never intends to smoke again. You congratulate her on having quit and tell her you will talk to your preceptor about the cardiologist.

Address the health care maintenance items unresolved from the last visit and review test results. You tell Ms. Carr that her mammogram was normal, as was her Pap smear. Her cholesterol is slightly elevated and you discuss a low cholesterol diet and give her some literature on this. Her stools for occult blood are negative. She still cannot decide about estrogen replacement therapy but says after she sees the cardiologist she might consider it.

It is important that as a student you never collaborate on plans with your patient until you have discussed them with your preceptor.

The follow-up visit includes an appropriate physical examination.

Recheck her pulse and blood pressure as her new medication is a beta blocker which can lower both blood pressure and pulse. You perform an examination of the heart and lungs remembering that beta blockers can cause wheezing. You examine her legs for swelling. Her pulse is 70 and her blood pressure is 110/80, both normal. There are no new findings on the

physical examination. You tell Ms. Carr that you need to discuss your findings with your preceptor and that you will mention her request to see the cardiologist. Once again, you explain you will both be back in a few minutes.

You present your findings to your preceptor and discuss referral to a cardiologist. The preceptor agrees that this is a reasonable plan.

On returning to the room, your preceptor tells Ms. Carr that indeed her medicines can make her feel tired. There is further discussion about cardiologist referral and an appointment is made for her for next week. As at the initial visit, you ask if there is anything else she wants to discuss and she says "no." You discuss follow-up in 1 month to review the cardiologist's recommendations. She is satisfied with the plan and repeats it back to you. In the interim she will stay on her current medications as she feels that they are controlling the pain and the fatigue is tolerable.

SOAP Notes

After Ms. Carr leaves, document your findings in the form of a progress note, often called a "SOAP" note. **SOAP** is the acronym for **subjective**, **objective**, **assessment** and **plan**.

- "Subjective" information includes what your patient told you as part of the history. **Symptoms** or "complaints" are examples of subjective information.
- "Objective" information is data you can measure or quantify. Physical findings are an example of objective information and are referred to as **signs**. Test results are also objective information.
- The "assessment" is a statement of the status of the problem. In Ms. Carr's case, her pain is improved but not resolved and she is tolerating her medicines with minimal side effects.
- The "Plan" documents treatment and diagnostic plans. You record that Ms. Carr's medicines will be continued as previously described and new diagnostic plans include a referral to cardiology.

Table 8-4 illustrates an example of a SOAP note. Notice that it is not necessary to use complete sentences in structuring your SOAP notes.

Table 8-4. Example of a SOAP Note (Ms. Carr's Follow-up Visit)

S   Ms. Carr's chest pain is less but she still cannot carry out strenuous tasks.

Hasn't tried any NTG (concerned about headache from it).

Has stopped smoking!

Taking meds regularly but wondering if they're making her feel tired; is willing to continue them as they help the pain. Friend has recently had angioplasty and is doing well. Ms. Carr now agrees to see the cardiologist who helped her friend.

O   Looks well. BP 110/80; P70, regular; Lungs clear. No leg edema.

Heart: S1, S2 normal. Regular rate, no murmurs, rubs or gallops.

Test results: Mammogram normal

Pap normal

Cholesterol—slightly elevated

Hemoccult stools—negative

A   Some symptomatic improvement of anginal pain but still has poor exercise tolerance.

At mild increased risk from slightly elevated cholesterol. Has decreased cardiac risk somewhat by stopping tobacco use.

Patient undecided on estrogen replacement.

P   Refer to cardiologist.

Low cholesterol diet plan given and discussed; will recheck lipids in three months.

Continue ASA and beta blocker.

RTC after cardiology evaluation.*

*RTC is a common abbreviation for "return to clinic." Also, sometimes expressed as "return to office" (RTO), or as "follow-up appointment" (F/U appt).

SUMMARY

We reviewed both an initial visit and a follow-up visit in this chapter. An initial visit may include a traditional medical history and physical examination and is intended to establish a database on your patient. It affords you an opportunity to establish rapport with your patient. A follow-up visit is much shorter and is used to re-assess old problems and discuss

any new problems that have occurred since the last visit. During the next few years you will do both of these types of interviews at various times under the guidance of your preceptors. Feel comfortable to establish appropriate goals with your preceptor and remember that they want to help you. If you are unsure of what to do, always ask. A good working relationship with your preceptor can pave an exciting and smooth pathway to acquiring the knowledge, skills and attitudes necessary to provide excellent patient care.

STUDY QUESTIONS*

1. Patients report many symptoms to you, such as pain, fatigue, and cough. To more fully evaluate these symptoms, always ask all the following questions *except*:
   A. What is the quality and severity of the symptom?
   B. Are there any exacerbating or relieving factors?
   C. What has your family told you about your symptoms?
   D. How long have you had the symptom and how often does it recur?

2. You are working with your mentor in her office for the first time and she tells you to "go see the new patient in exam room 2." You should:
   A. Go into the room and ask the patient why he came to the office.
   B. Ask the mentor to clarify what she means by "seeing" the patient, and then carry out her instructions.
   C. Ask the office nurse what the doctor usually does with her patients.
   D. Tell the patient you don't know what you're supposed to do, but you'll try to "do it right."

3. The History of Present Illness is a very important part of your adult examination. Key aspects of this part of the history include all the following *except*:
   A. It is good to begin with an open-ended question, such as "How would you describe your pain?"
   B. It is often valuable to inquire as to what the patient thinks is the cause of the symptom.
   C. A patient may have more than one "present illness."
   D. This section of the H&P is a good place to record family illnesses since so many medical problems are genetic.

4. Most office visits and hospital daily visits are documented as "SOAP" notes. Which definition is *incorrect*?

* For answers, see page 347.

A. "Subjective" information includes what the patient reports to you about their symptoms.

B. "Objective" information includes physical findings and test results.

C. The "Assessment" section is a list of the patient's diagnosis.

D. The "Plan" may include medications, tests and consultations you are ordering, and patient education services.

5. You are doing a history and physical exam on a 60-year-old man. All of the following items of information are documented correctly *except*:

A. In the Chief Complaint "Patient complains of nausea and occasional vomiting for 2 days."

B. In the Past Medical History "No history of any surgery. Has had well-controlled hypertension for 8 years."

C. In the Social History "Smokes ½ pack per day. No alcohol. Works regularly in insurance office. Wife of 30 years is his only sexual partner."

D. In the Review of Systems "Vomited small quantity of clear liquid material in the ER."

Suggested Reading

DeGowin, R.L.: DeGowin & DeGowin's Diagnostic Examination, 6th Edition, McGraw-Hill, Inc., New York, 1994.

Seidel, H.M, J. Ball, J.E. Dains, G.W. Benedict: Mosby's Guide to Physical Diagnosis, 3rd Edition. Chapter 1, The History and Interviewing Process, pages 1–33, Chapter 19, Putting It All Together, pages 775–804, Chapter 21, Recording Information, pages 828–851, C.V. Mosby, St Louis.

A Patient with Cough

9

Nancy J. Munn

INTRODUCTION

CASE PRESENTATION

A 45-year-old woman comes to the ambulatory care clinic with a complaint of a cough for the past 6 months. In her words: "This cough is worse at night and during cold weather, but I never do bring up anything". She could not relate its onset to any prior upper respiratory tract infection. She denied coughing up blood, shortness of breath, chest tightness, fever, chills, sweats, wheezing or weight loss. "I've never had any lung problems; I do not even have sinus trouble."

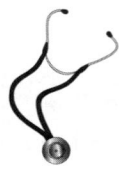

Cough is a common problem of patients treated in ambulatory care clinics; the prevalence of chronic cough is 14–23% of nonsmoking adults. Patients with cough seek treatment because it is an annoyance, or because of fear that a cough means serious underlying disease. Most patients will tolerate brief episodes of cough, but they usually seek medical attention when it persists for weeks to months.

Cough, a normal physiologic mechanism, acts as a defense for the respiratory system to clear secretions and foreign bodies. However, cough seldom occurs in the healthy adult, as clearance of respiratory tract secretions is usually accomplished by other mechanisms. Although a nonspecific symptom, cough often signifies serious respiratory tract disease. Patients respond differently to cough; some patients are aware and disturbed by coughing and others seem to hardly notice it.

> Cough is the fifth most common symptom in outpatient visits.

> Quantifying cough may be difficult depending on the patient's *awareness* of the cough.

DEFINITIONS

Cough: an explosive expiration that acts to protect the lungs from aspiration and to propel secretions and other materials upward through the airways.

Productive cough: a cough which produces purulent or mucoid sputum.

Nonproductive cough: a cough without production of purulent or mucoid sputum, usually because of persistent stimulation of irritant receptors.

Chronic cough: persistent or recurrent cough exceeding 3 weeks' duration.

Hemoptysis: coughing up blood.

Sputum: expectorated or mucopurulent secretion from the air passages.

Dyspnea: difficulty breathing (a subjective symptom); patients usually call this "being short of breath", and physicians often record this symptom by the abbreviation "SOB."

COUGH PATHOPHYSIOLOGY

Mechanics of the Cough Reflex

Cough can be initiated from receptor sites widely disseminated throughout the head, neck, and thorax.

Cough is triggered by stimulation of receptor sites which are widely distributed throughout the head, neck and thorax, including the pharynx, larynx, trachea, carina, major bronchi, lung parenchyma, pleura, esophagus, sinuses, diaphragm, tympanic membranes and pericardium. A variety of stimuli can trigger these receptors including inflammatory, mechanical, thermal, chemical, and neoplastic processes (Table 9-1). When stimulated, afferent impulses travel through the vagus and glossopharyngeal nerves to the cough center in the medulla. From the cough center, efferent impulses travel through the vagus, phrenic and spinal accessory nerves to effector organs (larynx, tracheobronchial tree, diaphragm, expiratory muscles) and cough ensues.

A cough consists of three phases:

- *Inspiratory phase* Cough begins with opening of the glottis with deep inspiration to obtain a high lung volume. The vertical and

Table 9-1.   Stimuli of the Cough Reflex

Category	Specific stimuli
Mechanical	Particulate matter (dust, foreign bodies)
	Compression from tumors/masses
	Tension from atelectasis/pneumonia
Inflammatory	Bacterial or viral bronchitis
(causing edema and	Colds
hyperemia of	Cigarette smoke
respiratory mucosa)	Postnasal drip
	Reflux of gastric acid
Chemical	Irritant gases
	Smoke
	Fumes
	Drugs
Thermal	Hot or cold weather or indoor environment

lateral dimensions of the chest increase as does the caliber of the bronchi.

- *Compressive phase* This phase includes closure of the glottis with active contraction of the expiratory muscles (both thoracic and abdominal) and subsequent increase in intrathoracic pressures.
- *Expiratory phase* During this phase, there is sudden opening of the glottis. Further contraction of the respiratory muscles leads to high intrathoracic pressures (50–100 mmHg or more). Airways become more narrow. There is rapid and forceful expulsion of air carrying particulate matter.

CLINICAL CAUSES OF COUGH

A vast majority of cases of chronic cough prove to be caused by the following four common illnesses which are discussed below:

1. Postnasal drip syndrome
2. Asthma
3. Gastroesophageal reflux disease
4. Chronic bronchitis.

A variety of conditions ranging from benign to extremely serious, and from common to relatively rare, cause the remaining few cases. Table 9-2 includes all causes of cough.

Postnasal drip syndrome is the most common cause of chronic cough in nonsmokers. Patients describe "feeling something dripping down the back of my throat" or complain of having copious nasal discharge and the need to clear their throat all the time. When you examine their throat, you may see secretions in the nasopharynx or oropharynx.

Asthma is the second most common cause of chronic cough and it *may be* the only manifestation of asthma. More typically, patients complain of episodes of shortness of breath or wheezing. Pulmonary function tests may demonstrate obstruction to airflow with reversibility; however, sometimes they are normal in asthma patients. Challenge testing with methacholine or other agents helps in the diagnosis of asthma in the setting of normal pulmonary function tests.

Gastroesophageal reflux disease (GERD) is the third most common reason for chronic cough. In GERD, cough may be generated by aspiration which stimulates tracheobronchial receptors, or in the absence of aspiration, stomach contents may stimulate receptors in the hypopharynx and larynx. Patients with hiatal hernia usually have a history of "heartburn" and coughing worse at night and after meals. Other symptoms of GERD include sour taste in the mouth and regurgitation of food.

The fourth most common cause of chronic cough is **chronic bronchitis**. Patients with chronic bronchitis produce excess mucus and have decreased mucociliary clearance. Dust, fumes, and smoke frequently cause irritation and stimulation of the cough reflex, leading in turn to inflammatory changes in the bronchial mucosa and hypersecretion of mucus. You can diagnose chronic bronchitis by history alone, if the patient reports *a cough which produces sputum daily for at least 3 months of the year for 2 years in a row.*

> The mucosa in the posterior pharynx may have a "cobblestone" appearance in cases of postnasal drip.

> Cough in asthma usually worsens with exposure to cold, dry air, perfumes, scents, or smoke.

COMPLICATIONS OF COUGH

Cough poses a problem to patients not only because its occurrence may represent serious disease, but also because its presence can cause a variety of secondary problems. Table 9-3 outlines several potential complications of cough. Importantly, the longer cough persists and the more forceful it is, the more likely complications will occur.

Table 9-2.   Causes of Cough

Category	Specific cause	Frequency*	Key signs or symptoms/ unique features
Acute and chronic infectious processes	• Viral respiratory infections	Common	• Cough usually transient but may be persistent; presumed due to damage to tracheal lining
	• Bacterial respiratory infections (bronchitis, pneumonia)	Common	• Most common cause of hemoptysis • May follow viral infections • Cough often produces heavy green or yellow sputum
	• Tuberculosis	Uncommon*	• Bloody sputum common • May be due to *M. tuberculosis* or an atypical mycobacterium
	• Mycoses	Rare	• Persistent cough for weeks to months
	• Mycoplasma	Common	• Paroxysmal cough
Environmental irritants	• Smoking	Very common	• The "smoker's cough" improves in 77% of those who quit, more than 50% within 4 weeks
	• Air pollution	Common	• Cough worsens during episodes of increased pollution with smog, sulfur dioxide, nitrous oxide
Airway obstruction	• Asthma	Very common	• Usually patients have wheezing or shortness of breath, but *cough may be the only manifestation*
	• Chronic bronchitis	Very common	• Always a productive cough • Often worsened by dust, fumes, and smoke
	• Foreign body	Uncommon	• Inhaled objects lodge in the airways and cause irritation
Neoplasm	• Inside or outside the bronchi; benign and malignant tumors	Common	• Cough is rarely the *only* symptom of neoplasm

Table 9-2.   Continued

Category	Specific cause	Frequency*	Key signs or symptoms/ unique features
Cardiovascular	• Left-sided congestive heart failure	Common	• The cough of CHF is sometimes relieved by standing up
	• Pulmonary embolism	Uncommon	• Cough frequently produces bloody mucus
	• Mitral stenosis	Uncommon	• Also a cause of bloody sputum
Infiltrative processes	• Pulmonary fibrosis/ interstitial lung disease	Uncommon	• Usually nonproductive cough
	• Sarcoidosis	Rare	• May have associated dyspnea and abnormal chest X-ray
	• Collagen vascular disorders	Rare	• Cough may be a symptom of these disorders but there are almost always other associated findings
ENT disorders	• Postnasal drip	Very common	• Patient feels need to clear the throat frequently
	• Sinusitis	Common	• When acute, causes headaches, facial pressure and tenderness
	• Epistaxis	Common	• Sometimes nose bleed is the true cause of "hemoptysis"
	• Foreign bodies in nose or touching tympanic membrane	Uncommon	• Ear examination in some patients is quite difficult due to the cough induced by irritation of the tympanic membrane
Diaphragmatic or pleural disorders	• Pleural effusion	Common	• May stimulate cough receptors in pleura or cause compression of underlying lung tissue
Psychogenic disorders	• Cough tics or "nervous" habit	Rare	• Nonproductive. Ceases at night. Diagnosis of exclusion. • Can be an attention getter

* Frequency with which this disorder is the cause of a chronic cough.

Table 9-2. Continued

Category	Specific cause	Frequency*	Key signs or symptoms/ unique features
Esophageal disorders	• Gastro-esophageal reflux disease	Very common	• Patients *may* have other symptoms of GERD, such as "heartburn" or sour taste in mouth
Drugs	• ACE inhibitors	Common	• Mechanism unknown, but about 2% of cases of chronic cough are due to these medications
	• Beta-blockers, including Timolol eye drops	Uncommon	• May "unmask" latent asthma
	• Inhaled steroids	Uncommon	• May cause irritant cough

*Tuberculosis must be strongly considered in patients with AIDS or other immuno-compromised states.

ACE, angiotensin converting enzyme.

Cough Syncope

Cough syncope, or loss of consciousness associated with coughing, is a frightening complication. Although generally benign, it may lead to an extensive (and expensive) evaluation.

Cough syncope most often occurs in middle-aged men who are moderately obese and large chested. Patients often have some degree of obstructive lung disease and also may have a history of excess alcohol and tobacco use. Usually cough syncope occurs when the patient is standing; it may develop when the person sits or lies down. No signs of seizure occur, i.e., the patient experiences no aura, incontinence, or convulsive movements, and does not lapse into a postictal state. Generally no sequelae occur after the patient regains consciousness.

The etiology of cough syncope is unknown. Several theories have been formulated. It is likely that at least part of the problem arises from development of positive intrathoracic pressure which decreases

Loss of consciousness in cough syncope occurs within a few seconds of the onset of a paroxysm of (usually) dry cough.

Table 9-3. Complications of Cough

Category	Specific problem	Key signs or symptoms/unique features
Musculoskeletal	Rib fracture	Usually one of the lower ribs involved; no underlying bone pathology necessary for fractures to occur
	Vertebral fracture	Unusual unless patient has osteoporosis or bone tumor
	Rupture of rectus abdominis	May mimic intraabdominal crisis
	Asymptomatic elevation of creatine phosphokinase (CPK)	Can confuse the diagnostic picture in patients with chest pain
Pulmonary	Pneumothorax or pneumomediastinum	May cause sudden chest pain and SOB; subcutaneous emphysema may develop
	Bronchial rupture	Rare, but a serious emergency
	Increased airway irritation	Creates a "vicious cycle" of continuing cough
Cardiovascular	Rupture of veins	Particularly common in subconjunctival, nasal and anal veins
	Dysrhythmias	Especially bradycardia and heart block due to reflex increase in vagal tone with cough
CNS	Headache	Very common
	Cerebral air embolism	Rare, but may be deadly
	Cough syncope	See discussion in text
Miscellaneous	Constitutional symptoms	Insomnia, anxiety, headache, vomiting, anorexia
	Urinary incontinence	Common cause of urine leakage in patients with stress incontinence
	Disruption of surgical wounds	Wound "dehiscence" is a very serious postoperative complication
	Hoarseness	Due to stress on vocal cords from cough
	Social implications	Patients are usually self-conscious; may make significant lifestyle changes because of cough

venous return to the heart and thereby decreases cardiac output. Cerebral hypoperfusion and an increase in cerebrospinal fluid (CSF) pressure follow, and these events contribute to the syncope. Decreased blood pressure and bradycardia, along with a reflex induced loss of peripheral resistance may occur also. A concussive effect of intrathoracic and intraabdominal pressures transmitted to the central nervous system (CNS) may be involved.

HISTORY AND PHYSICAL

Developing the HPI

As always, a thorough history forms the basis to approach a diagnosis. First you need an accurate description of the cough, including the following aspects:

- *Duration*—acute (very recent onset) or chronic (lasting 3 weeks or more)
- *Time of occurrence*—seasonal, day/night, relationship to meals, relationship to change in position
- *Sputum production and character of sputum*—color, consistency, odor, volume
- *Associated symptoms*—dyspnea, hemoptysis, wheezing, chest pain, fever, hoarseness
- *Previous episodes*—history of asthma, heartburn
- *Alleviating and relieving factors*—frequent need to clear throat, change in position
- *Quality or character of cough*—for example, cough of viral infection or cancer-related cough is usually dry; cough of congestive heart failure (CHF), asthma, or food aspiration is often paroxysmal or "spasmodic"; tracheal lesions may cause a "brassy" cough.
- *It is critically important to know the patient's smoking history* and *medications*.

Other Relevant History

Certain other points in the patient's history are especially relevant to evaluating cough. Has the patient been exposed to environmental or occupational hazards, such as dusts or chemicals? Is there a history of

previous upper respiratory infections, especially sinusitis? Does the patient have allergies?

Questions which are part of the Review of Systems may uncover a history of weight loss, fever, GI symptoms, or chest pain. Also, investigate the family history, especially for a history of asthma, tuberculosis, and malignancies.

Physical Examination

The most important aspects of the physical examination are:

- *Vital signs*, especially temperature, pulse, and respiratory rate.
- *ENT examination*
  - Look especially for a cobblestone appearance of the mucosa in the posterior pharynx, or secretions in nose or oropharynx
  - Evaluate for possible sinusitis—sinus tenderness or opacification
  - Examine for wax or foreign body on the tympanic membrane
- *Neck examination*—look for enlarged lymph nodes, tracheal deviation, jugular venous distension
- *Respiratory system*—listen for stridor or wheezes, rhonchi, and rales; examine the respiratory pattern, chest size and expansion.
- *Cardiovascular system*—listen for murmurs, rubs, and gallops. Look for edema.

Ancillary Tests

Laboratory tests

- *CBC*—high total WBC shows evidence of infection; a high eosinophil count supports a diagnosis of allergy
- *Sputum examination*—evaluate character of the sputum and when necessary, do Gram stain, culture for bacteria smears and cultures for acid-fast bacilli (AFB), fungal examination, and cytologic examination.

Imaging

- *Chest X-ray*—the pivotal study in the work-up of a patient with chronic cough. If abnormal, additional evaluation is mandatory.

- *Sinus X-rays*—not necessary for diagnosis of acute sinusitis; quite useful in chronic conditions.
- *Computed tomography (CT) scan of the chest or head*—very often needed to follow up abnormal chest X-rays or sinus films; can demonstrate hiatal hernia and support diagnosis of GERD.

Special Studies

Pulmonary

Pulmonary function tests—often important to evaluate patients for reversible airway obstruction, decreased lung volumes, or altered diffusing capacity

Bronchoscopy—may be a definitive diagnostic test, *but* only done if other tests are inconclusive.

Bronchography—contrast X-ray studies to outline bronchial tree if bronchiectasis suspected. However, it is rarely performed, as high resolution CT scanning also demonstrates bronchiectasis.

Cardiac

Echocardiogram—very important if mitral stenosis or other valve lesions are suspected

Other Special Tests

- *Arterial blood gases*—occasionally useful but not routine
- *Mantoux skin test using purified protein derivative (PPD)*—mandatory if tuberculosis (TB) suspected
- *Upper GI studies or 24 hour (esophageal) pH monitoring*—to evaluate for possible GERD.

CASE RESOLUTION

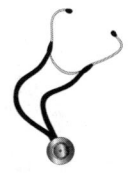

The following discussion illustrates resolution of the Case Presentation using the steps outlined in this chapter, namely a knowledge of diseases, a detailed history and physical examination, and the results of ancillary testing. An assessment and diagnosis can be made and treatment initiated.

A 45-year-old woman was seen in the ambulatory care clinic with a complaint of chronic cough for a 6-month period of time. The cough was nonproductive and more prominent at night and during cold weather. She could not relate its onset to any prior upper respiratory tract infection. She also denied any history of hemoptysis, dyspnea, chest tightness, fever, chills, sweats, wheezing or weight loss. She denied any prior cardiac or pulmonary disease. There was no history of sinusitis or postnasal drip.

At this point, you can organize the historical information. This woman's main complaint is persistent cough, without other associated symptoms.

You complete the patient's past history, family and social histories, and review of systems. You determine that she had a history of eczema as a child and previously smoked one pack of cigarettes per day but only for a 5-year period. She quit smoking entirely 10 years ago. Two sisters have asthma. She takes no medications at this time. Her physical examination was essentially normal including sinuses nontender to percussion, clear lungs and normal cardiac and abdominal examination. She had no evidence of peripheral edema, cyanosis or clubbing.

The woman is previously healthy, but now has a persistent cough, somewhat worse at night and during cold weather. She had eczema and two relatives have asthma. Although she smoked cigarettes previously, it was for a short time only, prior to the development of her current symptoms. She takes no medications that could cause her cough. She does not have signs or symptoms of postnasal drip or sinusitis. At this point, you inform the patient that further testing will be needed to determine the cause of her cough.

A CBC does not show evidence of eosinophilia which would have been consistent with an allergy. A PPD was negative, eliminating prior exposure to TB. Her chest X-ray was normal; it did not show any evidence of infection or tumor. Pulmonary function testing showed normal values. You order a methacholine challenge as an additional test and this shows a decrease in forced expiratory volume in 1 second (FEV_1) of 20%, consistent with a diagnosis of asthma.

You reassure the patient about the diagnosis of asthma and initiate therapy with bronchodilators and inhaled steroids. With therapy, her cough resolves.

SUMMARY

Cough is an important symptom and can signify either minor or serious disease. The cause of cough usually can be determined by a systematic approach to the history, physical examination and laboratory testing. If a specific etiology can be determined, then therapy directed towards it is usually successful. Cough can have multiple causes, which require a multifaceted approach to work-up and treatment.

STUDY QUESTIONS*

1. A 45-year-old man comes to your office complaining of cough. Which of the following aspects of his history is *least* important in assessing possible causes of the cough?
   A. He is employed as a bulldozer operator in road construction.
   B. His uncle has pneumoconiosis.
   C. He smokes one pack of cigarettes per day.
   D. He was diagnosed recently with gastroesophageal reflux disease.

2. You are caring for an 80-year-old man in a nursing home who developed a cough about 2 weeks ago. In addition to a physical examination, you may need to do all the following to evaluate his cough *except*:
   A. Review his medication list
   B. Obtain a chest X-ray
   C. Obtain a complete blood count
   D. Obtain air samples at the nursing home for analysis

3. The typical patient with cough syncope is:
   A. A middle-aged man with mild emphysema
   B. A thin, anxious appearing 28-year-old woman with a history of asthma
   C. An adolescent girl who has tried smoking for the first time
   D. A 70-year-old woman with newly diagnosed tuberculosis

4. The physical finding of "cobblestoning" in the posterior pharyngeal mucosa is most likely associated with which diagnosis?
   A. GERD
   B. Chronic bronchitis
   C. Asthma
   D. Postnasal drip

---

* For answers, see page 347.

5. A forceful cough may result in complications that include all of the following *except*:
    A.   Bruising of the skin
    B.   Cough syncope
    C.   Rib fractures
    D.   Urinary incontinence

Suggested Reading

Bramma, S. & Carras, W.: Chronic cough—diagnosis and treatment. J. Prim Care 12: 2; 1985.

Irwin, R.S., Corrao, W.M. & Pratter, M.R.: Chronic persistent cough in the adult. The spectrum and frequency of causes and successful outcome of specific therapy. Am Rev Respir Dis 123: 413–417; 1981.

Irwin, R.S., Curley, F.J. & French, C.L.: Chronic cough: The spectrum and frequency of causes, key components of the diagnostic evaluation and outcomes of specific therapy. Am Rev Respir Dis 141: 640–647; 1990.

Patrick, H. & Patrick, F.: Chronic cough. Med Cl North Am 79: 361–372; 1995.

Poe, R.H., Harder, R.V., Israel, R.H. *et al*.: Chronic persistent cough: Experience in diagnosis and outcome using an anatomic diagnostic protocol. Chest 95: 723–728; 1989.

A Patient with Acute Low Back Pain

Kevin W. Yingling and Ralph W. Webb

INTRODUCTION

CASE PRESENTATION

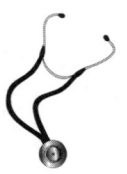

Mrs. R.B., a 62-year-old woman comes to your office with complaint of progressive low back pain for 3 days. "I can't really tell you when or why this pain started, but now its moving down the back of my right leg." She continues, "I've had back pain occasionally in the past, but I've never injured my back, at least I don't think I did, and I didn't do anything to it this time." She had a routine week prior to the onset of pain.

Low back pain ranks as one of the ten most frequent complaints to primary care physicians; approximately 80% of Americans seek relief of back pain at some time in their life. Acute low back pain, defined as pain lasting less than 3 weeks, has a peak incidence between ages 40 and 45. The natural history of acute low back pain is that one-third of patients will be free of pain within 1 week and nearly 90% will be free of pain by 2 months.

Goals of the evaluation of acute low back pain include:

- Identification of the cause of pain by proper use of diagnostic tests
- Alleviation of pain
- Education of the patient about contributing causes and prevention of recurrences.

The primary care physician should be able to make a working diagnosis for most patients with acute low back pain. A properly focused physical examination and judicious use of ancillary tests lead to cost effective care for acute low back pain.

DEFINITIONS

Analgesia:	relief of pain.
Cauda equina syndrome:	symptoms caused by a structure infringing upon the most distal part of the spinal cord and the nerves adjacent to it.
Hyperparathyroidism:	excess production of parathyroid hormone.
Kyphosis:	an exaggeration of the normal upper thoracic spinal curve. When severe, a "hump back" appearance develops.
Neoplasia:	literally means "new growth"; it encompasses all forms of malignancy (primary—at the site of origin; metastatic—having spread from somewhere else).
Nephrolithiasis:	stones in the kidney or urinary tract.
Osteomyelitis:	infection in the bone.
Osteoporosis:	porous or "thin" bones.
Paresthesia:	disturbance of sensation—most often refers to unpleasant tingling sensation or pain secondary to nerve damage.
Sciatica:	pain in the lower back and along the sciatic nerve distribution.
Scoliosis:	a side-to-side curvature in the spine.

CAUSES OF ACUTE LOW BACK PAIN

Several categories of disease may present clinically as acute low back pain. These include:

- mechanical acute low back pain
- osteoporosis with fracture
- neoplastic disease
- infectious disease
- secondary causes (processes not related to the spine or vertebral column which cause back pain) including abdominal aortic aneurysm, hyperparathyroidism, and nephrolithiasis.

Mechanical Low Back Pain

History and physical examination can identify most mechanical causes of low back pain (Table 10-1). While it is tempting to order imaging tests immediately, they offer *little diagnostic value in the initial evaluation* of a patient with low back pain.

Spondylolysis is a defect or break in the continuity of the pars interarticularis in the lamina. It is found in approximately 5% of the general population. When the defect permits one vertebral body to slide forward on its neighbor, then the diagnosis is **spondylolisthesis**.

Spondylolysis is a common radiographic finding, often discovered as a coincidental finding on X-rays of patients who do not have back pain. In patients who have pain related to spondylolysis, it is usually localized in the back; generally, radicular pain does not occur. No specific pharmacologic or surgical intervention is indicated for this finding.

Spinal stenosis is mechanical encroachment upon the spinal cord within the spinal canal or upon nerve roots exiting the foramina. It can produce "pseudoclaudication"—pain in the buttocks and legs that is precipitated by walking and relieved by rest—mimicking claudication due to arterial insufficiency. However, it occurs in patients who do not have circulatory disease. Flexion of the spine, e.g., leaning forward, relieves the pain, while extension of the spine intensifies it.

Ankylosing spondylitis, a rare cause of low back pain, is an inflammatory disease characterized by recurrent back pain, often beginning early in life. There may be a family history of this disease. Other findings include decreased chest expansion and poor spinal flexion. Sometimes the sedimentation rate is elevated. Sacroiliac joint films may show evidence of inflammatory changes early in this disease. Later, spinal X-rays show changes called the "bamboo spine."

Nucleus pulposus herniation, also called "herniated disk" or "slipped disk," commonly causes low back pain. It usually occurs in the third to fourth decade of life, and may be traumatic or degenerative in origin. *The most common level for disk herniation is the L4–5 area, accounting for >95% of cases.* The pain, characterized as a sharp, lancinating sensation originating in the low back, usually radiates to the lateral aspect of the leg past the knee.

Table 10-1. Mechanical Causes of Acute Low Back Pain

Diagnosis	Causes	Key signs and symptoms/ unique features
Spondylolysis	Defect in pars inter-articularis of vetebral body	No radicular pain Common X-ray finding even in absence of back pain
Spondylolisthesis	Displacement of one vetebral body upon another due to spondylolysis	Patient usually has exagger-ated lumbar curve and may have skin dimple at site of defect
Spinal stenosis	Narrowed spinal canal, usually caused by osteoarthritic changes	Buttock and leg pain upon walking relieved by sitting down (pseudoclaudication). Leaning forward usually relieves pain
Herniated nucleus pulposus	Degenerative or traumatic damage to an intervertebral disk, allowing pressure on nerve roots or cord by the extruded disk	Usually patient has radicular pain, sharp in nature, start-ing in back and radiating to lateral aspect of the involved leg

Syndromes associated with muscle or joint injury

Lumbosacral strain	Usually caused by a twisting injury or by repetitive lifting or bending	Paravertebral muscle spasm is prominent. Usually lag time of hours to days between the injury and the onset of pain
Pyriformis syndrome	Usually caused by a fall directly on the buttocks	Pyriformis muscle spasm with resulting sciatic nerve irritation
Facet joint arthropathy	Irritation of a facet joint in the spinal column	Pelvic crest pain
Quadratus lumborum syndrome	Direct injury to quadratus lumborum muscle	Worse with bending to side away from pain Pressure on 12th rib reproduces the pain

Trauma causes several kinds of mechanical low back pain, including lumbar strain, pyriformis syndrome, facet arthropathy, and quadratus lumborum syndrome.

The most common trauma-induced mechanical low back pain is **lumbosacral strain** caused by an acute twisting injury or by significant overuse for a short period of time. Such injury causes stretching or partial tears of paravertebral muscles, lumbar fascia, and interspinous ligaments. Pain may be felt in the involved paravertebral muscles and sometimes it radiates upward or into the buttock, but usually *not* into the leg, as occurs in sciatica. The straight leg raising test is negative.

The back or buttock pain of **pyriformis syndrome** radiates to the legs. It is usually caused by a fall directly on the buttocks. The pyriformis muscle goes into spasm and irritates the sciatic nerve.

Irritation of a facet joint causes pelvic crest pain, which occasionally radiates to the groin area. This process is caused by irritation to the iliohypogastric and the ilioinguinal nerve. Iliac crest tenderness is unusual in any other cause of low back pain.

The **quadratus lumborum syndrome** is characterized by worsening of pain when the patient bends to the side, away from the side of pain. It is usually caused by direct injury to the quadratus lumborum muscle. As the quadratus lumborum muscle extends from the ilium to the floating twelfth rib, pressure on this rib will produce pain.

Osteoporosis with Fracture

Osteoporosis, a common bone disease, most often occurs in women over the age of 65. However, it can occur at any age and in men. Steroid medications, smoking, and certain genetic factors increase the risk of developing osteoporosis.

Patients usually manifest no symptoms until a fracture occurs, after a seemingly trivial injury. Then the patient experiences severe pain. A plain X-ray of the spine often shows a compression fracture and on examination you can detect acute localized tenderness of the spine. Pain relief is the primary goal of treatment.

Primary prevention of osteoporosis is the goal of the primary care provider. It is estimated that a primary care physician with an average size practice will treat a dozen patients in any given week who have osteoporosis. Preventive interventions including calcium, vitamin D, and estrogen supplementation can be effective in limiting the disability of osteoporosis in postmenopausal women.

Table 10-2. Imaging Procedures Sometimes Useful in Evaluating Back Pain

Procedure	When the procedure is useful
Spinal X-rays ("plain films")	Adds important information in systemic illness, patients with risk of infection or prior malignancy, patients with serious injuries, and in elderly persons; not needed in every case
Bone scans	Tumors or infection suspected
Myelograms	Confirming suspicion of herniated disk, tumors, or nerve root compression prior to surgery
MRI	Define both soft tissue and bony lesions
CT scans	Define bony lesions
EMG/NCV	Nerve root injuries such as from herniated disks

Neoplasia—Metastatic or Primary

Back pain is occasionally the first symptom of cancer; other systemic signs such as weight loss may or may not occur. Usually cancers in the back are "metastatic." The primary tumor often arises in the breast, prostate, or colon, then spreads to the spinal bones or epidural area. The most common *primary* neoplasm of the spine is multiple myeloma, which usually involves other bony sites as well.

With cancer in the spinal column, the greatest risk is that impingement upon or infiltration of the spinal cord may occur, with the subsequent development of paralysis and other neurologic deficits.

A "sensory level" is a neurologic finding in which a patient has altered sensation in the entire body distal to an identifiable spinal cord level.

When back pain and neurologic deficits coexist, emergency evaluation and intervention are necessary. Such neurologic deficits as muscle weakness, paresthesias, a "sensory level," or acute urinary retention must be addressed immediately. *A sensory deficit at a specific dermatome level is a highly suggestive finding of acute spinal cord compression.* A true medical emergency, this finding requires emergent diagnostic imaging and pharmacologic and surgical intervention.

Infections

Various infections can localize to vertebral bone, usually in the lumbosacral area. Intervertebral disks can become infected also, and most seriously, infection may localize in the epidural space. Certain patient

populations are more susceptible, especially diabetics and the elderly, and alcoholics and intravenous (i.v.) drug abusers.

Patients who present with back pain and fever must be considered to have an infection until proven otherwise. Physical examination identifies local tenderness and sometimes skin erythema at the site of involvement. The infecting organisms can be bacterial, commonly *Staphylococcus aureus* or *Mycobacterium tuberculosis,* or, less commonly, fungal. Bone scans may help in the evaluation of such patients.

Other Secondary Causes of Acute Low Back Pain

Disease processes unrelated to the back can cause back pain. A thorough history and physical examination are necessary to evaluate these diseases.

Abdominal aortic aneurysm is the most critical of these diseases. It is an abnormal dilatation of the aorta, usually occurring below the renal arteries. It is more common in patients older than age 50 who are smokers and who have coronary artery disease. Physical examination may reveal an abdominal bruit and a pulsatile mass, and absent or very diminished lower extremity pulses. The case fatality rate in ruptured aneurysm is nearly 100%.

Nephrolithiasis, or stones within the upper urinary tract, can cause back pain, often colicky in nature. Gentle percussion of the flank region elicits pain; occasionally the pain will radiate into the groin or testicles. You must do a urinalysis to look for hematuria.

The mnemonic for hyperparathyroidism is "bones, moans, groans, and stones," representing the clinical features of bone pain, depression, abdominal pain and kidney stones.

Hyperparathyroidism, a rare cause of low back pain, is usually insidious in onset and associated with diffuse bone pain. Elevated blood pressure and hypercalcemia commonly occur.

HISTORY AND PHYSICAL EXAMINATION

Developing the HPI

As you must differentiate acute from chronic low back pain, it is critical to elicit a history along the following lines:

The combination of saddle anesthesia, progressive motor weakness in the lower extremities, and sphincter dysfunction are diagnostic of the "cauda equina syndrome."

The sphincter dysfunction of spinal cord compression is usually manifested as urinary retention.

- Details of the onset of the pain, e.g., abrupt, insidious
- The quality of the pain, e.g., dull,, sharp, stabbing
- Location of the pain
- Whether the pain is constant or intermittent
- Whether it radiates to the thighs or knees
- What time of the day is the pain worse
- What improves or worsens the pain, e.g., lying down, standing up, bending over
- Whether the patient recognizes a previous injury
- Whether systemic symptoms are present, e.g., fever or weight loss, or if there has been any recent infection disease occurred.

Ask specifically, and in detail, about neurologic symptoms including paresthesias, such as numbness, tingling, or burning sensation, loss of motor function in the lower extremities, or the presence of sphincter dysfunction.

Age and gender also provide clues as to the etiology of back pain. Some conditions, such as spinal stenosis, osteoporotic vertebral fracture, and metastatic and primary tumors, most often occur in older age groups. On the other hand, spondyloarthropathies, such as ankylosing spondylitis, generally occur in younger persons. Lumbosacral strain or osteoarthritis commonly cause back pain in all age groups. Women are more likely to develop osteoporosis, while men more likely develop ankylosing spondylitis.

Other Relevant History

Other historical data can contribute to defining back pain. A history of malignancy, arthritis, or use of medications that affect bone structure increases your suspicion of fracture or metastatic disease. Family history may give clues to osteoporosis, spinal stenosis, or other familial disorders.

Important data from the social history include cigarette smoking, consumption of alcohol, use of recreational drugs, and occupation. For example, if a patient has a history of intravenous drug use, the possibility of an underlying infection should be strongly considered.

Physical Examination

Your focused examination in a patient with low back pain should include assessment of anatomy, function, and neurologic status.

- Observe the **contour of the spine**. Look for scoliosis, loss of the normal lumbar curvature, and for kyphosis.
- Evaluate the appearance of the **pelvis**. Assess for pelvic tilt caused by a leg length discrepancy.
- Look for **swelling** or **erythema**. While infection of a vertebral body or disk is relatively rare, it may result in a palpable swelling or warmth of the affected area.
- Lumbar strain causes **tenderness** in the **paravertebral muscles**, and a spinal fracture may cause **point tenderness over the vertebral body itself**.
- You must check the **range of motion of the lumbar spine** in all patients complaining of lower back pain.

The "**Schober maneuver**" assesses forward flexion; perform this by marking the area overlying the fifth lumbar vertebra with a dot of ink (this position correlates with the level of the superior aspect of the posterior iliac crest). Measure 10 cm above this point and make another mark. Then have the patient bend as far forward as possible without bending the knees. The distance between the two marks should increase to at least 15 cm.

Decreased lumbar mobility can be evaluated also by checking lateral movement and hyperextension, but these movements are more difficult to measure objectively than is forward flexion. If you elicit pain with any of these maneuvers, spinal stenosis should be considered.

The neurologic examination is critical in the assessment of low back pain. Examine the patient's gait, strength, sensation, and reflexes.

Muscle weakness is the most reliable indicator of nerve compression. Sensory changes can be affected by several factors including patient fatigue and emotional state, rendering them less useful. Similarly, reflex changes may be affected by *prior* nerve compression; sometimes a loss of reflex may persist even if sensory and motor function recover from a previous insult. In older patients, the ankle reflexes are frequently absent as a normal finding. However, *acute* bilateral loss of lower extremity reflexes may represent impingement of the cauda equina.

The **straight leg raising test** is especially important in evaluating back pain. In this test, have your patient in the supine position on the examination table; then lift each leg, flexing at the hip as far as possible until pain occurs. If *sciatica-type* pain is produced, the test is "positive." It is *not* positive when the patient complains of only back discomfort, or of the pulling of tight hamstrings.

Lumbar nerve root functions include:

L2 hip flexion
    hip adduction

L3 hip abduction
    knee extension
    (knee jerk reflex)

L4 knee extension
    foot dorsiflexion
    foot inversion
    (knee jerk reflex)

L5 hip extension
    hip abduction
    knee flexion
    foot dorsiflexion
    (posterior tibial reflex)

S1 knee flexion
    foot plantar flexion
    foor eversion
    (ankle jerk reflex)

If you suspect that the patient's low back pain may be *referred* pain from a visceral process, then examine the abdomen, rectum, and genito-urinary organs.

If you suspect that a patient's symptoms are vascular in origin, you must examine the peripheral vasculature. Assess the pressure and equality of the femoral and more distal pulses of the lower extremities, and check for the presence of a pulsatile mass in the abdomen that might indicate an aneurysm.

Ancillary Investigations

Usually your clinical examination alone provides sufficient information to appropriately manage your patient with acute low back pain. Extensive ancillary investigations are seldom needed because:

- Most patients with acute mechanical low back pain do not have abnormalities in a single identifiable anatomic structure which can be proven to be the source of pain.
- Commonly available imaging techniques do not add much to the clinician's decision making process and do not change the patient's outcome. In fact, these tests will yield "abnormal" results in otherwise asymptomatic and healthy individuals (false positive findings).

At times you *will* need to do additional tests. Reasons to obtain X-rays or other tests include:

- The presence of a "red flag" in the history or the physical examination.
- Lack of resolution of complaints after an adequate period of conservative management, usually 4 to 8 weeks.

When indicated, some of the useful tests are (see also Table 10-2):

Spinal X-rays
Plain radiographs of the spine may sometimes be helpful. Criteria for obtaining plain films include:

- systemic illness
- neurologic deficits
- risks for infection (such as patients with alcohol or drug abuse)
- prior malignancy

"Red flags" indicating a need for furthur testing include:
- history of trauma
- history of malignancy
- constitutional complaints such as weight loss or fever
- neurologic signs such as paresthesias, motor deficits, bowel or bladder dysfunction
- abnormal laboratory tests such as low hemoglobin, high ESR, or hematuria

- significant trauma
- older age.

Bone scans

Radionuclide scintigraphy ("bone scanning") uses a radioactive isotope that is taken up by osteoblasts to detect increased bone turnover. It cannot distinguish between mechanical and nonmechanical lesions, so its use in the assessment of back symptoms should be selective, reserved for evaluation of suspected tumors or infection.

CT scan

Computed tomography (CT) scanning can identify many processes, such as sacroiliitis, before they appear on plain radiographs. Bony structures are best visualized by CT, and mechanical abnormalities such as spinal canal narrowing or neuroforaminal encroachment are usually demonstrated very well. Soft tissues *do not* show up as well on the CT as on magnetic resonance imaging (MRI), and intradural lesions require intrathecal contrast to be visualized.

Myelography

Myelography requires the injection of contrast media into the spinal column and has a number of potential drawbacks; it may cause headache or back pain, and there is a small risk of infection. Myelography can augment CT scanning to improve diagnostic accuracy; however, it should be used as a preoperative confirmatory assessment for suspected herniated disks, tumors, or compressed nerve roots.

MRI

MRI has many advantages over other imaging techniques, including the ability to visualize the entire spine in multiple planes, as well as to define soft tissue and bony structures *without* the injection of contrast. MRI is probably the single most useful modality for lumbar spine imaging, but its relatively high cost and lack of general availability limit its use.

MRI is especially useful for identifying spinal cord tumors, vascular abnormalities, infections of the bone and disks, occult fractures, and disk herniation.

Electromyograms (EMG)

Electrodiagnostic studies evaluate the electrical activity of muscle fibers at rest and during contraction. EMG will identify partially denervated muscle resulting from disc herniation. EMG abnormalities may not be apparent for about two to four weeks after the initial nerve root injury.

Nerve conduction velocities (NCV)

NCV tests can evaluate motor, somotosensory and sensorimotor nerve pathways. They differentiate purely superficial sensory abnormalities from radiculopathies.

Clinical Laboratory Testing

In most cases of low back pain, laboratory testing is not required. In some patients, e.g., the elderly, persons who have constitutional symptoms, or those who have failed conservative therapy, an erythrocyte sedimentation rate (ESR) and complete blood count (CBC) are useful. An elevated ESR suggests systemic inflammation. Abnormalities of the blood count, including the white blood cell count, hematocrit, and platelet count also indicate inflammatory disorders such as infection or neoplasm.

Depending on the patient's presentation, other laboratory studies *may* be needed. A urinalysis reveals hematuria in a patient with nephrolithiasis, and abnormalities of serum alkaline phosphatase and calcium suggest diffuse bone disease. An elevated prostate specific antigen is an indicator of prostate cancer.

CASE RESOLUTION

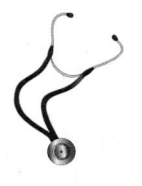

Mrs. R.B., a 62-year-old woman comes to your office with a complaint of progressive low back pain for 3 days. "I can't really tell you when or why this pain started, but now its moving down the back of my right leg." She continues, "I've had back pain occasionally in the past, but I've never injured my back, at least I don't think I did, and I didn't do anything to it this time." She had a routine week prior to the onset of pain.

This patient has come in for evaluation of a very common complaint, low back pain. You will need additional history.

She denied weakness of her legs. She was able to complete routine activities until this change occurred. Now she has difficulty arising from bed or chair without severe pain. She noted movement of pain down the back of her leg to the lateral distal calf. Physical examination revealed a woman in mild distress sitting with her right leg bent, flexed toward her chest. Her back is normal, without scoliosis. Percussion fails to elicit costovertebral angle tenderness, but mild pain to palpation over the right sciatic notch is noted.

Lower extremity deep tendon reflexes and sensation are intact. Dorsiflexion of foot is normal. Dorsiflexion of the right great toe is 4/5. Rectal examination is normal, as is skin sensation in that region. Straight leg raising on the right reproduced the radiating leg pain, to the level of the right lateral malleolus.

Strength is usually graded on a scale of 1 to 5/5 with "5/5" being normal strength.

This 62-year-old patient may be diagnosed with right L5 nerve compression. Since the only finding of nerve root compression was slight weakness in the right great toe, the patient was treated conservatively. No radiographic tests were ordered. The patient was advised to rest in bed for 24 hours and carry on only essential activities. She was prescribed a moderate dose of ibuprofen. Narcotic analgesics and muscle relaxants were avoided. She was encouraged to use local heat and she was given a regimen of low impact exercises for the low back and legs.

The patient was told that if her symptoms should progress, e.g. weakness of the great toe, dragging of the foot, decreased sensation of the leg, change in bowel or bladder function, then she should report for immediate re-evaluation.

The patient's pain gradually improved over the next week and by 2 weeks she had returned to her baseline functional status. On follow-up appointment, her pain had resolved and her examination was entirely normal. She was advised of the need for conditioning through progressive low back exercises to strengthen the back musculature, and on proper lifting and standing techniques to avoid irritation of her nerve roots or sciatic nerve.

SUMMARY

In most patients with acute low back pain, the focused history and physical examination will differentiate those patients who require additional testing from the patients who have nonspecific "mechanical" back pain. The latter group of patients does not require additional testing for at least 4 to 6 weeks, as the majority of these patients will have spontaneous resolution of symptoms regardless of treatment.

Patient education is paramount to reinforce the benign nature of back pain symptoms and to reassure the patient that complete recovery should be expected. Minimize the use of bed rest (no more than one to two days) and judiciously restrict usual activity. Increase mobilization as tolerated.

Because many cases of nonspecific back pain are related to relative deconditioning, progressive low back exercises to strengthen the back musculature may help

Occasionally, spinal manipulation or deep massage is employed early on in cases of pain limited to the lower back without leg symptoms.

prevent recurrences. Local heat *or* ice application, with or without topical salicylate preparations, also may enhance pain relief. Other physical therapy modalities are reserved for patients who have symptoms persisting more than one month. These other modalities include nerve stimulation units, trigger point or epidural injections, back traction, and back supports. The utility of some of these modalities is questionable.

Pharmacologic management can offer additional symptom relief. Acetaminophen is effective and safe in almost all patients, and it should be the first line medication. Aspirin and nonsteroidal antiinflammatory drugs (NSAIDs), such as ibuprofen or naproxen, are effective analgesics, but pose a risk of GI toxicity. Most NSAIDs cost more than acetaminophen. Opioid or narcotic analgesics should be employed *with great caution*. Muscle relaxants provide marginal benefit, and, like opiate analgesics, can result in undesirable cognitive or behavioral effects.

STUDY QUESTIONS*

1. All of the following are true *except*:
   A. Low back pain is a very common complaint to primary care physicians.
   B. The peak incidence of low back pain is in midlife.
   C. Most patients have persistent back pain symptoms, lasting more than 2 months.
   D. Primary care physicians should be able to establish a working diagnosis for the majority of patients with low back pain.

2. Which of the following statements is true regarding mechanical low back pain:
   A. Often imaging tests are helpful in the initial evaluation of the patient with low back pain.
   B. Spondylolysis is a common finding, seen in more than 50% of the general population.
   C. Proper history and physical examination will identify mechanical causes of low back pain in most cases.
   D. Bamboo spine and elevated sedimentation rates are common findings with spinal stenosis.

3. Which of the following statements is true:
   A. Saddle anesthesia, progressive motor loss in the lower extremities, and sphincter dysfunction are diagnostic of spinal stenosis.

---

* For answers, see page 347.

    B.   Ankylosing spondylitis is common in women.

    C.   Pyriformis syndrome is associated with pain which is worse upon bending side to side and with pressure on the 12th rib.

    D.   The pain associated with herniated nucleus pulposus is radicular, sharp in nature, and often extends down the lateral aspect of the involved leg.

4.   The following physical examination must be done in every patient with low back pain except:

    A.   Examination of the contour of the spine.

    B.   Observation for swelling or erythema.

    C.   Evaluation of the range of motion of the spine.

    D.   Examination of the peripheral vasculature.

Suggested Reading

Boyd, R.J. Evaluation of Back Pain, in Primary Care Medicine: Office Evaluation and Management of the Adult Patient, 3rd Edition, edited by A.H. Goroll, L.A. May, and A.G. Mulley, Jr. J.B. Lippincott Co., Philadelphia, 1995, pp. 742–751.

DeGowin, R.L. Diagnostic Examination, 6th edn., McGraw Hill Inc., New York, 1994, pp. 703–713.

A Patient with
Chest Pain

**Paulette S. Wehner, Shirley M. Neitch, and
Kevin W. Yingling**

INTRODUCTION

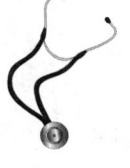

CASE PRESENTATION

Mr. C.J., a 55-year-old man, is brought to your office by his wife because of "severe and steady chest pain" for about 15 or 20 minutes earlier today. Both the patient and his wife report that he had brief chest pains several times in the past 2 or 3 months while working in the yard, but today the pain lasted more than 15 minutes and it was accompanied by indigestion.

Today, many public initiatives encourage patients who experience chest pain to see their doctor immediately. However, often the patient does so only after recurrent or prolonged episodes of pain, or at the insistence of a family member. Regardless of the patient's response to chest pain, you must promptly and aggressively evaluate the patient to identify the cause of their pain and when the problem is heart disease, to treat quickly to prevent or minimize cardiac injury.

Chest pain is categorized into three diagnostic groups defined by the quality of the pain. They include:

- angina (cardiac chest pain)
- atypical chest pain (chest pain believed to be angina but without typical features)
- noncardiac chest pain.

Using the features of the chest pain as the patient describes them and the age of the patient, you can assess the probability that atherosclerotic coronary artery disease is the etiology of their chest pain. Initially defin-

ing the patient's chest pain in this manner is critical to appropriate diagnostic and therapeutic intervention. For example, the patient who has an acute myocardial infarction may present with a clinical picture somewhat resembling a patient who has a duodenal ulcer, but needs very different treatment. The administration of a thrombolytic agent ("clot buster") to a patient with an acute myocardial infarction can be life-saving, but to do so to a patient with duodenal ulcer could be catastrophic.

After your initial assessment of the pain as cardiac or noncardiac in origin, you will need to further categorize your patient's chest pain as to which of five organ systems is involved. Ultimately a thorough history and physical examination and appropriate diagnostic testing will lead to a specific diagnosis.

The main categories of chest pain are:

- Cardiac diseases
- Gastrointestinal diseases
- Musculoskeletal diseases
- Pulmonary diseases
- Psychiatric disorders.

Each organ system presents unique diagnostic and therapeutic challenges. Nonetheless, most primary care physicians will make a working diagnosis and initiate proper interventions in a timely manner. In selected instances, the primary care physician will need to refer a particularly complicated patient to an appropriate specialist for consultation.

DEFINITIONS

Achalasia:	condition in which the lower esophageal sphincter does not relax to allow normal flow of food into the stomach. The esophagus usually dilates above the obstruction.
Atalectasis:	compressed lung tissue with collapsed alveolar air spaces.
Bruit:	sound produced by disturbance in laminar blood flow through an artery.
Cardiac enzymes:	proteins which are normal components of cardiac tissue. These are released into the circulation when heart tissue is damaged. The main cardiac enzymes are the "MB" fraction of crea-

	tine kinase or CK (also called creatine phosphokinase or CPK), LDH (lactate dehydrogenase), myoglobin, and troponin I.
Dissection:	in reference to the aorta, dissection occurs when the intimal layer of the vessel splits apart from the deeper muscle layers and blood flows into and tears apart the layers.
Ejection fraction:	the amount of blood expelled from the ventricular cavity when the heart contracts in systole.
Infarction:	death of tissue caused by cessation of blood flow.
Thrombolytic agent:	a drug given to dissolve a blood clot.

CATEGORIES OF DISEASES CAUSING CHEST PAIN

Cardiac Diseases

Stable angina

Angina can present as jaw pain and may be mistaken for a toothache.

Angina or anginal syndrome, is a clinical diagnosis of chest pain of cardiac origin. It is defined as retrosternal, pressure-type chest pain brought on by exertion and relieved by rest or the administration of nitroglycerin. It often radiates to and down the left arm, or to the jaw or neck. Physical activity and emotional stress can bring on anginal pain. Usually the patient knows how much activity they can tolerate before the pain predictably begins. ("It only hurts if I walk more than one block," or "I have discomfort every time I sweep my porch.")

Unstable angina

Angina or even acute MI can occur *without* the classic pain pattern occurring. "Silent MI" is especially common in diabetics and in the elderly.

Unstable angina, a symptom of acute life-threatening cardiac disease, exhibits a characteristic *pattern* of chest pain. Unstable angina is defined as

- pain of anginal quality occurring *at rest*
- pain of anginal quality occurring with *increased frequency*
- pain of anginal quality that *has changed from its previous pattern*.

Because about 15% of patients with unstable angina will develop an acute myocardial infarction (MI) soon after their pain begins, it is important to identify these patients promptly. Once you diagnose

unstable angina, you must hospitalize the patient and begin a specific therapeutic drug regimen designed to prevent acute MI, or to limit cardiac injury if an acute MI has occurred.

Acute myocardial infarction

Acute MI classically presents as crushing or squeezing mid-retrosternal chest pain or heaviness, associated with sweating, shortness of breath and often nausea. The pain may also involve the arms or jaws, especially on the left side. Not every patient manifests all of these symptoms at the same time. Some patients may have additional symptoms, such as frequent belching or palpitations. Patients experiencing acute myocardial infarction require emergent and aggressive intervention.

The diagnosis of acute MI depends upon meeting two of the following three criteria:

- Consistent history
- Diagnostic electrocardiographic (EKG) changes
- Confirmatory laboratory tests (i.e., "positive cardiac enzymes").

Up to 8% of patients presenting to the physician for evaluation of chest pain will be inappropriately discharged to home even though they have sustained an acute myocardial infarction. These missed MIs are associated with high short-term morbidity or even death. They also cause major medicolegal burdens for the physician. Litigation for missed MI accounts for the largest financial loss category in medical malpractice.

> The sensitivity of physician evaluations in predicting myocardial infarction is approximately 85%, whereas the specificity is only about 70%.

Pericarditis

Acute chest pain can be caused by pericarditis or inflammation of the fibrous tissue encasing the heart. Several unique features characterize the pain of pericarditis:

- it is usually continuous
- it is not relieved by anti-anginal medications such as nitroglycerin
- it is often enhanced by movement
- it may be worsened when the patient sits up.

The hallmark of pericarditis on the physical examination is a **pericardial friction rub**. A rub sounds similar to the sound made by the friction of leather when one sits on a new saddle. Pericarditis is usually caused by a viral infection, but may be associated with other diseases, such as renal failure or metastatic cancer.

> A patient suffering from pericarditis tends to sit very still, as movement worsens the pain.

Aortic dissection

Aortic dissection, a life-threatening event, causes severe pain described as tearing or shearing, with radiation towards the arms. It requires emergency surgical intervention. The chest X-ray often demonstrates a widening of the mediastinum (the central structures of the chest).

Gastrointestinal Causes of Chest Pain

Esophagitis/esophageal dysmotility

Candida (a yeast) and CMV (cytomegalovirus) are common opportunistic infections of immunosuppressed patients.

Pain of esophageal spasm may be relieved by nitroglycerin.

The most common source of chest pain of gastrointestinal etiology is **esophagitis** or inflammation of the esophagus caused by reflux of acid from the stomach. Patients with esophagitis usually have indigestion and heartburn symptoms. Esophagitis can be due to infection, especially in patients with AIDS who suffer candidal or CMV esophagitis.

Disorders of esophageal motility also cause chest pain; these include esophageal spasm and achalasia. Esophageal spasm causes sudden inability to swallow food or liquids. Achalasia causes mild pain or fullness while the patient is eating; later there is regurgitation of undigested food.

Gastric or duodenal ulcer

Patients with peptic ulcers often say their pain is in the chest. When asked to point to the area of pain, usually they indicate the epigastric or lower retrosternal area. Frequently of a "burning" quality, their pain is often relieved with eating and returns quickly after they stop eating.

Acute cholecystitis

The pain of gallbladder inflammation sometimes mimics angina, which complicates its recognition. Typically, it begins in the right upper quadrant of the abdomen and radiates to the right shoulder or between the scapulae. Nausea and a low grade fever accompany this pain.

The pain of pancreatitis is improved when the patient folds his knees toward him and leans forward.

Pancreatitis

The pain of pancreatitis is usually in the abdomen but it may radiate to the lower chest or back. Nausea, vomiting, and fever are common. Inflammation of the pancreas may be acute or chronic. Its causes are

varied, and include excessive alcohol intake, hypertriglyceridemia, infection, and gallstones. Very severe hemorrhagic pancreatitis may present with two signs rarely seen in any other condition: Cullen's sign (blue area around umbilicus) and Turner's sign (discoloration of the patient's flanks).

Pulmonary Causes of Chest Pain

Vague, poorly localized chest pain occurs in patients with chronic obstructive pulmonary disease, asthma, or pulmonary hypertension. It is often described as "tightness" in the chest, especially with asthma. When lung cancers are located deep in the lung tissue without involving the pleural surface, they cause a dull ache or a "full" sensation.

Pain of pleural irritation differs significantly from this tightness or dull ache. Pleural pain is severe and sharp, and worsened by deep breathing or other movements of the chest wall. It occurs in several conditions, including:

- *Pleurisy*—infection or inflammation of the pleura
- *Pneumothorax*—a "collapsed lung"
- *Pulmonary embolism*—a blood clot in the pulmonary circulation. Emboli cause pleuritic chest pain when they have been present long enough to infarct lung tissue
- *Pneumonia*—infection in the air spaces, which irritates adjacent pleural tissue
- *Lung cancers*—when they involve the pleural surfaces.

Musculoskeletal Causes of Chest Pain

Musculoskeletal disorders, a very common cause of chest pain, should be readily distinguishable from angina or gastrointestinal problems (but they are not always!).

Costochondritis, inflammation of the costochondral junction, is very painful. You can elicit the pain by palpating along the edge of the sternum or along the ribs. Deep inspiration, which moves the inflamed joints, also exacerbates the pain of costochondritis.

Strain of the intercostal muscles can be caused by severe coughing, injury, or exercise. As with any muscle strain, there may be a lag of a few hours or days before pain appears and peaks; then it gradually resolves

Rib fractures are most commonly secondary to trauma but may occur with other problems such as metastatic tumors or osteoporosis. Occasionally, a rib fracture may occur spontaneously from a very heavy cough.

over time. The pain of intercostal muscle strain is, like pleuritic pain, worse with deep inspiration and exacerbated by movement.

An often overlooked source of chest pain is rib fracture. The pain is worse with inspiration, and it becomes quite severe when you palpate the area over the fracture. Complications of rib fracture include pneumonia and atelectasis; these occur because the patient finds it too painful to breathe deeply or to cough when they should to clear pulmonary secretions.

Arthritic changes in the cervical spine (cervical spondylosis) cause neck, upper chest, and arm pain which may be very similar to anginal pain. An episode of arthritic pain lasts longer than an anginal attack, and it does not improve with nitroglycerin.

Psychiatric Disorders

"Somatization," defined as "converting anxiety into physical symptoms," is common. Very often, chest pain is the physical symptom experienced by the patient. Somatization occurs commonly in anxiety disorders particularly panic attacks, and in depression.

Considerable clinical skill is required with patients who exhibit somatization. You must be careful to exclude physical disease. However, when the initial evaluation does not suggest *any* physical disease, you must resist the temptation to order every conceivable test to "rule out" every possible disorder. Not only is it unnecessary to utilize resources in this way, but often the patient's anxiety intensifies with each additional test you order. Patients seem to think, "I have such a bad problem the doctor can't even find out what it is."

There is a second important aspect of the psychiatric dimension of chest pain. Patients who *do* have serious medical problems need your clinical skills to help them to cope with their problems without excess fear. We may inadvertently contribute to a patient becoming a "cardiac cripple", i.e., excessively disabled by a minimal heart problem, if we overreact to every minor new symptom or if we overly restrict their activity.

HISTORY AND PHYSICAL EXAMINATION

Developing the HPI

Since chest pain is caused by very serious medical problems, a rapid and accurate assessment of a patient with this complaint is critical.

The most important questions about the pain itself are:

- What is the quality of the pain? (stabbing, pressure-like, tingling, squeezing, etc.)
- What is the degree of pain? (e.g., "On a scale of 1–10, how bad is this pain?")
- Where is the pain?
- Does the pain get worse when you breathe deeply?
- Do you have any other symptom? (such as shortness of breath or nausea)
- Have you tried anything to relieve the pain? (rest, position change, medication)

In evaluation of chest pain, *certain aspects of the past history are important to the present illness:*

- Does the patient have any known cardiac disease, especially coronary artery disease?
- If so, is the pain similar to what the patient experienced before?
- Does the patient have hypertension?

And always, inquire about the presence of the main *risk factors for coronary atherosclerosis*:

- Smoking
- Hyperlipidemia
- Diabetes mellitus
- Family history of atherosclerosis (especially if it occurred at younger ages)
- Advancing age
- Estrogen deficiency in women (due to hysterectomy or menopause)

Relevant Other History

You will want to ask the patient about their past history and do a review of systems for symptoms related to noncardiac causes of chest pain. For example:

- Does the patient a past history of anxiety?
- Does the patient have any abdominal pain accompanying their chest pain?
- Has the patient noticed any bright red or dark blood in their stool or have they vomited any blood?
- Has the patient had any cough or shortness of breath?

Physical Examination

If the patient is stable and pain-free at the time of your examination, you should do a thorough and systematic examination. On the other hand, *if the patient is experiencing pain at the time of your visit*, concentrate on the following aspects of the physical examination:

- Vital signs: **blood pressure**, respiratory rate, temperature and **pulse rate** and **rhythm**
- Cardiac examination
  - ▸ Inspect the chest wall for heaves or lifts
  - ▸ Palpate for the point of maximum impulse, thrills, rate, and rhythm
  - ▸ Auscultate for rate and rhythm, for normal heart sounds (S1 and S2), for any abnormal heart sounds (S3, S4, clicks, or snaps), and for murmurs, rubs, and gallops.
- Lung examination
  - ▸ Inspect for respiratory pattern, use of accessory muscles of respiration, and contour of the chest
  - ▸ Percuss the chest to evaluate any area of dullness which may represent pneumonia or neoplasm
  - ▸ Auscultate for breath sounds; are they normal or diminished?
  - ▸ Listen carefully for pleural friction rubs.
- Abdominal examination
  - ▸ A brief examination of the abdomen is indicated in the evaluation of chest pain; look especially for epigastric tenderness, masses, and bowel sounds.
- Peripheral pulse examination

▶ Auscultate the carotid, renal and femoral arteries for bruits, and palpate the lower extremity pulses.

Laboratory Tests

The extent of laboratory tests you order for your patient depends upon their stability at the time of your evaluation, and how much you know about their past history.

All patients with unstable anginal pain need laboratory tests to rule out myocardial infarction ("R/O MI"). This usually includes three sets of "cardiac enzymes" obtained at intervals over 24 hours. Stable angina which has not changed recently does not demand this testing.

> Most laboratories' cardiac enzyme profiles include CPK, CPK-MB fraction and index, myoglobin, and sometimes troponin.

CBC (complete blood count)
Increased white blood cell counts may signify infection. Decreased hemoglobin and hematocrit may point to blood loss or chronic disease

ESR (erythrocyte sedimentation rate)
An elevated ESR indicates inflammation and may be especially useful in evaluating patients in whom you suspect somatization symptoms.

Lipid profile
Patients with any other risk factors, or with pain consistent with angina *must* have lipid profiles checked.

Imaging

Chest X-ray
A chest X-ray is frequently needed to evaluate chest pain; it will demonstrate pneumonia, pneumothorax, cardiac enlargement and may give supporting evidence for aortic aneurysm or hiatal hernia.

Cervical spine X-rays
Cervical arthritis frequently causes neck and arm pain, which can mimic angina.

Special Studies

- *Electrocardiogram* (EKG or ECG)—an electrical tracing of the heart which may indicate ischemia, infarction or dysrhythmia.
- *Echocardiogram*—an ultrasound of the heart which is frequently used to evaluate cardiac wall motion, ejection fraction, and valve regurgitation or stenosis.
- *Stress tests*—some form of stress testing will be necessary for most clinically stable patients with chest pain of anginal quality.
  - *Exercise stress test*—patients exercise on a treadmill or bicycle ergometer and ECGs are recorded during the test.
  - *Exercise thallium stress test*—thallium imaging of the heart is added to the stress test; the image is completed immediately after excerise and a few hours later at rest; these images are compared for differences.
  - *Dobutamine thallium*—medication is used to "stress" the heart when a patient cannot exercise. Thallium images are again obtained at rest and after heart rate is sufficiently increased using dobutamine.
  - *Persantine thallium*—medication is used to selectively vasodilate nondiseased arteries and cause abnormal images in areas of diseased arteries. Adenosine may also be used for this purpose.
  - *Stress echocardiography*—an ultrasound of the heart is performed both during exercise and rest. The images are ivaluated for loss of wall motion during stress which indicates ischemia. If a patient is unable to ambulate, this study may be completed using dobutamine to pharmacologically increase the heart rate.

Invasive Imaging

Cardiac catheterization may be needed for definitive visualization of the coronary circulation in patients with a history strongly suggestive of angina, a positive stress test, or a history of MI, *if* the patient will consider any invasive treatment.

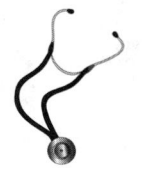

CASE RESOLUTION

Mr. C.J., a 55-year-old man is brought to your office by his wife, because of "severe and steady chest pain" for about 15 or 20 minutes earlier today. Both the patient and his wife report that he had brief chest pains several

times in the past two or three months while working in the yard, but today the pain lasted more than 15 minutes and it was accompanied by indigestion.

Quickly, ask a few additional relevant questions.

"Mr. J., tell me how that pain felt; on a scale of 1 to 10, how bad was it?"
"Well, Doctor, it felt like an anchor had been set down on my chest, and at the worst, it hurt badly, at least an 8 out of 10."
"Does the pain go anywhere else, Mr. J.?"
"Yes, for about 5 minutes when it was the worst, it seemed to be in my jaw and left arm."

This patient describes classic anginal pain. He has two risk factors: he smokes over a pack per day; and his father died of a "heart attack" at age 63. However, his cholesterol has been normal. With this risk profile and his typical anginal symptoms, you must consider coronary atherosclerosis as the most likely diagnosis, and immediately obtain an EKG.

His EKG is normal; but you admit him to the hospital with a diagnosis of "Unstable Angina, R/O MI". Serial EKGs and three sets of cardiac enzymes confirm that the patient has *not* had a myocardial infarction.

While you are happy to inform your patient that this episode of pain was not a "heart attack", you recognize that he may still have life-threatening coronary artery disease. The patient agrees to further testing.

Mr. J. agrees to a stress test, but tells you that he does not want to have a "heart cath" unless you *really* insist on it. He has arthritis in his right hip and cannot exercise enough for an exercise stress test. He undergoes a persantine thallium stress test. The test shows reversible defects in the area of the heart supplied by the right coronary artery which indicates ischemia. You discuss these findings with him and explain why you want a more complete picture of the anatomy of his coronary circulation. He then agrees to catheterization, which shows a 90% occlusion of his right coronary artery, a 70% occlusion of his left anterior descending artery, and a 90% occlusion of his left circumflex artery. Left ventricular ejection fraction is calculated at 40%, which is diminished. You suggest that he undergo coronary artery bypass grafting because of significant three vessel atherosclerotic coronary artery disease and mild to moderately impaired left ventricular function. Mr. J. agrees and has a successful operation.

SUMMARY

Chest pain is a common problem often reflecting serious underlying disease. A systematic evaluation will lead to a diagnosis. You must be attentive to the emotional and symbolic aspects of this problem.

STUDY QUESTIONS*

1. The pain pattern most consistent with myocardial infarction is:
   A. Vague upper chest and neck pain which has occurred every morning for the past week.
   B. Shearing or tearing mid chest pain associated with rapidly dropping blood pressure.
   C. Crushing midsternal chest pressure associated with jaw pain, sweating, and nausea.
   D. Left lower chest pain of a stabbing quality, worse with each deep breath.

2. Chest pain which you can reproduce in the patient by pressing on the chest wall is most consistent with which diagnosis?
   A. Esophagitis
   B. Intercostal muscle strain
   C. Costochondritis
   D. Pneumonia

3. All of the following are significant risk factors for coronary atherosclerosis except:
   A. Hyperlipidemia
   B. Connective tissue disorders
   C. Smoking
   D. Positive family history

4. Which statement is true concerning chest pain?
   A. Public service advertising campaigns have been so successful that patients nearly always come to the doctor when they have chest pain.
   B. Nearly all pulmonary diseases cause pleuritic chest pain.
   C. Anginal pain is always described as dull or heavy.
   D. Rib fractures are not always apparent to patients at the moment they occur.

5. Which statement is true regarding the evaluation of patients with chest pain?

* For answers, see page 347.

A. Anyone with chest pain must have an EKG done at the time of every recurrence of pain.
B. Three sets of "cardiac enzymes" are a usual part of the R/O MI protocol.
C. Every patient who has an MI must have cardiac catheterization.
D. Patients with chest pain usually have cardiac disease and seldom need chest X-rays.

6. Which of the following tests may be used to evaluate a patient with chest pain who is unable to walk?
A. Persantine thallium
B. Dobutamine thallium
C. Dobutamine echo
D. All of the above

Suggested Reading

DeGowin, R. The Thorax and Cardiovascular System, in Diagnostic Examination 6th edn. McGraw-Hill, New York, 1994.

Goroll, A., L. May and A. Mulley (eds) Evaluation of Chest Pain, in Primary Care Medicine 3rd edn. J.B. Lippincott Co., Philadelphia, 1995.

A Patient with Abdominal Pain

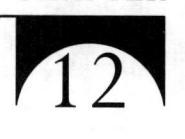

Marc A. Subik

INTRODUCTION

CASE PRESENTATION

Mr. T.G., a 75-year-old man, comes to your office because of acute onset of poorly localized abdominal pain that seems to be worse around his umbilicus. He states that the pain began about 3 hours ago and that he has vomited repeatedly without relief of his pain. He has episodes of severe, crampy pain that comes and goes at 5 or 10 minutes intervals. Walking or changing body position neither relieves nor worsens the pain.

Acute abdominal pain requires immediate evaluation because it may mean an "acute abdomen." This is a general term for a number of intra-abdominal conditions that require rapid surgical interventions. When abdominal pain is the presenting complaint, you must thoroughly evaluate it by quickly obtaining a history, performing a physical examination, and evaluating laboratory and X-ray data. Not all abdominal pain signals an acute abdomen; however, without a detailed examination and laboratory data, you cannot differentiate an acute abdomen from other causes of abdominal pain. In this chapter, we discuss a process for determining the cause of abdominal pain and establishing a specific diagnosis.

DEFINITIONS

Abscess:	localized collection of pus
Anorexia:	loss of appetite
Arteriogram:	X-ray study in which dye is injected into blood vessels

Barium enema:	X-ray of the large bowel after barium has been inserted
Computerized (CT or CAT) scan:	
	Computer-enhanced X-rays which produce cross-sectional images of the body highlighting different tissue densities
Colitis:	inflammation of the large bowel
Distention:	swelling or stretching
Diverticula:	small pouches usually found extending from the wall of the colon
Endoscopy:	process of using a flexible tube to visually inspect the lining of the upper or lower gastrointestinal tract
Enteritis:	inflammation of the small bowel
Epigastrium:	upper middle portion of the abdomen
Fibrosis:	scarring
Flatulence:	gas
Gastroscopy:	visualization of the esophagus, stomach, and proximal duodenum with a lighted tube
Hematemesis:	vomiting of blood
Hepatitis:	inflammation of the liver
Infarction:	death of tissue caused by loss of blood flow
Inflammation:	reaction of body tissues to injury as manifested by swelling, warmth, pain
Ischemia:	temporary lack of blood flow to tissue
MRI (Magnetic resonance imaging):	
	image produced by measuring nuclear magnetic resonance signals in body tissues after subjecting patients to a magnetic field
Pancreatitis:	inflammation of the pancreas
Peritoneum:	space between the bowels and the abdominal wall
Rectum:	the lower portion of the large bowel
Renal:	pertaining to the kidneys
Sign:	objective evidence of disease as found on physical exam
Sonogram (Ultrasound):	image produced by reflection of sound waves at tissue interfaces; especially useful

	for examining fluid-filled structures such as the gallbladder
Symptom:	an alteration in health status which the patient perceives and expresses; elicited during the history
Vascular:	involving blood vessels

COMMON MECHANISMS OF GASTROINTESTINAL DISEASE

Symptoms of gastrointestinal (GI) disease can be varied and complex. Many features of GI disease are reflected in nonspecific symptoms, often influenced by psychological and environmental factors. Some symptoms of GI tract malfunction include nausea, vomiting, anorexia, weight loss, bloating, diarrhea, hematemesis, rectal bleeding, melena, and pain. These symptoms arise from a variety of diseases. In this chapter we focus mainly on abdominal pain as a presenting symptom of GI tract disease.

The Sensation of Pain

Sensory information regarding pain travels along sympathetic pathways to spinal sensory neurons. Visceral afferent fibers mediating pain travel with the sympathetic nerves, except those from the pelvic organs which follow the parasympathetic pelvic nerves. The afferent endings are located in the smooth muscle layers of the hollow organs, in organ capsules, in the peritoneum, and in the walls of the intra-abdominal blood vessels.

The gastrointestinal tract is *insensitive to many stimuli* that produce pain in other organs, such as cutting, tearing, and burning. The intestine can be cut or crushed without pain. Mucosal biopsies of the gastrointestinal tract may produce an ulcer but never pain. The *principal forces that do produce pain in the GI tract* are stretching of the gut wall, ischemia, and inflammation of the peritoneum.

Stretching the Gut Wall

Abdominal pain can be produced by stretching the wall of a hollow organ or the outer surface capsule of a solid organ. Only when the

stretching develops rapidly will pain be produced. Gradual distention, such as common bile duct obstruction from a slow growing cancer, may be completely painless.

Tubular organs stretch when lesions obstruct flow of material through them. Such obstruction may be caused by a process within the lumen (intraluminal), within the muscle wall of the organ (intramural), or outside of the organ (extramural). **Intraluminal** lesions include stones or foreign bodies. **Intramural** abnormalities include tumors or fibrous strictures. **Extramural** processes compress externally; these abnormalities may be tumors or fibrotic changes also. Other obstructing lesions include volvulus (twisting of the gut), and intussusception (which occurs when one part of the gut inverts and is pulled further into the lumen by peristalsis).

> Volvulus is especially common in the cecal and sigmoid regions.

Ischemia

Ischemia of tissue occurs when local blood flow is reduced because of either blood vessel blockage or lessened systemic perfusion caused by hypotension. Acute severe ischemia produces death of tissue (infarction); lesser degrees of ischemia produce less damage. For example, ischemia affecting just the mucosal lining of the gut will cause ulceration, or ischemia of deeper muscle layers of the bowel wall may cause an encircling scar called a stricture, which narrows the lumen.

Ischemia of visceral tissue produces intense, continuous pain owing to release of tissue metabolites and to traction on blood vessels supplied with pain fibers. The most common cause of intestinal ischemia is circulatory blockage; this can result from hernia, or volvulus, or from direct blood vessel blockage caused by atherosclerosis or embolus.

Hernia

Normally, the abdominal viscera are contained within the parietal peritoneum by layers of fascia and strong muscles. If defects develop in the fascia or are congenitally present, peritoneum and internal organs can bulge through the opening, i.e., "herniate". Often hernias are of no clinical significance. However, if the fascial defect is narrow, herniated viscera may become trapped or "incarcerated". Then the blood supply to the organ can be compromised resulting in edema, swelling, pain, and ultimately infarction.

Inflammation produces pain by the release of mediators such as prostaglandins, histamine, serotonin, and leukotrienes.

Inflammation and tissue swelling sensitize the nerve endings and lower the threshold to pain from other stimuli.

Inflammation

Inflammation of the peritoneum is the third major cause of abdominal pain. Initially, inflammation will be limited to the covering of a diseased organ, e.g., appendix or gallbladder. If undetected or untreated, the inflammation will extend to the adjacent parietal peritoneum and produce "peritoneal signs" on physical examination. These include guarding, tenderness to palpation, and rebound tenderness.

Inflammation of damaged peritoneum usually resolves without scarring. However, if two inflamed surfaces remain in contact, they may adhere to each other by scar tissue. These scars, termed **adhesions,** infrequently cause obstruction years after healing of the inflammatory process because loops of bowel can become trapped by them.

Inflammation from disruption of the gut

Disruption of the gut or "perforation" allows spillage of its contents into the peritoneal cavity. This invariably leads to bacterial contamination of the peritoneum, termed **peritonitis**. If this infection becomes walled off and contained, it is termed an **abscess**. **Fistulas** are chronic persistent tracts connecting the intestine to another organ. Fistulas result when trauma, inflammation, infection, or cancer disrupt the intestinal wall. They can occur between the gut and skin (enterocutaneous), or between two organs in the peritoneal cavity, such as colon and bladder (colovesical).

Diverticula

Diverticula, or outpouchings of the wall of a hollow organ, may involve all layers of the bowel wall (true diverticulum), or the mucosa and submucosa alone may push through the muscle wall (false diverticulum). The presence of diverticula (a condition called **diverticulosis**) is common and generally asymptomatic. When one or more diverticula perforate or become inflamed, the patient experiences all the problems associated with peritoneal inflammation. This condition is called **diverticulitis**.

TYPES OF ABDOMINAL PAIN

Abdominal pain may be classified into three categories: visceral (including colic), parietal, and referred pain. Colic can be a specific diagnostic sign.

Visceral pain originates in abdominal organs covered by visceral peritoneum. Such viscera are innervated by afferent sympathetic fibers

of the autonomic nervous system and are sensitive to stretch, ischemia, and inflammation, but insensitive to burns and cuts. Visceral pain localizes poorly because of overlapping segmental innervation and because the involved nerves are usually dormant. When severe visceral pain occurs, count on the patient experiencing anxiety, nausea, vomiting, sweating, and low blood pressure.

Colic is crampy pain that arises from a hollow organ when its muscle layers are stretched by obstruction, or become fatigued by repeated spasms attempting to overcome the blockage. The intensity of the pain and the intraluminal pressure are inversely proportional to the diameter of the involved hollow organ. Colic is much more severe when the ureter is involved than when the stomach is involved.

Parietal pain arises from irritation of the parietal peritoneum. Pain impulses from the parietal peritoneum reach the central nervous system via the intercostal nerves. Thus, parietal pain can be localized more precisely than visceral pain. Movement or coughing aggravates parietal pain and contracting the abdominal muscles diminishes it.

Referred pain is produced by pathology at one location, but felt at another location. Pain from internal organs often will be referred to more superficial areas, sometimes at substantial distance from the involved organ, because both are supplied by the same spinal nerve and share central pathways for afferent neurons. Examples of referred pain are pain at the right scapula as a result of gallbladder disease and pain at the top of the shoulder produced by a subdiaphragmatic abscess.

CAUSES OF ABDOMINAL PAIN

Clinical Clues

The differential diagnosis of abdominal pain encompasses many diverse illnesses, including: acute appendicitis, cholecystitis, pancreatitis, kidney stone, intestinal obstruction and perforation, intestinal infarction, diverticulitis, and ruptured aortic aneurysm. *Importantly, nonabdominal and/or systemic diseases also cause acute abdominal pain.* These include: pneumonia, pneumothorax, hepatitis, sickle cell crisis, and acute porphyria.

The severity of the patient's pain may be disproportionate to the severity of their illness, complicating the evaluation of these patients. Some conditions which produce an acute abdomen are potentially lethal unless treated promptly. By contrast, some relatively benign problems may present in an equally acute fashion.

In distinguishing among the causes of abdominal pain, many features need to be considered. The most critical are determination of the *mode of onset of pain* and its *location*.

Onset of pain

The severe pain of a ruptured aortic aneurysm, a perforated viscus, passage of a kidney stone, or ruptured ectopic pregnancy characteristically is of abrupt onset, easily recalled by the patient. Obstruction or inflammation of a hollow viscus may cause pain of rapid, but not instantaneous onset, developing over one to several hours. Examples of this type of pain include appendicitis, acute cholecystitis, pancreatitis, bowel obstruction, and diverticulitis. Disorders which cause pain of very gradual or vague onset include malignant diseases and hepatitis.

Locality of pain

The location of the pain may be an important diagnostic clue. Pursue questions which help the patient to show you where their pain localizes. **Upper abdominal pain** usually is caused by cholecystitis, pancreatitis, or perforated ulcer. **Midabdominal** pain results from small intestinal disorders, early stages of appendicitis, and pancreatitis. **Lower abdominal pain** may be caused by diverticulitis, kidney stones, ectopic pregnancy, ruptured ovarian cyst, or late stages of appendicitis (Figure 12-1).

Common Acute Pain Syndromes

The most common and most serious causes of acute abdominal pain are acute appendicitis, diverticulitis, cholecystitis, pancreatitis, perforated gastric or duodenal ulcer, intestinal obstruction, intestinal infarction, ruptured or leaking abdominal aortic aneurysm, and several gynecological disorders (Table 12-1).

Atypical presentation of appendicitis is especially common in the elderly.

Prompt and accurate diagnosis of **appendicitis** decreases complications. Delay in diagnosis greatly increases the risk of perforation. Pain usually begins in the epigastric or periumbilical area, and progresses to the right lower quadrant. Its onset is gradual and increases hourly, accompanied by a low-grade fever (less than 101°F, 38.3°C) and tenderness in the right lower quadrant. Rebound tenderness, pain when the examiner releases their fingers from deep palpation of the abdomen, is characteristic. Unfortunately, only 20–30% of patients with acute appendicitis follow this typical or classic pattern.

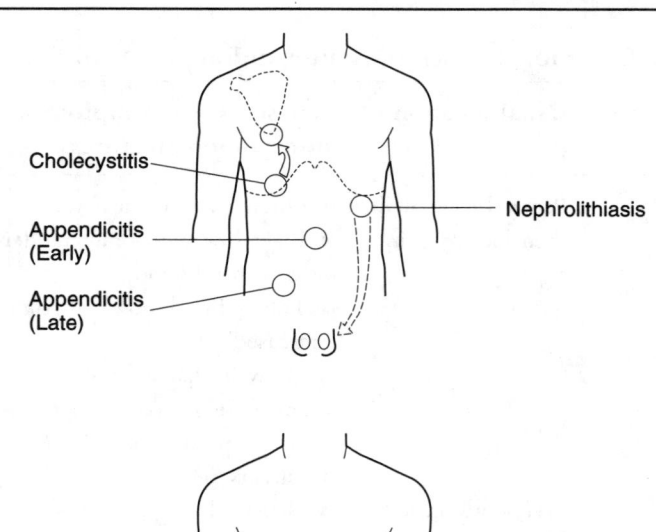

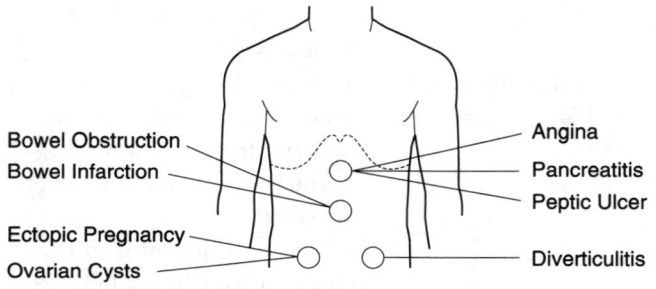

Figure 12-1. Locations of common types of abdominal pain. (Adapted from DeGowin and DeGowin, *Diagnostic Examination*, 6th ed. McGraw-Hill, New York, 1994, pp. 528 and 535.)

Other physical findings which occur occassionally in appendicitis include the **psoas sign**, namely right lower quadrant pain on hyperextension of the right hip, and the **obturator sign**, right lower quadrant pain on internal rotation of the right hip.

Acute **diverticulitis** occurs when diverticula become inflamed. Diverticular disease may involve the entire colon but acute diverticulitis most often involves only the sigmoid region. It may develop in the absence of prior symptoms or it may be superimposed on chronic constipation and mild lower left quadrant discomfort. The primary symptoms of diverticulitis are pain, nausea, occasionally vomiting, and GI bleeding, sometimes with accompanying low-grade fever, left lower quadrant tenderness and a mass discernable on physical examination. Bowel sounds are decreased and localized peritoneal signs may be present. The total white blood cell count is usually elevated. Treatment for bouts of acute diverticulitis consists of antibiotics and i.v. fluids. If the

Table 12-1. Common Causes of Acute Abdominal Pain

Disorder	Usual location of pain	Key signs and symptoms and other unique features
Appendicitis	Periumbilical at first, then localizing in right lower quadrant	• Often a low grade fever • Right lower quadrant tenderness with rebound • Total white blood cell count increased • Delay in diagnosis or treatment increases risk of perforation and peritonitis • Surgery required
Diverticulitis	Frequently in left lower quadrant	• Often a low grade fever • Left lower quadrant tenderness and frequently a mass • Total white blood cell count increased • Can try treatment with i.v. fluids and antibiotics, but surgery often needed
Cholecystitis	Right upper quadrant, sometimes right shoulder	• Low grade to moderate fever • Tender right upper quadrant sometimes with Murphy's sign (see text, page 188) • Caused by gallstones obstructing the cystic duct, sometimes with bacterial infection and rarely with infarction of the gallbladder.
Acute pancreatitis	Upper abdomen, often radiating to the back; may be eased by leaning forward	• Variable degree of pain, often very severe • Usually associated with nausea and vomiting • Sometimes epigastric or periumbilical tenderness

Table 12-1. Continued

Disorder	Usual location of pain	Key signs and symptoms and other unique features
Perforated stomach or bowel	Usually diffuse throughout abdomen	• Rigid, board-like abdomen with rebound tenderness • Low blood pressure, diaphoresis, shallow breathing • Increased total white blood cell count; often increased amylase • Upright chest X-ray shows free air under diaphragm
Small bowel obstruction	Variable	• Pain, vomiting, distention, inability to pass gas or stool • Early stage—high pitched bowel sounds; later stage—absent bowel sounds
Intestinal infarction	Diffuse	• Intense visceral pain out of proportion to degree of abdominal tenderness • Patient appears very ill with diaphoresis, tachycardia, elevated total white blood cell count, and hypotension
Ruptured aortic aneurysm	Usually back and epigastrium	• Pulsatile abdominal mass • Often hypertensive patient with a precipitous drop in BP as intra-abdominal bleeding progresses • Surgical repair mandatory
Gynecologic disorders	Twisted or ruptured ovarian cysts	• Abrupt onset of pain in one lower quadrant • Tender mass on examination
	Ectopic pregnancy	• May occur before patient knows she is pregnant

The two most common causes of pancreatitis are alcohol and gallstone disease.

Most gallstones are *not* calcified and cannot be seen on plain X-rays. The opposite is true of kidney stones.

diverticulitis does not resolve completely or if the inflammation recurs, surgical removal of the inflamed colonic segments is the next step.

Acute **cholecystitis** begins with colicky, or rhythmically recurring, pain in the epigastric or right upper quadrant area. The pain becomes steady and increases in intensity over several hours, occasionally radiating to the right scapula. Many patients develop nausea, vomiting, and fever. On examination, some patients exhibit **Murphy's sign**, which is right upper quadrant tenderness aggravated by deep inspiration. The diagnosis is confirmed by finding gallstones on an ultrasound. The pain results from cystic duct obstruction by a gallstone, which interferes with gallbladder emptying and leads to distention and ischemia of the gallbladder. Sometimes secondary bacterial infection ensues. Treatment includes antibiotics to treat the infection and surgical removal of the gallbladder.

The clinical presentation of acute **pancreatitis** varies, ranging from mild epigastric discomfort to sudden and severe abdominal distress. Typically the pain of pancreatitis is located in the upper abdomen and radiates to the back. It may be mild or severe, is usually continuous over several hours, and it is associated with nausea or vomiting. Sitting up or leaning forward eases the pain. On physical examination, periumbilical tenderness can be detected as well as low blood pressure, sweating, and pallor. Patients may be jaundiced, have an elevated total white blood cell count or low serum calcium. Serum and urine amylase and lipase levels are elevated during an acute episode.

Patients with mild pancreatitis recover spontaneously in 1–2 days. However, severe and complicated cases require supportive care consisting of "resting the pancreas" by prohibiting oral intake and administration of intravenous fluids, pain medications, and antibiotics.

Perforation of a gastric or duodenal ulcer causes sudden, severe pain beginning in the epigastrium and soon spreading to the entire abdomen. Patients appear very ill with low blood pressure, sweating, and shallow breathing. On physical examination, they have a rigid, board-like abdomen with rebound tenderness. The total white blood cell count and amylase levels are usually elevated. The diagnosis is confirmed by identifying a perforated ulcer at the time of surgery.

Upright chest X-rays can help diagnose perforated organs, as free air can be seen under the diaphragm.

In patients with **intestinal obstruction,** common features are pain, distention, vomiting, and inability to pass gas or stool. These symptoms vary depending on the location and degree of obstruction. Stomach and small bowel obstructions more often cause pain and vomiting, while colonic obstruction is associated with more distention and constipation. Symptoms may be present for weeks in a partial bowel obstruction or only 1–2 days in a more complete obstruction.

On examination, patients in an early stage of bowel obstruction may have high-pitched, active bowel sounds. Later, these sounds diminish or disappear and peritonitis develops as the bowel becomes ischemic. Colon obstruction may be distinguished from small bowel obstruction by flat and upright X-rays of the abdomen. If there is no air in the colon and the small bowel is distended, the small bowel is obstructed. If there is no air in the rectum and the colon above it is distended, the colon is obstructed. Once bowel obstruction is diagnosed, consult a surgeon promptly.

Intestinal infarction or "**ischemic gut,**" an uncommon, but serious cause of abdominal pain, can be caused by either arterial or venous occlusion. Pain of **arterial** occlusion is colicky at first, and soon becomes constant as tissue sustains further damage. *The characteristic feature of ischemic gut is intense visceral pain out of proportion to any tenderness elicited on physical examination.* Patients have hypotension, pallor, diaphoresis, and rapid heart rate. The total white blood cell count is usually elevated. Initially, medical care consists of supportive measures, with i.v. fluids. Most patients will need a diagnostic arteriogram or exploratory surgery. Ischemic gut is a life-threatening condition and survival of the patient requires the physician to apply a high index of suspicion.

> Bowel infarction usually occurs in older patients, 60 years old or more.

The symptoms of mesenteric **venous** occlusion are more subtle and evolve slowly, often being present for weeks. It can be diagnosed by CT scan or arteriogram with special attention to the venous phase. Treatment requires anticoagulation, heparin acutely and coumadin later on a chronic basis.

A **ruptured or leaking abdominal aortic aneurysm** causes acute and constant back and epigastric pain. Physical examination reveals a pulsatile abdominal mass or enlarged tender aorta. Patients usually have a history of hypertension, though after the vessel ruptures, the blood pressure is usually low and femoral pulses may be asymmetric. An ultrasound or CT scan may show an enlarged aorta. If the patient is stable, a diagnostic arteriogram can be done. Treatment is resection and repair of the aneurysm.

Gynecologic disorders also cause substantial abdominal pain. A twisted or **ruptured ovarian cyst** can cause an abrupt onset of pain in *one lower quadrant*. A tender mass in the region of the ovary can be felt and seen on ultrasound. Treatment is surgical removal of the ovary. Acute **salpingitis** or Fallopian tube infection presents with abdominal and pelvic tenderness, which is *bilateral* in most cases. Palpation of the cervix is very painful. Fever is typically present. With antibiotic treatment, recovery is usually rapid. **Ectopic pregnancy** in which a fertilized ovum implants itself outside the uterus, may cause very severe

abdominal pain. In such an abnormal site, only limited growth of the embryo can occur before significant pain and bleeding begin and surgery is mandatory.

An **acute abdomen during pregnancy** poses unique problems because the enlarged uterus displaces abdominal organs from their usual position, limits the extent of the abdominal examination, and alters otherwise typical clinical manifestations. When an acute surgical condition is suspected, surgery should proceed; exploratory surgery is well tolerated by the pregnant woman and fetus. Appendicitis and ruptured ovarian cysts are the most common indications for laparotomy.

Chronic Pain Syndromes

Of the many causes of chronic and recurrent abdominal pain, four require particular attention. They are irritable bowel syndrome, gallstones, chronic pancreatitis, and cancer of the pancreas (Table 12-2).

Irritable bowel syndrome, the most common cause of chronic abdominal pain, occurs slightly more often in women, appearing usually in early to mid adulthood, and rarely after the age of 60. Symptoms include bloating, belching, recurrent nonlocalized abdominal pain of a vague and sometimes crampy nature, alternating diarrhea and constipation, mucus in the stools, and pain relief with defecation. Stress, anxiety, and certain foods can aggravate these symptoms.

Patients with irritable bowel syndrome generally appear well, and their physical examination is normal except for scattered areas of mild abdominal tenderness on palpation. The results of laboratory tests are normal; stool studies for infection are negative. Endoscopy and X-rays are normal. Treatment consists of your reassuring the patient of the absence of a life-threatening problem, and explaining the nature of irritable bowel syndrome as a lifelong motility disorder. Mainstays of therapy include increasing the fiber content of the patient's diet, avoiding foods that incite or worsen their symptoms, antispasmodic medicines, and antidiarrhea medicines and/or laxatives as indicated.

Gallstones may intermittently obstruct the cystic duct producing inflammation of the gallbladder. Often, symptoms are nonspecific; however, the simultaneous occurrence of fever, jaundice, and colicky right upper quadrant pain is virtually diagnostic. The pain of gallstones may occasionally localize in the epigastrium or the left upper quadrant. The diagnosis of chronic cholecystitis is based on a history of pain occurring several hours after meals or awakening the patient from sleep, and the demonstration of gallstones on an ultrasound. Belching, gas, and cramp-

---

Symptoms of irritable bowel syndrome are attributed to spastic and uncoordinated muscle contractions of the bowel. Patients appear to be hypersensitive to gut distention.

Ultrasound is the most accurate test to document the presence of stones in the gallbladder. It is not as accurate in detecting stones in the common bile duct.

Table 12-2. Common Causes of Chronic Abdominal Pain

Disorder	Usual location of pain	Key signs and symptoms and other unique features
Irritable bowel syndrome	Vague, nonlocalized	• Bloating and belching • Alternating diarrhea and constipation • Much mucus in stool • Normal physical examination and laboratory tests
Gallstones (cholelithiasis)	Usually right upper quadrant and epigastric	• Pain several hours after eating • Cramping and bloating *may* be induced by fatty foods
Chronic pancreatitis	Epigastric and sometimes mid-back	• Dull intermittent pain, much less intense than with acute pancreatitis • Progressive loss of pancreatic enzyme secretions occur
Pancreatic cancer	Epigastrium and occasionally mid-back	• Common cause of cancer deaths • Often diagnosed late due to nonspecific symptoms • Dull achy pain and weight loss usually occur

ing caused by fatty foods, onions, broccoli, and other "gas-producing" foods *may* occur *but these symptoms are not specific for gallbladder disease.* The treatment is surgical removal of the gallbladder.

Alcohol abuse causes more than 90% of cases of **chronic pancreatitis.** The pain is dull, intermittent, usually lasting several hours, located primarily in the epigastric area, and occasionally radiating to the mid-back. As progressive destruction of the pancreas occurs, protein plugs calcify and they can be identified on abdominal X-rays in 20% of patients. Loss of pancreatic enzyme secretion may occur and then patients will not absorb fats and protein normally.

Several imaging techniques show the characteristic changes of alternate dilation and constriction (beading) of the pancreatic duct. CT of the abdomen and endoscopic retrograde cholangiopancreatography (ERCP), an endoscopic procedure in which dye is injected into the

Pain of chronic pancreatitis *will not* be relieved if the patient continues to drink alcohol.

pancreatic duct, are used in establishing the diagnosis of chronic pancreatitis.

Treatment of chronic pancreatitis consists mainly of pain control, which may be difficult to accomplish. Surgical resection of portions of the pancreas may be tried to relieve ductal obstruction. Oral pancreatic enzyme supplements are often necessary.

Cancer of the pancreas is the fifth most common cause of cancer death. Typically, the diagnosis is made late in the disease, and consequently the 5-year survival rate is less than 5%. Pain, the most common initial symptom, is a dull epigastric ache, occasionally radiating to the back. Weight loss and depression are common. As most of these cancers involve the head of the pancreas, they frequently present with jaundice caused by bile duct obstruction. Currently, any possibility for long-term survival rests in a pancreatic resection, but unfortunately, most patients are diagnosed late, beyond the time surgery might help. Moreover, the tumor responds poorly to chemotherapy or radiation therapy.

Abdominal CT scan is the best test to visualize a pancreatic tumor.

HISTORY AND PHYSICAL EXAMINATION

As with all medical conditions, a careful and accurate history provides critical clues for determining the etiology of acute and chronic abdominal pain. The information obtained from the history, physical examination, laboratory test results, and X-rays, considered together in a meaningful way, can lead to the diagnosis. Then you can develop a therapeutic plan. Laboratory tests and other diagnostic studies should be used selectively. Every laboratory test has the potential to generate clinically misleading information; for this reason, avoid the "shotgun" approach of ordering a multitude of laboratory tests and X-rays.

Developing the HPI

Key questions must be asked of each patient with abdominal pain.

- The **onset** of pain may help to distinguish its etiology. Ask, "When did your pain begin?" For example, pain of a perforated ulcer can be precisely timed, but the exact time of onset of pain from bowel obstruction is seldom known.
- A **qualitative** description relates how the pain feels. Ask, "Is your pain sharp, stabbing, burning, squeezing, crampy, dull, or aching?" Sharp, stabbing pain is parietal, while vague pressure or cramping pain is visceral.

- The severity or **intensity** of the pain is loosely related to the magnitude of the offending stimulus, though estimates of severity are often unreliable. Ask, "Tell me how much your abdomen hurts."
- Ask, "Does the pain come and go with a certain **rhythm**?" Does it occur, for example, every 10–15 minutes, or predictably on a weekly or monthly basis?
- Pinpointing the **location** is important. Ask "Point with one finger where your abdomen hurts the most." Visceral pain tends to be poorly localized but, parietal pain can sometimes be localized by the patient pointing to it with one finger.
- Ask, "Does the pain travel (Is it **referred**) to any other location?" Gallbladder disease causes right upper quadrant pain with referred pain to the scapula; pancreatic cancer causes epigastric pain with referred pain to the back.
- Ask "What is the **duration** of your pain? Seconds, minutes, or hours?" Duodenal ulcer pain is present for minutes at a time, while ischemic gut pain is steady for hours.
- Ask "Does anything **aggravate** or **relieve** the pain?" Is eating, moving into certain positions, taking particular medications, or moving the bowels associated with any change in the pain?

Other History

Ask about other associated symptoms such as nausea, vomiting, poor appetite, constipation, diarrhea, weight loss, and bleeding. Certain questions about family history are important, as gallstone disease and atherosclerosis tends to be familiar. Ask about alcohol abuse and emotional stress and other social history.

Physical Examination

Proper positioning is critical. The patient should be supine and the entire abdomen should be exposed, and they should be as comfortable as possible. The sequence of physical examination steps is: inspection, auscultation, percussion, and palpation.

Inspection is the process of critically looking at the abdomen. Note its shape or contour. Is it "scooped out," or scaphoid? Is it distended, is it asymmetric? Other abnormalities to look for include scars, hernias, dilated veins, visible peristalsis, bruises on the skin, and rashes. If the abdomen appears distended, think of the "five f's:" fat, fluid, flatus, feces, fetus.

You should stand on the patient's right side to do your abdominal exam.

Auscultation detects and characterizes bowel sounds and identifies bruits. Normal bowel sounds are intermittent and gurgly and usually heard within 15 seconds of your starting to auscultate. They may be absent, as in ileus or late in the course of bowel obstruction, or they may be continuous and hyperactive suggesting enteritis. Tinkling, high-pitched sounds suggest small bowel obstruction.

Percussion of the abdomen discriminates liquids and solid tissues from gas-filled bowel. Gas is resonant to percussion and liquid/solid tissue dull to percussion. The liver borders or a distended bladder can be identified by the differing sounds of percussion. Ascites (fluid in the abdomen) can be determined by noting the resonance of air-filled loops of bowel floating on top of the ascitic fluid, while the fluid-laden flanks are dull to percussion.

Palpation of the abdomen using the pads of the fingertips may elicit diffuse or localized tenderness, or identify an enlarged liver or spleen, and abnormal masses. As a rule, inflammatory diseases produce tenderness, neoplastic diseases do not. Palpate the abdomen gently at first then apply somewhat greater pressure; palpate lower quadrants first then the right and left upper quadrants. The liver edge may normally be felt on deep inspiration. The normal spleen will *not* be palpable.

Gentle palpation of inflamed parietal peritoneum evokes localized tenderness, accompanied by **guarding**, an involuntary spasm of the abdominal muscles. **Rebound tenderness** is diagnostic of parietal irritation. Tenderness in the abdominal wall is exacerbated by having the patient lift the head off the pillow which increases the tension in the muscles. During deep palpation in a thin patient, you may palpate a normal aorta.

A **rectal examination** is part of every complete physical examination. Inspect the perianal skin looking for warts, hemorrhoids, infection, or fistulas. Then gently insert your gloved and lubricated index finger into the rectum, and assess for tenderness and sphincter tone. Move your finger circumferentially, feeling for any masses, and in the male evaluate the size and consistency of the prostate. You may detect tenderness in adjacent structures, such as the appendix, and in the female uterus and Fallopian tubes.

LABORATORY TESTS

Certain tests are routinely done in the evaluation of a patient with abdominal pain.

- *Urinalysis*—A urinalysis helps assess the presence of a kidney stone, infection, or tumor.
- *Complete blood count*—A low hemoglobin reveals evidence of blood loss and an increased hemoglobin may indicate dehydration. An elevated total white blood cell count suggests infection, sepsis, inflammation, or infarction.
- *Additional blood tests*—The level of amylase and lipase in the serum are normally increased in pancreatic and biliary diseases. However, remember that disorders unrelated to the pancreas can cause an elevated amylase. Other liver function tests are often necessary.

DIAGNOSTIC STUDIES

Imaging

Plain X-rays (upright and supine abdomen) can show specific gas patterns associated with certain causes of abdominal pain, as well as free intraabdominal air which occurs from a perforated viscus. **Contrast studies** with barium outline the esophagus, stomach, and duodenum (upper GI series) or the colon (barium enema).

   Ultrasound is the best way to diagnose gallstones. It is extremely useful in identifying cystic lesions in the abdomen, evaluating the pelvis, and scanning for a dilated bile duct system and for dilated ureters. **CT scanning** provides the best imaging of soft tissue structures in the abdominal cavity, especially for evaluating suspected pancreatic disorders.

Endoscopy

Endoscopy, visual evaluation of the upper GI tract or colon with fiberoptic instruments, is rarely indicated in *acute* abdominal pain. A cautious sigmoidoscopy, however, is appropriate occasionally to reveal colon ischemia, acute ulcerative or infectious colitis.

CASE RESOLUTION

A 75-year-old man comes to your office because of acute onset of poorly localized abdominal pain that seems to be worse around his umbilicus. He states that the pain began about 3 hours ago and that he has vomited repeatedly without relief of his pain. He has episodes of severe, crampy pain, that comes and goes at intervals of 5 or 10 minutes. Walking or changing body position neither relieves nor worsens the pain.

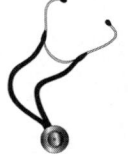

Your patient has poorly localized, colicky pain; your initial thought is that this is likely visceral pain. Probably, the peritoneum is not involved since movement does not make it worse. You proceed by obtaining additional history.

The patient has been healthy, except for two abdominal operations that he required several years ago after a car accident which caused "internal bleeding". He abstains from alcohol, eats a regular diet, and is retired and living a relatively stress-free life.

Except for his previous abdominal surgery, he has few risk factors for his current episode of pain. You proceed with your physical examination.

The patient's examination reveals a rapid heart rate of about 104 beats per minute, and a slightly increased respiratory rate of 28 per minute. He has no fever. Chest examination is normal. His abdomen is mildly diffusely tender but no masses are palpable. Bowel sounds are high-pitched with a "tinkling" quality.

Now you are highly suspicious of an intestinal obstruction. You proceed by ordering a CBC and abdominal X-rays.

The patient has a normal hemoglobin and a slightly increased total white blood cell count. The X-rays show a distended small bowel with no air in the colon.

At this point, you wisely refer your patient to a surgeon for treatment of small bowel obstruction. Exploratory surgery shows obstruction due to adhesions from his previous abdominal trauma; the surgeon lyses them. Following surgery, the patient recovers without sequelae.

STUDY QUESTIONS*

1. Which is *not* true regarding appendicitis?
   A. Patients usually have periumbilical pain early, and right lower quadrant pain later on.
   B. Appendectomy is nearly always necessary.
   C. Elderly people with appendicitis usually have a very typical presentation.
   D. The psoas sign and the obturator sign are seen sometimes in appendicitis.

---

*For answers, see page 347.

2. The primary forces that cause pain in the gastrointestinal tract include all except:
    A. Ischemia
    B. Inflammation
    C. Heat
    D. Tension

3. A 32-year-old man comes to your office complaining of vague abdominal pains, bloating, and alternating diarrhea and constipation. He believes that the stress of his new job makes his symptoms worse. His physical examination is entirely normal. The most likely diagnosis is:
    A. Chronic cholecystitis
    B. Irritable bowel syndrome
    C. Pancreatic cancer
    D. Intestinal obstruction

4. Types of abdominal pain include all of the following except:
    A. Visceral
    B. Referred
    C. Parietal
    D. Omental

5. Which statement regarding gynecologic causes of abdominal pain is true?
    A. Surgery for an acute abdominal disorder during pregnancy is very dangerous for the fetus
    B. Ruptured ovarian cysts cause chronic pain.
    C. Ectopic pregnancy usually causes pain beginning at around 4 months' gestation.
    D. Salpingitis or infection of the Fallopian tubes often causes bilateral lower quadrant pain.

Suggested Reading

Goroll, A., L. May, and A. Mulley (eds). Primary Care Medicine: Office Evaluation and Management of the Adult Patient, 3rd edn, Chapters 55–76, 116, 135. J.B. Lippincott Co., Philadelphia, 1994.

DeGowin, R.L. ed. Diagnostic Examination, 6th edn, pp. 463–566. McGraw-Hill Inc., New York, 1994.

A Patient with Hypertension

Sachin T. Dave and Jayson L. Yap

INTRODUCTION

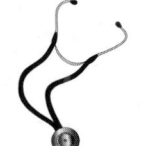

CASE PRESENTATION

Mr. N.T., a 50-year-old man, comes to your office for his regular appointment. "It's time to get my blood pressure checked again. I'm feeling fine," he reports to your nurse. She records today's BP as 162/100.

Blood pressure is defined as the pressure through the circulatory bed which maintains blood flow to meet metabolic demands of the body. Excessively high blood pressure in the arterial system, known as **hypertension,** is that level of pressure beyond which a very high likelihood exists of sustaining end organ damage, either acutely or chronically.

The Sixth Joint National Committee (JNC-6) has developed criteria for classification of hypertension in adults aged 18 years and older (1). Based on the average of *two or more blood pressure readings taken at each of two or more visits after an initial screening visit*, hypertension is classified according to the JNC-6 criteria in Table 13-1.

DEFINITIONS

SBP: systolic blood pressure ("the top number")
DBP: diastolic blood pressure ("the bottom number")
End-organ: also called "target organ"—the organ on which a substance or process exerts its influence or action. In reference to hypertension, "end organs" are those

Table 13-1. JNC-6 Criteria for Classifying Hypertension

Category	Systolic (SBP) (mmHg)	Diastolic (DBP) (mmHg)
Optimal	<120	<80
Normal	<130	<85
High normal	130–139	85–89
Hypertension		
Stage 1	140–159	90–99
Stage 2	160–179	100–109
Stage 3	≥180	≥110

which are most sensitive to the effects of hypertension such as the kidneys, heart, and eyes.

Exudates: funduscopic changes seen when material exudes from damaged retinal blood vessels.

HBP, HTN: common abbreviations for hypertension

ISH: isolated systolic hypertension

Labile: unpredictably changeable

Left ventricular hypertrophy:
thickening of the muscle of the left ventricle

Manometer: a pressure measuring device

NSAIDs: nonsteroidal antiinflammatory drugs

METHOD OF BLOOD PRESSURE MEASUREMENT

The Blood Pressure Cuff (Sphygmomanometer)

A **mercury manometer** is the standard to which other devices (aneroid manometers or automated home devices) are calibrated for accuracy. Use an arm cuff whose width is approximately two thirds the distance from the axilla to the antecubital space, with the inflatable bladder encircling 80% of the arm. A 15 × 35 cm bladder ("large" cuff) is recommended for most adults. For obese arms (arm circumference greater than 41 cm) use a "thigh" cuff (18 × 36–42 cm).

Seat your patient in a quiet environment at a moderate temperature for about 10 minutes. Then take readings in both arms, and when indicated to rule out coarctation of the aorta, in one leg. Take two or

The auscultatory gap is the occasional disappearance of sounds at a pressure below the true systolic level. This gap may mislead one into recording a much lower systolic pressure.

Deflating the cuff too fast may cause misreading when bradycardia or tachycardia is present, as cardiac output may vary considerably from beat to beat; deflating too slowly will falsely elevate the readings.

more readings in quick succession until the measurements are within 5 mmHg of each other.

Apply the cuff so that it is in a horizontal plane level with the heart, and inflate it until the radial pulse disappears. This establishes the approximate level of systolic pressure and avoids the "auscultatory gap." Deflate rapidly, then inflate the cuff again to 20 mmHg *above* your estimated systolic level and slowly deflate, allowing a pressure drop of 2–4 mmHg/second. Listen for the pulse (Korotkoff) sounds. The initial sound is recorded as "systolic" while the disappearance of all sounds is the "diastolic"reading.

Variability in BP Measurement

Both systolic and diastolic blood pressures vary with every heart beat and with the respiratory cycle. Blood pressure varies minute-to-minute by about 4 mmHg systolic and 2–3 mmHg diastolic. Day-to-day variation is even more striking, as much as 5–12 mmHg systolic and 6–8 mmHg diastolic. Blood pressure falls by an average of 30% during sleep.

Certain other circumstances may cause BP readings to vary.

Patients show a progressive fall in BP after being admitted to the hospital.

- Systolic BP typically rises during isotonic exercise.
- Both SBP and DBP rise after isometric exercise.
- Chronic alcohol intake beyond 2 ounces a day *can* result in considerable long-term rise in BP (may be the most common cause of reversible hypertension.)
- Habitual intake of caffeine does *not* raise BP, as tolerance to its effects develops.
- Smokers exhibit no more hypertension than nonsmokers. *Use of smokeless tobacco is associated with higher BP* (which may be related to its very high sodium content).

About 30% of patients with high BP in the office will be found to have white coat hypertension. Young, non-obese women are especially prone to this.

Because so many factors cause variability in readings, the *standard recommendation is to obtain two or three measurements at separate office visits (and more, if the readings are borderline) before an individual is labeled as having hypertension.*

Ambulatory Blood Pressure Measurement

One additional external factor known to influence BP readings is the person taking the reading. Having the pressure checked by a physician, especially a man, can lead to a substantial rise in BP reading compared to

having the procedure done by other medical professionals, including women physicians. This phenomenon is known as "white coat hypertension."

This BP variability engendered by the office visit has stimulated interest in home blood pressure monitoring. Ambulatory blood pressure monitors which record multiple readings over 24 hours are available. These monitors' readings are more consistent and reproducible than office measurements. Their correlation to target organ damage and mortality is also better than for office readings.

However, electronic 24-hours-per-day monitoring devices are expensive and inconvenient; we encourage patients to take BP readings at home with standard aneroid or mercury manometers. BP readings average slightly higher when manual BP cuffs are used for home monitoring (compared to electronic monitors), because no nighttime recordings are done. Nevertheless, reproducibility and consistency are still better than office readings.

> Educate patients who are monitoring BP's at home as to expected variability. Encourage them *not* to take their blood pressures too often.

RATIONALE FOR TREATMENT OF HYPERTENSION

Treatment of any medical condition is justified if you can show a reduction in morbidity and mortality in response to the therapy. Justification for treatment of hypertension comes from several comprehensive trials. These have shown conclusively that control of BP slows or prevents the complications of HTN and reduces mortality. Importantly, *all* levels of hypertension can be successfully treated and complications lessened.

Complications of hypertension can be divided into two groups:

> Very severe ("malignant") hypertension has an extremely poor prognosis if untreated (only a 10–20% one year survival).

- direct damage to the blood vessels by the elevated pressure, e.g.:
  - ▸ retinopathy
  - ▸ encephalopathy
  - ▸ cerebral hemorrhage
  - ▸ left ventricular hypertrophy
  - ▸ congestive heart failure
  - ▸ renal insufficiency
  - ▸ aortic dissection
- damage caused by acceleration of atherosclerotic disease, including:
  - ▸ cerebral thrombosis ("stroke")

► coronary artery disease syndromes, including myocardial infarction

► peripheral vascular disease.

Clinical trials have shown that antihypertensive treatment is effective in reducing stroke, cardiac failure, left ventricular hypertrophy, progression of renal disease, and overall mortality. However, reduction in rates of myocardial infarction have not been demonstrated; this may be because of the multifactorial etiology of coronary artery disease, short follow-up periods in the studies, or perhaps, the adverse effects on lipid profile of the antihypertensives used in the studies.

In elderly patients, the presence of **isolated systolic hypertension** (ISH) is common because of loss of arterial compliance. ISH, as well as elevations of *both* SBP and DBP, is correlated with increased risk of cardiovascular events and should be treated.

Secondary Hypertension

The vast majority (95%) of patients with high blood pressure have primary or "essential" hypertension.

Primary or "essential" hypertension is diagnosed after excluding diseases in which hypertension is only one manifestation of the disease. The latter disorders are collectively known as causes of "secondary" hypertension, and the more common ones are listed in Table 13-2. In the general population, more than 95% of all individuals with hypertension have "essential" hypertension. Uncovering patients with "secondary" hypertension is important, as successful treatment prevents complications and averts the need for lifelong medical therapy. Your diagnostic process, however, needs to be selective and cost effective.

Features of the patient's history, physical examination, or clinical course which *indicate a higher likelihood of a secondary cause of hypertension* include:

- Age of onset of hypertension before age 20 or after age 50
- Severe hypertension or sudden worsening of previously stable hypertension
- Evidence of end-organ damage (e.g., funduscopic changes greater than Grade II, renal insufficiency, or left ventricular hypertrophy) existing *at the time the hypertension is diagnosed*
- Hypokalemia (potassium level less than 3.5 mg/dl or less than 3.0 mg/dl while on diuretics)
- Abdominal bruits or evidence of other peripheral vascular disease
- Labile pressures especially if tachycardia, sweating, and tremors occur
- Poor response to appropriate antihypertensive therapy.

Table 13-2. Important Causes of Secondary Hypertension

Cause	Pathology or clinical signs	Confirmation of diagnosis
Renal parenchymal disease	Glomerular filtration low, leading to sodium retention and peripheral vasoconstriction.	Elevated serum creatinine and an abnormal urinalysis
Renovascular disease	Renal arteries develop atherosclerosis or fibromuscular dysplasia. Decreased blood flow to the kidney leads to activation of the renin–angiotensin–aldosterone system. Angiotensin causes vasoconstriction while aldosterone leads to sodium retention.	Nuclear renal scanning or arteriography of the renal arteries.
Coarctation of the aorta	Congenital condition in which a constriction is present in the aorta, typically distal to the origin of the left subclavian. The examination may reveal systolic ejection murmur or click (of bicuspid aortic valve).	Confirmed through X-rays, Doppler ultrasound and arteriographic examination.
Primary hyperaldosteronism	Caused by adrenal adenomas or bilateral hypertrophy of the zona glomerulosa. Increased aldosterone leads to hypertension, hypokalemia and metabolic alkalosis.	Confirmed through metabolic testing.
Pheochromocytoma	Catecholamine-producing tumor usually located in the adrenal medulla. A syndrome of paroxysmal or sustained hypertension associated with headache, fever, sweating, and tachycardia may be seen.	Radiologic exams and measurement of urine or plasma catecholamines.
Cushing's syndrome	Oversecretion of cortisol leads to hypertension. The patient presents with truncal obesity, myopathy, bruising and plethora.	Measurement of plasma cortisol after dexamethasone suppression.

Syndrome X

Essential hypertension coexists with three other common medical conditions in many patients. These conditions—obesity, hyperinsulinism and hyperlipidemia—have pathophysiologic links with each other, and with hypertension, which are not fully understood. For example, measures to control one of the disorders will often have a positive impact on other elements of this quadrad. While we still have much to learn about this interrelationship, clinicians acknowledge its existence by referring to patients with all four disorders as having Syndrome X.

APPROACH TO A PATIENT WITH HYPERTENSION

Earlier, we discussed criteria for diagnosing hypertension. After you have established a definite diagnosis of hypertension your patient will return to your office for continuing evaluation, treatment, and follow-up. The goals of your ongoing evaluation are to:

- Delineate the underlying cause of hypertension
- Evaluate any target organ damage resulting from the hypertension
- Identify and control any coexisting (comorbid) medical illnesses (e.g., diabetes mellitus)
- Determine the patient's ability to understand his/her disease, and examine aspects of psychosocial status that may have an impact on therapeutic options.

HISTORY AND PHYSICAL EXAMINATION

Developing the HPI

Many patients with hypertension have *no* symptoms; if any symptoms do occur, they are usually headache, dizziness, flushing, or a feeling of fullness in the head.

Salient questions include:

- When was the last time you had your blood pressure taken? Was it normal?
- What symptoms or signs led to diagnosis of hypertension?
- What symptoms do you have currently?
- Are you taking all your prescribed medications as directed?
- Ask about side effects of medications. Side effects vary by class of medication, but common to a number of antihypertensives are fatigue, fluid retention, and impotence.

- Are you taking any over-the-counter medicines? Ask especially about decongestants, antihistamines, NSAIDs.

Relevant Other History

- Review the patient's social history, including sexual history
- Review your female patients' ob–gyn history
- Ask about symptoms of complications of hypertension (see Table 13-3)
- If you are suspicious that your patient may have secondary rather than essential hypertension, than you will need to inquire about symptoms of the diseases which cause secondary hypertension (review Table 13-2)
- Finally it is important to know about any of the patient's comorbid illnesses which might affect your choice of medication (e.g., prostatic hypertrophy, bronchospasm, lipid abnormalities or diabetes).

Physical Examination

If you have a patient *newly diagnosed with hypertension, a complete physical examination is necessary to rule out a variety of causes of secondary hypertension*.

Table 13-3. Symptoms of Target Organ Damage

Target organ	Symptoms
Eyes	Blurring of vision, new visual field defects
Heart	Symptoms of heart failure such as shortness of breath on exertion, paroxysmal nocturnal dyspnea, orthopnea, nocturia, pink frothy sputum, leg edema
Kidneys	Hematuria, oliguria, nocturia, leg edema, periorbital puffiness
CNS	Change in mental status, new weakness of extremities, new sensory symptoms, gait disturbances
Peripheral vascular disease	Claudication, skin discoloration or hair loss on extremities

On the other hand, if you are seeing a patient in follow-up for *documented* essential hypertension, then emphasis should be placed on assessing end-organ damage resulting from HTN. Particularly important are:

Examination of fundus
Carefully assess for hypertensive retinopathy, classified in Table 13-4.

Neck
Listen for carotid bruits or transmitted murmurs.

Heart
- Evaluate heart size by location of apical impulse
- Look for heaving or hyperdynamic apical impulse suggestive of left ventricular hypertrophy (LVH)
- Listen for third heart sound (S_3) which also suggests LVH
- Listen for fourth heart sound (S_4), common in hypertension
- Listen for murmurs indicating valve lesions.

Table 13-4. Hypertensive Retinopathy

Grade	Findings on funduscopic examination	Duration or severity of HTN
I	Arteriolar spasm leading to "copper wire" or "silver wire" appearance of vessels	Recent onset of hypertension
II	Changes of Grade I, plus arterio-venous nicking ("A-V nicking")—impingement of a vein by sclerotic arteriole	Hypertension for many months, probably years
III	Changes of Grade I and II, plus hemorrhages (diffuse or flame-shaped) and exudates: Soft exudates or "cotton wool" spots—fibrinoid changes Hard exudates—lipoid deposits from healing of old lesions	Severe or accelerated hypertension
IV	Papilledema: Blurred optic disk margins, especially on temporal side	Hypertensive emergency

Lungs

Evaluate for basilar crackles (rales) suggesting congestive heart failure.

Extremities

Evaluate for edema, loss of hair, skin pigmentation changes, diminished pulses.

Nervous system

Evaluate for isolated extremity weakness, reflex abnormalities, sensory loss.

Laboratory Testing in Hypertension

The role of laboratory tests is to:

- identify those individuals with potentially curable (secondary) hypertension (see Secondary Hypertension), and
- evaluate the risk profile of those with essential hypertension (by identifying end-organ damage and coexisting disease).

Initial tests for all hypertensive patients include a *complete blood count, urinalysis, electrolytes, blood urea nitrogen (BUN), creatinine, and lipid profile.* These tests identify renal disease, hyperlipidemia, electrolyte abnormalities and also will rule out anemia and infection. Measurement of 24-hour urine for protein identifies microalbuminuria (urine protein 30–300 mg/day) which estimates the degree of renal damage.

After this initial evaluation, patients whom you suspect of having secondary hypertension should undergo further testing. Several forms of secondary hypertension have characteristic renin–aldosterone profiles. Therefore, characterization of this profile is central to classifying these patients. Serum renin, aldosterone, and urinary sodium are collected after antihypertensive medications are discontinued. Renovascular hypertension, for example, shows high renin–high aldosterone levels, while primary hyperaldosteronism (Conn's syndrome) has a low renin–high aldosterone pattern. Urinary potassium measurement in the presence of serum hypokalemia may be needed.

Thyroid hormone should be checked if there is suspicion of thyroid disease.

Measurements of serum and urinary catecholamines and their metabolites can identify a pheochromocytoma.

Imaging/Other Tests

A chest X-ray will identify heart size and may show the radiographic correlate of coarctation of the aorta, i.e., notching of the inferior border of the ribs.

An EKG may reveal LVH which is characteristic of hypertensive heart disease; it will define the heart rhythm and can provide evidence of ischemia. An *echocardiogram* affords even greater sensitivity for evaluating LVH.

TREATMENT OF HYPERTENSION

Initial nonpharmacologic therapy consists of:

- weight reduction
- moderation of sodium, fat, and alcohol intake
- increase in potassium, magnesium, and calcium intake
- smoking cessation (this has only a short-lived effect on blood pressure, but greatly decreases overall cardiovascular risk)
- discontinuation of all smokeless tobacco products.

Nondrug therapies do not consistently reduce blood pressure as well as medications, but they should be tried because of lack of side-effects and their positive benefits on the overall well being of the patient. In some patients, they *may* obviate the need for medication altogether. Nondrug measures also have promise as **primary prevention strategies** and public education efforts should focus on them.

Eventually, drug therapy is required for most patients with essential hypertension. The goal of therapy is to reduce blood pressure to as nearly normal as possible with the fewest side effects. Even the best drug is useless if not taken correctly, so maximizing compliance is important. Factors which affect compliance include cost, number of required doses in a day, side effects, and the patient's attitude toward their illness; it can be challenging to choose medicines with good compliance profiles that are still effective.

Several classes of drugs may be successfully used to control hypertension. These include the following.

Diuretics, which act by inducing salt loss. They are grouped, according to their mechanism of action in the renal tubule:

- thiazides (such as hydrochlorothiazide)
- loop diuretics (e.g., furosemide)
- potassium sparing agents (e.g., spironolactone).

Adrenergic inhibitors, which act upon the sympathetic nervous system. These are divided into peripherally acting agents (e.g., reserpine); centrally acting agents (e.g., methyldopa); alpha-adrenergic receptor blockers (e.g., prazosin); and beta-adrenergic receptor blockers (cardioselective, e.g., atenolol, or noncardioselective, e.g., propranolol).

Vasodilators, which directly relax smooth muscle. Examples include hydralazine and minoxidil.

Calcium channel blockers, which interfere with calcium-dependent contractions of vascular smooth muscle. Commonly used ones include nifedipine, verapamil and diltiazem.

Angiotensin converting enzyme (ACE) inhibitors, which work by reducing levels of angiotensin in circulation and in tissue. (e.g., captopril).

Angiotensin receptor antagonists which block angiotensin effects. This class includes losartan.

CASE RESOLUTION

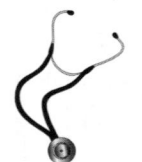

Mr. N.T., a 50-year-old man, comes to your office for his regular appointment. "It's time to get my blood pressure checked again. I'm feeling fine," he reports to your nurse. She records today's BP as 162/100.

This is your patient's regular visit. On reviewing the chart, you note that he has been hypertensive for 7 years, and since he was originally stabilized on his medication, blood pressure readings have been near normal. Immediately you begin considering what might be causing his BP to be higher today.

You repeat the BP and get a reading of 165/105. Having confirmed the nurse's finding, you expand on the history. "Well, Mr. T, your BP reading is higher than usual. How have you been feeling?"

"Like I told your nurse, I am really feeling fine. I may get tired quicker than I used to; but I work every day and I am really OK."

You ask several additional questions and determine that the patient's fatigue is not very significant. He has not changed his diet or had any other symptoms which would have suggested onset of any new medical problems. He takes no over-the-counter medicines. You will need more history to determine the problem.

"Are you taking your medication on schedule like always, Mr. T.?"

"Well, Doc, you caught me there. I have been skipping quite a few doses lately, and
only taking the pills when I feel like my pressure may be going up."
"Why did you start missing your medication doses? You have always taken it faithfully before."
"To be truthful, Doc, it is because I heard guys at work talking about their blood pressure pills causing trouble with, well, you know, their sex life. Since I have noticed a little trouble there myself, I thought I would try doing without the pills. And I *am* better without them."

With careful questioning, you have determined the cause of the patient's loss of blood pressure control. You perform a relevant physical examination, and then decide how to help him overcome his nonadherence problem.

Mr. N.T.'s examination is normal except for the elevated blood pressure reading. You also checked his blood count and chemistry profile. He is not anemic and has normal kidney function, plasma glucose, and electrolytes. He had been taking propranolol (a beta-blocker) at a dose of 20 mg four times daily.

Upon review, you realize that a better medication regimen may now be available for this patient. Many newer drugs cause less impotence, and many can be given once daily which facilitates patient compliance.

"Well Mr. T, let's try a new medication. It will be easier to take, and much less likely to cause you any sexual dysfunction. Try this medication; it's one of the new "ACE inhibitors"."
You discuss the medication with Mr. T. and have him return to be rechecked in 2 weeks. On examination then, his BP is 130/88.
"I am doing great, Doc. I should have called you sooner. I don't have my problem any more."

SUMMARY

Hypertension is an extremely common disorder. We have to be very careful in establishing a diagnosis of HTN as we may be committing a person to life-long medical therapy. A primary care physician plays the central role in providing appropriate treatment of hypertension and preventing serious complications. It is very important to develop sound skills for diagnosis and management of HTN which you will use for a lifetime.

STUDY QUESTIONS*

1. A 25-year-old construction worker had a job-related injury and was sent for evaluation to the nearest emergency department. During treatment there, his blood pressure was 160/100. All of the following are true *except*:
   A. This patient should be diagnosed as definitely having hypertension.
   B. Repeated readings may show variability in blood pressure readings.
   C. The reading by the ER physician is no more valid than that taken by the nurse.
   D. If the patient is a smoker it may not have any impact on his BP.

2. The patient in question 1 was sent to your office for evaluation. In your initial assessment, the history reveals the following points. All have a direct bearing on the finding of elevated blood pressure in this patient *except*:
   A. The patient states he was in pain when the reading was taken.
   B. The patient states he had his usual two cups of coffee that morning before work.
   C. The patient states that he goes out with his friends and has a few beers nightly.
   D. The patient states that his father had hypertension and died of a heart attack at the age of 50.

3. In the treatment of hypertension, which of the following statements is *not* true?
   A. Patients may be told that losing weight and reducing alcohol intake may help reduce blood pressure and make medications unnecessary.
   B. Patients may be told that if they are at Stage 2 hypertension or less, no treatment is necessary.
   C. Older medications compared to newer ones tend to be less costly but usually need to be taken several times a day.
   D. Sometimes blood pressure needs to be monitored outside the medical office setting.

4. Which of the following historical points makes you most suspicious of a secondary cause of hypertension in a 50-year-old woman?
   A. Patient states her high BP began when she was 40 years old.
   B. Patient states her doctors always find her potassium level low.
   C. Patient states her eye examination is always normal though her BP has been high for 10 years.
   D. Patient states that her father is being treated for hypertension.

*For answers, see page 347.

5. Which of the following is *not* an important cause of secondary hypertension?

A.   Renovascular atherosclerosis

B.   Pheochromocytoma

C.   Cushings syndrome

D.   Irritable bowel syndrome

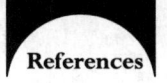

References

1. Archives of Internal Medicine, Vol. 157, 24 Nov. 1997 (entire issue).

Suggested Reading

Braunwald, E. (ed). A Textbook of Cardiovascular Medicine, 5th edn., W.B. Saunders, Philadelphia, 1997.

Iszo, J. and H. Black (eds). Hypertension Primer. American Heart Association, 1993.

Kaplan, N. (ed). Clinical Hypertension, 5th edn., William and Wilkins, Baltimore, 1990.

A Patient with a Red Eye

W. Michael Skeens

INTRODUCTION

CASE PRESENTATION

A 60-year-old man comes to your office with a complaint of redness and pain in his left eye which started abruptly this morning. Except for needing glasses for reading, he has never had eye problems. Since his red eye developed, he has felt a deep throbbing pain in his left eye and his vision has not been as clear as usual. He does not know of trauma to the eye region.

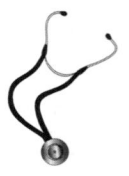

The many causes of red eye may be divided into two broad categories, problems extrinsic to the eye and problems intrinsic to the eye (Table 14-1). Those etiologies which are extrinsic to the eye may be extrinsic or intrinsic to the body itself. The most important point a primary care doctor must learn about treating patients with inflamed-appearing eyes is when to refer the patient to an ophthalmologist. Whenever you are uncertain, err on the safe side by seeking early the opinion of an ophthalmologist. This chapter describes a framework for evaluating red eye.

DEFINITIONS

Angle closure: Narrowing of the angle formed inside the lateral aspects of the anterior chamber where aqueous humor drains

Anterior chamber:	Portion of the eye anterior to the iris
Ciliary body:	Tissue which lies behind the iris, secretes aqueous humor, and controls thinning of the lens of the eye
Conjunctiva:	Thin membrane covering the inner eyelid and anterior sclera
Cornea:	Clear anterior portion of the eye; the terminal edge is the **limbus**
Glaucoma:	Elevated intraocular pressure (IOP) resulting in atrophy of the optic nerve head and visual field deficits
Globe:	The eye
Keratitis:	Corneal inflammation
Posterior chamber:	Portion of the eye posterior to the iris
Sclera:	White appearing tissue forming the outer coat of the eye, excluding the cornea
Snellen chart:	A chart of test objects (optotypes) all of which subtend an angle of 5 minutes of an arc at various distances; measurements are recorded in terms of the distance from the chart (top number) and the distance at which a person with normal vision could read it (bottom number)
Subconjunctival hemorrhage:	Bleeding from conjunctival vessels into the space between the conjunctiva and sclera
Systemic disease:	Disease process involving multiple organ systems in the body
Uveal tract:	Middle layer of the eye consisting of the iris, ciliary body and choroid
Uveitis:	Inflammation of the uveal tract (may be anterior, posterior, or panuveitis)
Vasculitis:	Inflammation of the arteries
Visual acuity:	Measurement of a person's vision recorded from a Snellen chart (20/20, 20/40, etc.)

Table 14-1. Conjunctivitis ("Pink Eye")

Cause	Key signs or symptoms or unique features
Bacterial infection	• Usually *Staph. aureus*, *Strep. pneumoniae*, or *Haemophilus influenzae* • Antibiotic eye drops usually effective
Neisseria gonorrhea	• "Hyper acute" conjunctivitis requiring systemic antibiotics
"Inclusion conjunctivitis"	• Due to *Chlamydia trachomatis* infection acquired at birth • Requires systemic antibiotic
Viral infection	• Most commonly due to adenovirus • Extremely contagious • Symptomatic treament
Allergic	• Due to a variety of allergens, usually affecting other body systems (especially upper respiratory tract) • Symptomatic treatment

COMMON ABBREVIATIONS

OS:	left eye
OD:	right eye
OU:	both eyes
gtts:	drops
EOM:	extraocular muscles
V/A:	visual acuity
Pinhole V/A:	visual acuity test done with the patient looking through a small pinhole in a heavy piece of paper, to check the vision without interference by refractive errors in the patient's eye. This is a good way of measuring best corrected vision without using lenses.

PRIMARY (INTRINSIC) EYE DISORDERS

Recognition of the primary or intrinsic eye disorders is most important, because you most likely will need the assistance of an ophthalmologist in the care of these patients. Infections, glaucoma, and inflammatory conditions are the primary eye disorders most often encountered in a generalist's office practice.

Eye Infections

Bacterial conjunctivitis, the most common disorder causing red eye in the ambulatory care setting, is usually due to *Staphylococcus aureus*, *Pneumococcus*, or *Haemophilus influenzae*. *Neisseria gonorrhea* causes a "hyperacute" conjunctivitis necessitating systemic antibiotic treatment. "Inclusion conjunctivitis" of newborns is due to an infection with *Chlamydia trachomatis* acquired during birth.

Viral conjunctivitis, mainly caused by adenovirus, is commonly seen in ambulatory care. Treatment is symptomatic including cool compresses. Frequently, it is difficult to differentiate on clinical grounds alone between viral and bacterial conjunctivitis. Therefore, antibiotic drops will be prescribed. *It is important to be aware of the ease of spread of conjunctivitis and to educate patients about this problem. Table 14-1 outlines the most important causes of conjunctivitis.*

Previously quite rare in developed nations, fungal and parasitic infections must now be considered in the differential diagnosis of red eye due to the increasing numbers of patients who are immunosuppressed because of acquired immune deficiency syndrome (AIDS) or to chemotherapy. These infections may present as more invasive forms of "ophthalmitis," not confined to the conjunctival tissue.

Herpes zoster infection of the eye is particularly common in the elderly as a part of "shingles." This illness represents reactivation of latent herpes zoster virus in the distribution of the fifth cranial nerve. Evaluation by an ophthalmologist is mandatory. Herpes zoster may cause ophthalmitis or "lightning bolt" corneal ulcers.

> Hand washing is of paramount importance to limit the spread of the infection.

> If your patient with shingles develops a vesicle on the end of their nose, they frequently go on to have ophthalmic herpes.

Glaucoma

Acute angle closure glaucoma can cause red eye and is a medical emergency. Besides redness, the patient has eye pain and sudden blurring of vision. The patient may be acutely ill with nausea and vomiting. On examination, you find very high pressure within the globe, which will close the anterior chamber angle and block aqueous outflow. A "hazy" or "steamy" cornea frequently occurs.

The more chronic and more common "open-angle" glaucoma does not cause red eye. Chronic glaucoma, also a serious eye disorder, does not cause intraocular pressure (IOP) to *suddenly* increase and therefore the aqueous outflow does not become acutely blocked.

Inflammatory Eye Disorders

The iris, ciliary body, and choroid, collectively referred to as the "uveal tract," can be sites of a variety of inflammatory disorders, both localized and systemic. *Any form of uveitis requires definitive ophthalmologic evaluation.* Localized uveitis may be caused by infection, especially tuberculosis or toxoplasmosis, or may be of unknown cause. If the uveitis is thought to be secondary to a systemic disorder such as a connective tissue disease, you will need to evaluate the patient's other organ systems.

SECONDARY (EXTRINSIC) DISORDERS

Other causes of red eye which are not primarily ophthalmologic disorders include trauma (to which the eye may randomly fall victim) and several systemic diseases, which routinely affect the eye along with other organ systems.

Trauma

Eye injuries are particularly frightening to patients because of the threat of blindness. Fortunately, many injuries prove to be superficial and the generalist physician can adequately handle them. Conjunctival abrasions are common, and many patients do not seek medical care for them because they are self-limited. If an abrasion occurs on the *cornea*, or if a foreign body remains in the eye after an injury, pain and redness persist, leading the patient to come in for an evaluation.

When a foreign body in the eye is suspected, a thorough search must be undertaken including an examination of the lower cul-de-sac and eversion of the upper eyelid. Fluorescein staining of the cornea to search for abrasion must be done. If only an abrasion is found, treatment is relatively easy and usually successful; it consists of application of a pressure dressing plus antibiotic ointment. If a foreign body is present, ophthalmologic referral is mandatory.

When red eye is caused by chemical exposure, intense irrigation of the eye is the most important initial step in treatment, including irrigating underneath the upper eyelid. Check the pH in the lower cul-de-sac with litmus paper to verify that it is neutral (pH = 7.0) before discontinuing irrigation.

If there is any evidence of penetration of the eyeball or fracture of the orbit, the patient must be seen by an ophthalmologist.

Allergies

Allergic reactions cause red eye commonly. Allergens induce a conjunctivitis which, although annoying, does not progress to any permanent damage.

Allergic conjunctivitis is generally treated symptomatically with cool compresses. Topical or oral antihistamines may be necessary. Mast cell stabilizing medications (such as cromolyn) may be useful.

Systemic Inflammatory Disorders

Patients with systemic inflammatory disease do not often come to you with a complaint of red eye; however, they do experience it. Systemic disorders which may cause red eye are rheumatoid arthritis, ankylosing spondylitis, and sarcoidosis, as well as certain infections such as toxoplasmosis or histoplasmosis. Red eye in these disorders derives from a uveitis, not conjunctivitis.

Subconjunctival Hemorrhage

Subconjunctival hemorrhage deserves special mention because of its dramatic appearance. A variably sized patch of bright red blood appearing on the sclera alarms most people, and they will quickly call their physician. Fortunately it is almost entirely benign, and it resolves without treatment. It is usually caused by a spontaneous rupture of a tiny conjunctival vessel and less often by extrinsic factors. Although the hemorrhage is benign and it gradually resolves, as would a bruise, the underlying cause *may* need investigation and treatment. Underlying disorders include blood clotting disorders, hypertension, and occasionally trauma.

Recurrent subconjunctival hemorrhages over a short time period should prompt a workup for an underlying cause. Coagulation disorders, thrombocytopenia or a recurrently rupturing vessel are the most likely causes. *If the subconjunctival hemorrhage follows trauma, you must exclude posterior globe rupture or a fracture of an orbital bone.*

HISTORY AND PHYSICAL EXAMINATION

A thorough history will help you in differentiating the myriad causes of red eye. The *time frame of the development of symptoms* and the *sequence of changes* is extremely important. You should not fail to ask whether any *perceived change in visual acuity* has occurred and quantify visual acuity using a Snellen chart.

Developing the HPI

You should pay particular attention to **pain** or **discomfort** accompanying red eye. Deep or severe pain in the eye/orbit indicates more dangerous pathology, such as angle-closure glaucoma. Sensations such as **itching** or **burning**, generally suggest more minor problems like allergies.

Additionally, you must collect information regarding systemic diseases, especially the connective tissue diseases. *Always include a review of the patient's current medications.*

Physical Examination

You will need to do a complete eye examination to determine a diagnosis and to follow the patient's clinical course.

- Measure visual acuity with a Snellen chart.
- Carefully examine the pattern of vessel injection. A **ciliary** (central) pattern of vessel injection resembles a sunburst in the sclera around the cornea. It is more worrisome than the **conjunctival** (peripheral) pattern seen with less severe disease processes (Table 14-2). The conjunctival pattern looks more red than the ciliary pattern, which may appear slightly violaceous.
- An area of diffuse bright redness on the sclera is seen in subconjunctival hemorrhages.
- Examine the pupil and cornea closely. An irregular or nonreacting pupil suggests more severe eye disease. A cloudy appearing cornea results from angle closure glaucoma or occasionally from anterior uveitis. Fluorescein staining will reveal an ulcer or abrasion.
- Assess extraocular muscle actions, especially when you examine a patient with subconjunctival hemorrhage associated with trauma, to exclude muscle entrapment due to fracture.

Table 14-2. Comparison of Pattern of Vessel Injection

Feature	Ciliary (central)	Conjunctival (peripheral)
Involved arteries	Anterior ciliary arteries	Peripheral marginal arcade vessels
Structures inflamed	The cornea, iris, ciliary body	The conjunctivae
Color	Violaceous	Red
Effect on acuity	Decreased	No change
Pain	Severe deep pain	Mild discomfort
Effect of epinephrine	Epinephrine (1:1000) does not affect injection	Epinephrine clears the injection
Condition of cornea	May be cloudy if vessels injected because of angle closure glaucoma	Clear
Condition of iris	Muddled in appearance	Normal
Condition of pupil	May be distorted or nonreactive	Normal
Pupillary light response	Poor in uveitis and absent in angle closure glaucoma	Normal
Intraocular pressure (IOP)	Increased in angle closure glaucoma	Normal

- Sometimes the patient's pupils need to be dilated for a full examination, but when you do this, you must avoid precipitating angle closure glaucoma. Patients with advanced cataracts should *not* generally be dilated in a primary care setting as the angle may be compromised by the cataract pushing forward. To check for adequate anterior chamber depth (open angle), hold a penlight at the lateral aspect of the eye and observe for a crescent shadow medially (Fig. 14-1). If a crescent shadow is present *do not* dilate as it suggests that the angle may already be narrowed.

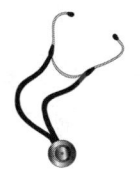

CASE RESOLUTION

A 60-year-old white man comes to your office with a complaint of redness and pain in his left eye which started abruptly this morning. Except for needing glasses for reading, he has never had eye problems. Since his red eye developed, he has felt a deep throbbing pain in his left eye and his

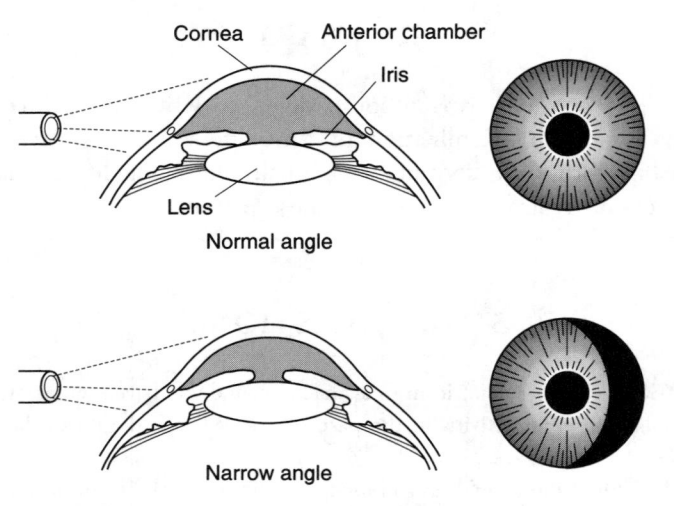

Figure 14-1. Assessing anterior chamber depth by looking for the crescent shadow. (Reprinted with permission from Swartz, *Textbook of Physical Diagnosis: History and Examination*, 2nd ed. W.B. Saunders Co., Philadelphia, 1994, p. 135.)

vision has not been as clear as usual. He does not know of trauma to the eye region.

At this point you know that the patient has pain, a visual change and a red eye. You will need more history and a full eye examination.

He has no other medical problems and he has been well except for a recent "cold," for which he has been taking an over-the-counter cold medicine. After your questioning, he tells you about some slight difficulty in initiating urination since his "cold" began. On examination, the patient's left eye is red, mostly in a "sunburst" pattern around the cornea. The cornea appears slightly cloudy. His visual acuity by the Snellen chart is 20/70 on the left and 20/20 on the right. Last year for an insurance physical, you had recorded 20/20 vision in both eyes.

You now have enough evidence to make a presumptive diagnosis of acute angle-closure glaucoma. You telephone an ophthalmologist who asks you to have the patient come to her office immediately. She determines the patient has greatly increased intraocular pressure in the right eye. Treatment is started immediately and the patient improves.

You ask the patient to return to your office because you note the medication which precipitated his glaucoma also caused him problems urinating. You discover that he has prostatic hypertrophy, for which you initiate treatment.

SUMMARY

Red eye is a common reason for patients to visit their primary care physician. A careful examination of the patient and a good working relationship with your consultant ophthalmologist facilitates diagnosis and successful treatment of most of these patients.

STUDY QUESTIONS*

1. You are a busy pediatrician in a small city, and you have seen eight 5-year-olds with conjunctivitis in the past 2 days. What is the most likely situation?
   A. All of these children had inclusion conjunctivitis as newborns and it is reoccurring.
   B. A chemical factory in your community has released a toxin which causes childhood glaucoma.
   C. All of these children have had eye injuries.
   D. One child with "pink eye" due to adenovirus went with the children on the kindergarten field trip last week.

2. A 23-year-old man presents with a subconjunctival hemorrhage after being involved in a motor vehicle accident. His right eye is affected and he is unable to elevate that eye. This would suggest:
   A. Toxoplasmosis
   B. Acute angle closure glaucoma
   C. Orbit fracture
   D. Conjunctivitis

3. Your old college physics professor comes by your office to have you check his painless red eye which he noted upon arising this morning. He is generally healthy and he has no other bleeding or bruising problems. On examination, his blood pressure is normal and he has subconjunctival hemorrhage. You decide the best treatment would be:
   A. Gentamicin ophthalmic drops
   B. Cool compresses
   C. Observe
   D. i.m. injection of ceftriaxone

4. A 38-year-old woman comes to your office with a red eye after being struck in the left eye with a golf ball. She complains of only mild discomfort. You see a subconjunctival hemorrhage in the left eye. The

*For answers, see page 347.

remainder of her eye examination is limited due to eyelid swelling. You are not sure that the extraocular movements are normal. Visual acuity is difficult to ascertain due to the swelling and tears. Your primary concern should be to rule out:

A.   Conjunctivitis
B.   Glaucoma
C.   Globe rupture
D.   Tear duct obstruction

5.   A 50-year-old machinist developed a painful right eye after some metal shavings blew into his face. On examination, you see a small metal fragment in the lateral cornea which has developed a "rust ring" around it. You should:

A.   Refer to an ophthalmologist as you can not be sure of the depth of penetration and the rust ring should be removed.
B.   Patch the eye and apply antibiotic ointment.
C.   Leave it alone since it is not in the direct visual axis.
D.   Gently remove the fragment.

Suggested Reading

Paton, D., B. Hyman, and J. Justice (eds). Introduction to Ophthalmoscopy: A Scope Publication. The Upjohn Co., Kalamazoo, MI, 1976.

Steinert, R.F. Evaluation of the red eye, in Goroll, A.H., L.A. May, and A.G. Mullery (eds). Primary Care Medicine, 3rd edn, pp. 956–960, J.B. Lippincott Co., Philadelphia, 1995.

A Patient with Congestive Heart Failure

15

Lynne J. Goebel

INTRODUCTION

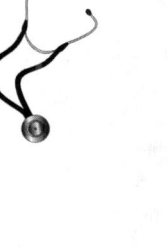

CASE PRESENTATION

An 87-year-old woman comes to your office with the chief complaint of being unable to catch her breath. Her symptoms have increased gradually over the past few weeks. The shortness of breath is worse with exertion. She has trouble especially when she lies down to sleep. She wakes up short of breath several times each night, and for the past week she has been sleeping in her reclining chair. She denies chest pain, but does note palpitations on occasion. The patient also has swelling in her feet and legs. She never had these symptoms before. She has a history of a heart murmur and high blood pressure, but no history of coronary artery disease or rheumatic fever. She never smoked cigarettes or drank alcohol.

Congestive heart failure (CHF) is a common disorder which can present in a number of different ways. Usually patients are older and have coronary artery disease or high blood pressure. But the diagnosis may also be CHF in the younger postpartum patient who appears as if she has pneumonia when she really has postpartum cardiomyopathy. An astute clinician should be able to use the history and physical examination to arrive at a diagnosis of congestive heart failure. Laboratory tests, X-rays and other imaging studies are used to confirm your clinical impression, determine the etiology of heart failure, and guide treatment decisions.

DEFINITIONS

Afterload: the resistance to flow encountered in the systemic circulation.

Ascites: fluid in the abdominal cavity which may be caused by right-sided heart failure. Liver disease such as cirrhosis, kidney disease with fluid overload, and ovarian cancer are other possible causes of ascites.

Constrictive pericarditis: a condition in which the outer layer of the heart restricts the heart's contractility. This can occur in conditions such as tuberculosis, postradiation therapy, postcoronary artery bypass surgery, and infiltration of the pericardium by tumor.

Diastolic dysfunction: stiffening or poor relaxation of the left ventricle which causes inefficient filling. This is seen in hypertension and hypertrophic or restrictive cardiomyopathies.

Ejection fraction: the amount of blood ejected from the ventricle during systole. Normally this is greater than 50%.

Gallops: extra heart sounds in addition to S1 and S2. An S3 gallop occurs *after the second heart sound* and sounds like "Ken-tuck-y" ("Ken" = S1, "tuck" = S2, "y" = S3). It is indicative of heart failure. An S4 gallop occurs *before the first heart sound* and sounds like "Ten-nes-see" ("Ten" = S4, "nes" = S1, "see" = S2). It indicates atrial contraction into a stiffened ventricle such as in hypertension. Gallops may be normal in young children.

Hepatojugular reflux (HJR): sustained distention of jugular veins seen when, on physical examination, you press just under the liver for 20–30 seconds.

Jugular venous distention (JVD):

engorged appearance of jugular veins seen when pressure on the right side of the heart is elevated. JVD can be estimated by laying the patient down and raising the head of the bed 45°. Draw an imaginary horizontal line from the top of the jugular venous pulsations to the sternal angle. The vertical distance from this line to the sternal angle is the jugular venous pressure measured in centimeters (Figure 15-1). A normal reading is less than 5 cm.

Left-sided heart failure:

weakness of the left ventricle leading to elevated end diastolic pressure and back-up of fluid into the lungs (called pulmonary edema).

Orthopnea:

a need to sleep sitting up or propped up on several pillows. It is usually described by the number of pillows, e.g., two pillow orthopnea.

Paroxysmal nocturnal dyspnea (PND):

waking up from sleep with sudden shortness of breath. Patients sometimes say that they need to sit up or go to an open window in order to breathe.

Pedal edema:

swelling of the feet.

Pericardial tamponade:

restriction of cardiac filling and emptying by fluid surrounding the heart in the pericardial sac.

Preload:

filling pressure of the heart.

Pulse pressure:

the difference between systolic and diastolic blood pressure. If blood pressure is 140/80, the pulse pressure would be 140–80 = 60 mmHg.

Rales:

wet crackling sounds heard on auscultation when interstitial or alveolar lung space is filled with fluid. Dry rales are crackles that are heard with some

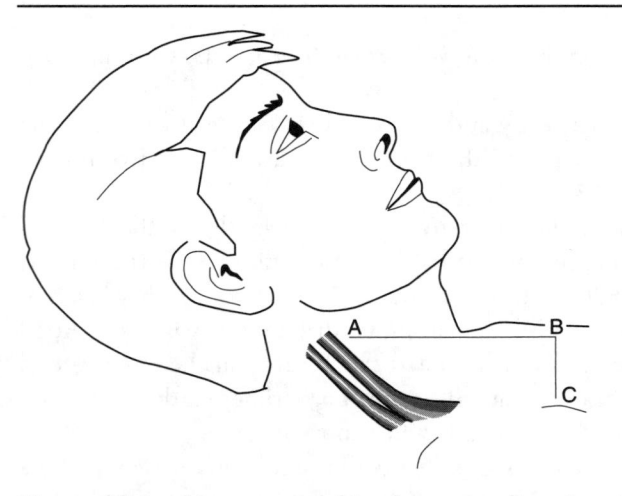

Figure 15-1. Measurement of jugular venous distension. A, top of jugular pulsation; C, sternal angle; B–C, jugular venous pressure (cm). (Illustrated by the author.)

interstitial lung diseases such as pulmonary fibrosis.

Right-sided heart failure: weakness of the right ventricle causing fluid to back up into the abdomen and feet.

CAUSES OF CONGESTIVE HEART FAILURE

Left-sided Heart Failure

When the left ventricle is weakened it becomes an inefficient pump, causing blood to "back up" *into the lungs*. The high back pressure placed on the pulmonary circulation by the failing left ventricle causes fluid to leak from the vessels into the interstitial spaces of the lung (pulmonary edema). Symptoms of shortness of breath, paroxysmal nocturnal dyspnea (PND), and orthopnea predominate in left-sided heart failure. The most common cause is **coronary artery disease**. An acute heart attack may certainly cause heart failure, but even transient ischemia may create enough myocardial dysfunction to allow pulmonary edema to occur.

Another fairly common cause of left-sided CHF is **valvular heart disease** such as aortic stenosis or mitral regurgitation. This diagnosis is usually apparent by the presence of a heart murmur on examination.

Uncontrolled **hypertension** can make the left ventricle "stiff" and lead to poor diastolic filling. This is referred to as *diastolic dysfunction*. The

left ventricular ejection fraction is normal in patients with diastolic dysfunction.

Dilated cardiomyopathy and **myocarditis** can lead to CHF. The history should provide clues to the many etiologies of these two potential disorders (Table 15-1).

Arrhythmias cause the heart to work inefficiently. If the heart is beating too fast such as in rapid atrial fibrillation, filling time is too short and cardiac output falls. Similarly, if the heart beats too slowly, such as in sick sinus syndrome with long pauses, cardiac output will drop. Atrial fibrillation can cause symptomatic heart failure even in the absence of a rapid heart rate because patients with borderline cardiac function depend on the atrial "kick" to assist in ventricular filling.

High-output heart failure is less commonly seen. So far we have been discussing causes of low-output heart failure. Patients with low-output failure have constricted peripheral blood vessels and a narrow pulse pressure. In contrast, patients with high-output heart failure have warm extremities and wide or normal pulse pressure. In high-output failure there is a normally functioning heart but such a large myocardial demand that a relative state of inadequate cardiac output exists. Some causes of high-output failure are **anemia, thyrotoxicosis, Paget's disease, multiple arteriovenous fistulas,** and **beriberi** (thiamine

Table 15-1. Some Causes of Cardiomyopathy and Myocarditis

Coronary artery disease	Toxins
Infections	Adriamycin
Viral	Bleomycin
Parasitic (Chagas)	Cyclophosphamide
Mycobacterial	Alcohol
Collagen vascular disease	Radiation
Infiltrative disease	Muscular dystrophy
Sarcoidosis	Rheumatic fever
Amyloidosis	Sickle cell anemia
Hemochromatosis	Hypersensitivity
Glycogen storage disorders	Nutritional
Gaucher's disease	Beriberi
Whipple's disease	Postpartum
Sphingolipidoses	Hyperthyroidism
Fabry's disease	Hypothyroidism
Mucopolysaccharidosis	Idiopathic

deficiency). Patients are more likely to develop symptoms of high-output CHF when the underlying disease is sudden in onset such as acute blood loss anemia or thyroid storm, than with slowly developing diseases such as Paget's disease.

Right-sided Heart Failure

Weakness of the right side of the heart causes blood to "back up" *into the abdomen and feet*. Fluid leaks from the capillaries because of back pressure and this causes the main signs of right-sided CHF, pedal edema and ascites. The most common cause of right-sided heart failure is **left-sided heart failure**. High pressures on the left side of the heart are transmitted backward through the pulmonary circulation, eventually causing the right ventricle to weaken.

Chronic lung disease such as emphysema, asthma, chronic bronchitis or cystic fibrosis can cause right-sided heart failure by causing pulmonary hypertension. Pulmonary hypertension is elevation of the normally low pressures in the arteries of the lungs. In a separate disease called **primary pulmonary hypertension**, the cause of the elevated pressure is not known.

Pulmonic valve stenosis and **tricuspid insufficiency** can lead to elevated right heart pressure and symptoms of right heart failure. Rheumatic heart disease is one of the main causes of these valve disorders.

Any of the congenital heart conditions which result in **left to right shunt** can cause right ventricular fluid overload and failure as blood flows from the high pressure on the left side of the circulation to the low pressure on the right side. An example would be a ventricular septal defect.

Pericardial disease can lead to inadequate filling, as in constrictive pericarditis or pericardial tamponade; this will cause breathlessness, but usually no rales. The predominant physical examination findings are those of right heart failure with jugular venous distention and peripheral edema.

In **restrictive cardiomyopathies** such as amyloidosis, infiltrates in the myocardium cause predominantly right-sided symptoms; there may be left-sided symptoms if the stiff left ventricle does not fill well (diastolic dysfunction).

HISTORY AND PHYSICAL EXAMINATION

Developing the HPI (Table 15-2)

Left-sided heart failure

Symptoms of congestive heart failure can develop acutely or subacutely depending on the etiology. Acute heart failure often requires intensive care unit or telemetry monitoring, therefore it is important to know *when symptoms began*. Include questions about shortness of breath, dyspnea on exertion, paroxysmal nocturnal dyspnea (PND), orthopnea, pedal edema, chest pain, cough, frothy blood-tinged sputum, wheezing, and palpitations. Be sure to ask about diet and medication compliance.

Right-sided heart failure

Patients generally complain of swelling in their legs and sometimes in their abdomen. If they have concurrent left-sided failure then the symptoms listed above will also be present.

Relevant Other History

Left-sided heart failure

Ask about past diagnoses such as coronary artery disease, hypertension, diabetes mellitus, rheumatic fever, and atrial fibrillation. Recent illnesses such as a viral infection, excessive menstrual bleeding, or heavy bleeding from any cause may be relevant. Note any symptoms of thyroid disease such as heat or cold intolerance. Keep in mind the myriad causes of dilated cardiomyopathy and ask about a of history of toxin exposure such as alcohol, chemotherapy, or radiation therapy.

Table 15-2. CHF: Important Elements of History

Symptom	Left-sided failure	Right-sided failure
Shortness of breath	Yes	Sometimes, due to lung disease
Paroxysmal nocturnal dyspnea	Yes	No
Orthopnea	Yes	No
Swelling in feet or abdomen	No	Yes

Right-sided heart failure

Chronic lung disease is the most important diagnosis to explore in patients with right-sided heart failure. Cancers which spread to the pericardium such as breast, lung, and lymphoma may cause right-sided heart failure. A history of using appetite suppressants such as dexfenfluramine is important if primary pulmonary hypertension is suspected.

Ask the patient if they have used "diet pills."

Physical Examination (see Table 15-3)

Pertinent physical examination includes:

- *Vital signs*—Look especially for slow, rapid or irregular pulse, rapid respirations, wide or narrow pulse pressure, high blood pressure, jugular venous pressure above 5 cm, hepatojugular reflux or ascites
- *Lung exam*—Examine for rales (wet or dry), wheezes, dullness at the bases
- *Heart exam*—Listen especially for mitral or aortic murmurs (left), pulmonic or tricuspid murmurs (right), gallops (S3 or S4)
- *Peripheral edema*—Foot, ankle and leg swelling are important clues.

Edema is graded from trace to 4+ depending on how deeply you can press your finger into the edematous area. It is also described according to the height of the edema on the leg and whether or not it is "pitting" edema. Edema is pitting if, when you press your finger into it, a depression is left in the skin. For example, a patient may have "2+ pitting edema to the level of the knees."

Table 15-3. CHF: Important Elements of Physical Examination

Physical finding	Left-sided failure	Right-sided failure
Jugular venous distention	Yes	Yes
Hepatojugular reflux	Sometimes	Yes
Rales	Yes (wet)	Sometimes (dry)
Wheezes	Occasionally	Often, due to lung disease
S3 at apex	Yes	No
Pedal edema	No	Yes
Ascites	No	Often

ANCILLARY TESTING

Chest X-ray

This can be helpful in evaluating heart size. In CHF the heart will be large and possibly globular appearing on the PA (posteroanterior view) chest X-ray. In addition, there are some classic findings on X-ray in pulmonary edema secondary to **left-sided heart failure**: Kerley B lines which are horizontal lines in the lung periphery indicating interstitial fluid; cephalization-engorged blood vessels in the upper part of the lung fields; and a fluid-filled minor fissure. A largely right-sided or bilateral pleural effusion may be seen (Figure 15-2).

With **right-sided heart failure** the chest X-ray can help diagnose and quantify chronic lung disease. With emphysema and asthma you see over-inflation of the lungs and flattening of the diaphragms. In emphysema there may be "bullous" changes which show up on X-ray as large dark spaces devoid of normal lung tissue. Cystic fibrosis has a characteristic honeycomb appearance on X-ray. Also in right-sided CHF, the right ventricle becomes enlarged and takes up more of the retrosternal space on the lateral chest X-ray. Table 15-4 summarizes the X-ray findings in CHF.

Electrocardiogram (EKG)

The EKG can provide electrical evidence of ischemia or an acute myocardial infarction; it shows the heart rate and rhythm.

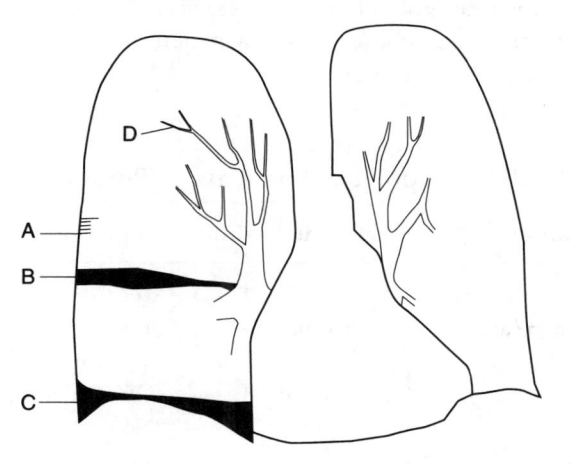

Figure 15-2. X-ray findings in CHF. A, Kerley B lines; B, fluid in minor fissure; C, pleural effusion; D, cephalization.

Table 15-4. X-ray Findings in CHF

Finding	Left-sided failure	Right-sided failure
Kerley B lines	Yes	No
Cephalization	Yes	No
Pleural effusion	Yes	No
Overinflation/flat diaphragms	No	Sometimes
Bullous disease/honeycomb pattern	No	Sometimes
Decreased retrosternal air space on lateral film	No	Sometimes
Enlarged heart on PA film	Yes	No

Arterial Blood Gas (ABG)

Although not necessarily a diagnostic tool, in the patient who is short of breath, ABGs can guide oxygen therapy and document the need for ventilator support. Pulse oximetry, which noninvasively measures oxygen saturation in the blood, may be sufficient monitoring in the patient who is not acutely ill.

Blood Tests

Complete blood count, liver function and kidney function tests, electrolytes, calcium, magnesium and phosphorus, and thyroid stimulating hormone are the usual initial blood tests ordered to evaluate the cause of congestive heart failure. If acute myocardial infarction is suspected, cardiac enzymes are ordered (see Chapter 11). Other tests may be needed to evaluate the patient for cardiomyopathy and myositis.

Echocardiogram

This is an ultrasound examination of the heart. It is especially helpful in assessing wall motion abnormalities which may indicate coronary artery disease. The echocardiogram aids in evaluating the heart valves. It is *not* the best test for determining the overall function of the heart, but you can get an estimate of the ejection fraction to guide therapy for heart failure. For example, afterload reduction is beneficial in patients with

low ejection fractions and calcium channel blockers may be better in patients with diastolic dysfunction. Because the quality of an echocardiogram is compromised in patients with bullous lung disease or obesity, a MUGA scan (see below) is the preferred test to measure ejection fraction.

Multigated Scan (MUGA)

This nuclear medicine scan of the heart uses tagged red blood cells to get a picture of the inside of the heart rather than the walls or valves. *The MUGA scan is the best test to determine the ejection fraction*. It is also called radionuclide cineangiography or RNCA.

Cardiac Catheterization

In cardiac catheterization a catheter is placed in the femoral artery and threaded up the aorta to the coronary arteries. Dye is injected to delineate the anatomy and any blockages that may be present in the coronary arteries. This test is not routinely ordered for all patients with heart failure.

Cardiac Muscle Biopsy

A catheter can be inserted into the subclavian vein on the right and threaded into the heart to biopsy the heart muscle. This can be helpful in determining the etiology of a cardiomyopathy thought to be due to, for example, infiltrating diseases, granulomatous diseases, or myositis.

Holter Monitor

This is a continuous electrocardiographic record of the heart rhythm. It is done over a period of 24–48 hours. This test detects brady- or tachyarrhythmias.

PUTTING IT ALL TOGETHER

Your history and physical should guide you to the most likely diagnosis. The laboratory data will be confirmatory for the most part. Special studies such as the echocardiogram and MUGA tests may be performed to help to tailor the patient's therapy. For example, patients with CHF and normal ejection fractions usually have diastolic dysfunction and require aggressive treatment of their hypertension. Patients with reduced ejection fraction may benefit from afterload reduction with angiotensin-converting enzyme inhibitors. In addition, patients with a low ejection fraction may improve on diuretics and digitalis. In cases where the ejection fraction is below 15%, anticoagulation would be considered to prevent blood clots from forming in the heart.

CASE RESOLUTION

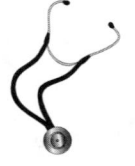

An 87-year-old woman comes to your office with the chief complaint of being unable to catch her breath. Her symptoms have increased gradually over the past few weeks. The shortness of breath is worse with exertion. She has trouble especially when she lies down to sleep. She wakes up short of breath several times each night, and for the past week she has been sleeping in her reclining chair. She denies chest pain, but does note palpitations on occasion. The patient also has swelling in her feet and legs. She never had these symptoms before. She has a history of a heart murmur and high blood pressure, but no history of coronary artery disease or rheumatic fever. She never smoked cigarettes or drank alcohol.

You have an 87-year-old woman with gradual onset of shortness of breath over a few weeks. She has PND, orthopnea and pedal edema. She denies chest pain or known history of coronary artery disease, but admits to palpitations. She has a history of a heart murmur and high blood pressure.

Your impression is that she has symptoms of left-sided heart failure which could be caused by either arrhythmia, valvular heart disease, or hypertensive heart disease. Given her age she certainly could have coronary artery disease as well. Her social history is negative for alcohol, cigarettes, or illicit drug use. Her past medical history is negative for cancer, anemia, or thyroid disease. Her medications are hydrochlorothiazide 25 mg which she takes for her blood pressure once daily.

On physical exam you find the following:

- General appearance: thin white female with mildly increased respirations
- Vital signs: Blood pressure normal at 130/85, pulse tachycardic at 120 and irregular, respirations elevated at 28, temperature 98 °F
- Jugular venous distention to 8 cm at 45 degrees
- No thyromegaly
- Rales heard from the lung bases to half way up the chest bilaterally, dullness at both lung bases
- Heart sounds, irregularly irregular with an S3 heard at the apex and a grade III/VI holosystolic murmur heard best at the apex, radiating to the axilla
- Abdominal examination, slightly tender liver, mildly enlarged at 13 cm in the midclavicular line; positive hepatojugular reflux
- Extremities, cool dry skin, intact pulses, and 2+ pitting edema to the midcalf bilaterally.

The examination confirms your suspicion of left-sided heart failure with some features of right-sided failure as well. The irregular rapid heart beat needs further evaluation with an EKG (Figure 15-3).

The EKG shows an irregularly irregular rhythm consistent with atrial fibrillation. There are some nonspecific ST–T wave abnormalities and evidence of left ventricular hypertrophy.

Atrial fibrillation may be the etiology for heart failure in an elderly patient who has borderline heart function from longstanding hypertension and is dependent on the atrial "kick" to preserve cardiac output. Rapid heart rate can cause heart failure secondary to inadequate time for diastolic filling. Rheumatic heart disease is a diagnostic possibility with her murmur which sounds like mitral regurgitation. (The regurgitation causes stretching of the left atrium which can lead to atrial fibrillation.) In addition, myocardial infarction is still in the differential diagnosis, since it too can cause atrial fibrillation and heart failure. Don't forget

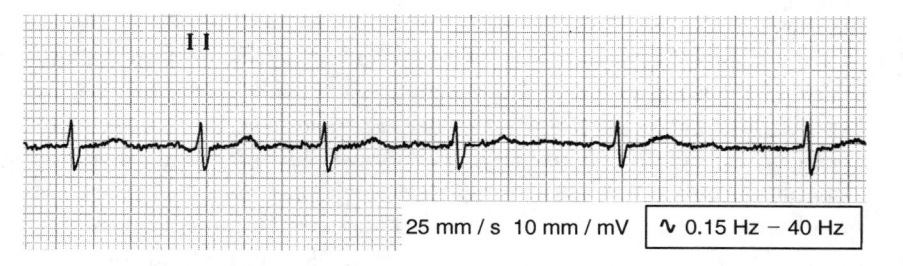

Figure 15-3. EKG rhythm strip of atrial fibrillation.

hyperthyroidism which can present in the elderly with atrial fibrillation and congestive heart failure.

You order a chest X-ray, pulse oximetry, complete blood count, electrolytes, liver function, kidney function, calcium, magnesium, phosphorus, and thyroid stimulating hormone.

The chest X-ray confirms an enlarged heart, cephalization, and small bilateral pleural effusions. The pulse oximetry shows 91% (slightly low). The other studies are normal.

You decide to admit the patient to the hospital for treatment of her rapid atrial fibrillation and heart failure. You put her on the telemetry unit where they can monitor her heart. You order an echocardiogram to assess valvular function, wall motion abnormalities, size of the left atrium and the ejection fraction.

The echocardiogram shows moderate to severe mitral regurgitation with an enlarged left atrium. The left ventricle is thickened and has a moderately decreased ejection fraction of 40%. There are no regional wall motion abnormalities.

Given the patient's age you decide to try medical management with digoxin, diuretics and afterload reduction with angiotensin converting enzyme inhibitor. The patient will likely remain in atrial fibrillation and consideration will be given to anticoagulation or aspirin to help prevent embolic stroke.

STUDY QUESTIONS*

1. A 23-year-old woman presents with shortness of breath and wheezing. She has no history of asthma. She has PND and orthopnea, but no pedal edema. Her only medical history is that she delivered a healthy baby boy two weeks ago. At this point you suspect that she has:
   A. Right-sided heart failure
   B. Postpartum cardiomyopathy
   C. Pneumonia
   D. Lupus

2. A 55-year-old man is being followed for hypertension in your office. He could not afford his medication and therefore has not taken any pills for

---

*For answers, see page 347.

two weeks. He is complaining of shortness of breath. His blood pressure is 200/120. He likely has all of the following *except*:

A. An S4 heard on cardiac exam
B. Diastolic dysfunction
C. Tricuspid valve regurgitation
D. Left ventricular hypertrophy on EKG

3. A 72-year-old woman presents with shortness of breath and severe crushing chest pain of three hour's duration. She has rales at both lung bases and an S3 on cardiac examination. There is no pedal edema. Your impression is:
    A. Coronary artery disease and high output failure
    B. Coronary artery disease and left-sided heart failure
    C. Coronary artery disease and right-sided heart failure
    D. Noncardiac chest pain

4. A 65-year-old man with a 100 pack per year smoking history presents with gradual onset of swelling in his legs over the past few weeks. He has a chronic cough productive of clear sputum and chronic dyspnea on exertion. A chest X-ray shows flattening of the diaphragms and over-inflation of the lungs.
    Your clinical impression is:
    A. Chronic lung disease with right-sided heart failure
    B. Left-sided congestive heart failure
    C. Pneumonia
    D. Cystic fibrosis

5. A 60-year-old obese female presents with left-sided heart failure of acute onset. You decide to admit her to the hospital for further evaluation and treatment. After you rule out myocardial infarction the most appropriate noninvasive test to evaluate her left ventricular ejection fraction would be:
    A. Electrocardiogram
    B. Echocardiogram
    C. Cardiac catheterization
    D. Multigated scan (MUGA)

A Patient with  16
Diabetes Mellitus

Henry K. Driscoll, John W. Leidy, Jr. and
Bruce S. Chertow

INTRODUCTION

CASE PRESENTATION

A 60-year-old man came to the office because of an abnormal laboratory test found during health screening at his work place. A nonfasting blood sugar (or "plasma glucose") was found to be 230 mg/dl (which is quite high). His previous health care had been intermittent, with occasional visits to an emergency room for sore throats, bronchitis, and muscle strain. He reports to you, "I feel fine for a man my age, but the nurse at work told me I had better see a doctor right away."

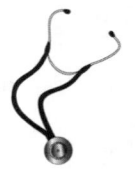

The American Diabetes Association's Expert Committee on the Diagnosis and Classification of Diabetes Mellitus has defined diabetes as "a group of metabolic diseases characterized by hyperglycemia resulting from defects in insulin secretion, insulin action, or both. The chronic hyperglycemia of diabetes is associated with longterm damage, dysfunction, and failure of various organs, especially the eyes, kidneys, nerves, heart, and blood vessels." This chapter introduces this extremely important disease which you will see frequently in your clinical experiences.

DEFINITIONS

Diabetic complications: damage to tissues resulting from chronic hyperglycemia. Usually the term refers to damage to the eyes (retinopathy), damage

to the kidneys (nephropathy), damage to nerves (neuropathy), and damage to blood vessels (vasculopathy).

Macrovascular complications:

damage to organs resulting from athero- sclerosis of the large and medium size arteries supplying the organ. These compli- cations include injuries from occlusion of vessels supplying the brain (cerebrovascular disease), the heart (cardiovascular disease), and the extremities (peripheral vascular dis- ease).

Microvascular complications:

damage to organs or tissues resulting from blood vessel damage that is apparent at a microscopic level. These complications include damage to the retina, with leakage, bleeding, and formation of new vessels. In kidney damage (nephropathy) the glomeruli are primarily affected. In damage to nerves (neuropathy) there is impairment of circula- tion at the microscopic level, but derange- ments of the metabolism inside the neuron may be more important in damaging the nerves.

Fasting: no caloric intake for at least 8 hours.

Obesity: a condition in which the weight is greater than 20% above ideal body weight. Alternatively a body mass index (BMI) can be calculated by dividing the body mass (kg) by the height squared (meters^2). Obesity is defined as BMI $\geq 27\,kg/m^2$.

Impaired glucose tolerance and impaired fasting glucose:

a metabolic stage where blood sugars are not completely normal but do not meet the cri- teria for diagnosing diabetes.

IGT refers to a patient who has a plasma glucose $\geq 140\,mg/dl$ but $< 200\,mg/dl$ 2 hours after a 75 g glucose "meal."

IFG refers to patients with fasting glucose $\geq 110\,mg/dl$ but $< 126\,mg/dl$

CLASSIFICATION AND DEMOGRAPHICS OF DIABETES MELLITUS

Diabetes mellitus can be classified into several types based on the etiology or clinical features. In **type 1 diabetes** there is destruction of the insulin-secreting beta cells of the pancreatic islets, usually by autoimmune mechanisms. Typically, type 1 diabetes occurs in children and young adults. It frequently begins suddenly with severe symptoms of insulin deficiency and the development of diabetic ketoacidosis. In this condition the *level of insulin is very low*, and the body is in a state similar to severe starvation. As glucose cannot be utilized normally, stored energy from fat is broken down to ketone bodies. Because ketone bodies are acidic, a metabolic acidosis results which can be life threatening. Patients with type 1 diabetes require lifelong insulin replacement.

> Type 1 diabetes mellitus has previously been called insulin-dependent diabetes and juvenile diabetes.

The most common type of diabetes mellitus is **type 2**. In this condition hyperglycemia develops because of a *combination of defects in insulin secretion and resistance to its action*. Approximately 90% of diabetic patients have type 2 diabetes mellitus. It occurs with increasing frequency with advancing age, and it runs strongly in families. The risk of developing type 2 diabetes for a person who has a first-degree relative with type 2 diabetes varies widely in differing populations, but averages 15–35%. In contrast, in type 1 diabetes the risk is about 5%. Obesity is a major risk factor in the development of type 2 diabetes.

> Type 2 diabetes was previously called non-insulin-dependent diabetes mellitus or adult-onset diabetes mellitus.

Other specific types of diabetes develop in patients who:

- have pancreatic disease or surgery
- use drugs which cause hyperglycemia
- have infections which result in loss of insulin-producing cells
- have defects in the receptors which mediate insulin action
- have defects in the mechanisms of insulin secretion
- are pregnant; most frequently this diabetic state develops in the third trimester, and is called **gestational diabetes mellitus**.

Insulin resistance is prominent in pregnancy due to the gestational hormones, especially human placental lactogen and estrogens. Screening for the presence of gestational diabetes is important, as control of blood sugar has clearly been shown to avoid perinatal complications and improve fetal, neonatal, and maternal outcomes.

Diabetes occurs commonly in the United States; approximately 8% of persons in the US aged 40 to 74 years carry a diagnosis of diabetes. At least as many more persons may have the disease but remain undiagnosed. Risk of developing diabetes varies among population groups. Risk

of type 2 diabetes is higher among African Americans, Latinos, and Native Americans. Type 1 diabetes also varies among differing populations. The highest prevalence is in Finland, Sardinia, and Scandinavia, and the lowest rates occur in Korea, Mexico, China, Japan, and among Native Americans.

The *estimated cost of diabetes in the United States exceeds $90 billion annually*. Approximately one-half the costs are direct costs for hospital, nursing home, and outpatient treatment of patients with diabetes. *This amount represents nearly 12% of total US health care expenditures.* No other single disease compares to diabetes mellitus in this respect.

DIAGNOSIS OF DIABETES

Current criteria for the diagnosis of diabetes mellitus are:

- the presence of symptoms (polyuria, polydipsia, unexplained weight loss) and a random plasma glucose concentration ≥ 200 mg/dl **or**
- fasting plasma glucose ≥ 126 mg/dl, with fasting defined as no caloric intake for at least 8 hours **or**
- a 2-hour postglucose load plasma glucose level ≥ 200 mg/dl during an oral glucose tolerance test in which the patient ingests 75 g of glucose.

These criteria should be confirmed by repeat testing before firmly establishing the diagnosis. In practice the diagnosis is not usually in question, and the criteria of fasting plasma glucose or random plasma glucose are easy to obtain, so oral glucose tolerance testing is not generally required.

COMPLICATIONS OF DIABETES MELLITUS

Good blood sugar control can definitely slow the complications of diabetes.

The complications of diabetes mellitus include retinopathy (damage to the retina), nephropathy (damage to the kidneys), neuropathy (damage to the nerves), and vasculopathy (damage to the blood vessels, particularly the arterial circulation). In 1993 the Diabetes Control and Complications Trial, a comprehensive 9-year study of 1441 patients with type 1 diabetes, demonstrated clearly that reduction of hyperglycemia can prevent and slow the progression of the complications of retinopathy, nephropathy, and neuropathy. Therefore, these complications are believed to be secondary to the hyperglycemic state. Further

studies are in progress to link reduction of hyperglycemia conclusively with prevention of vasculopathy.

Retinopathy is the most frequent and often the earliest complication to develop in diabetes (Table 16-1). In patients with type 2 diabetes retinopathy can be present at the time of first diagnosis. In this case, it is likely that the disease was present but clinically inapparent for several years prior to the diagnosis. Diabetic retinopathy initially develops as **nonproliferative (background) retinopathy** manifested by dot and blot hemorrhages, microaneurysms, and soft and hard exudates in the retina (See Figure 16-1). Most often, nonproliferative changes do not seriously threaten vision unless the background changes involve the macula.

With continuing hyperglycemia growth of new blood vessels develops, a process termed **proliferative diabetic retinopathy**. The most severe visual loss associated with diabetes mellitus results from this form of retinopathy; patients are prone to hemorrhage with subsequent scarring, retinal detachment, and severe visual loss. Laser photocoagulation of proliferative retinopathy, swelling around the macula (macular edema) and background changes around the macula has proven very beneficial in reducing severe visual loss.

> Early detection by frequent ophthalmologic exams and prompt treatment are the keys to avoid severe visual loss from diabetes mellitus.

Nephropathy is another serious complication of diabetes mellitus (Table 16-2). The appearance of protein in the urine is the earliest hallmark of diabetic nephropathy, reflecting damage to the glomeruli. In the early stages "microalbuminuria" occurs—protein excretion of 30–300 mg per day—and in the later advanced stages "frank proteinuria" occurs, excretion of 300 mg or more per day.

> Early in the course of diabetic nephropathy, both protein and blood may be excreted in the urine.

Several interventions prevent the progression of diabetic nephropathy. These should be initiated early in the disease when only microalbuminuria is present. They are:

- *Most important, strict control of hypertension*. The target blood pressure for diabetic patients should be 120/80 (rather than the target of 140/90 for the general population).
- *Restriction of protein intake*. The current diet recommended for patients with diabetes mellitus includes 0.8 g protein per kg ideal body weight, per day (sufficient protein for maintenance, but little enough to reduce the progression of nephropathy).

> Routine urinalysis dipstick checks for protein are insensitive as a screen for early nephropathy.

- *Administration of angiotensin-converting-enzyme (ACE) inhibitors*. These drugs reduce proteinuria and limit the progression of diabetic nephropathy independent of their antihypertensive effects. If the patient can tolerate an ACE inhibitor, one should be prescribed for patients with diabetic nephropathy.

Table 16-1. Diabetic Retinopathy

Type	Frequency	Visual changes	Key signs and symptoms/ unique features
Non-proliferative (background)	Very common	• Usually no symptoms unless changes are at the macula and lead to visual loss	• Microaneurysms, dot and blot hemorrhages, and soft and hard exudates may be present • Laser photocoagulation may help prevent visual loss from background changes involving the macula • Periodic eye examinations by ophthalmologist recommended.
Advanced non-proliferative	Common	• Visual loss *can* occur	• Intraretinal microvascular abnormalities, macular edema, larger hemorrhages, and more soft exudates (indicating ischemia) may be present • No new vessel formation • Laser photocoagulation can help prevent visual loss • More frequent ophthalmologic examinations necessary
Proliferative	Common	• Visual loss is common, especially from hemorrhage	• New vessels grow on the retina, into the vitreous, or on the iris • Glaucoma can occur from new vessels or hemorrhage • Bleeding and scarring can lead to blindness • Laser photocoagulation generally used, and other surgical procedures (such as vitrectomy) may be helpful • Requires immediate referral to ophthalmologist when detected

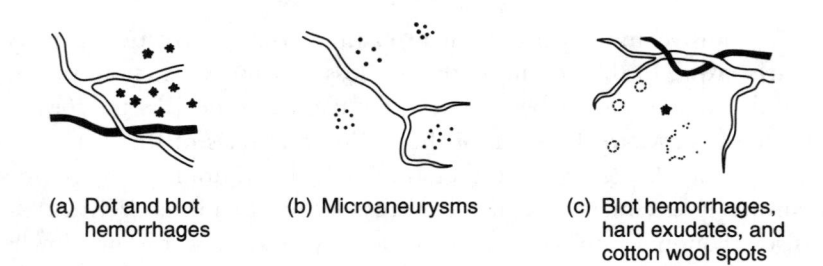

Figure 16-1. Patterns of diabetic retinopathy. (Adapted from DeGowin and DeGowin, *Diagnostic Examination*, 6th edn., McGraw-Hill, New York, 1994, p. 118.)

Table 16-2. Diabetic Nephropathy

Stage	Amount of protein	Symptoms	Blood pressure	Progression
Micro-albuminuria	30–300 mg/24hr	• None	• May or may not be elevated	• Patients are at risk of progression to more advanced nephropathy
Frank protei-nuria	>300 mg/24hr	• Symptoms related to specific syndromes, e.g., severe hypertension, nephrotic syndrome, or end-stage renal disease	• Usually elevated	• Patients likely to progress to end-stage renal disease if not treated

- *Hyperglycemia reduction*. Strict glucose control reduces the progression of diabetic nephropathy.

Neuropathy is a third diabetic complication (Table 16-3). Nerve damage is caused by both interruption of the blood supply to the nerves and the accumulation of metabolic products within the nerve cells which eventually are toxic to nerve function.

Most patients experience burning or shooting pain especially on the bottom of the feet which may keep them awake at night.

The most common diabetic neuropathy is **distal symmetric poly-neuropathy**. In this condition there is loss of sensory function, starting with the longest nerve fibers. Hence, the feet and especially the toes are affected first. Motor function of the intrinsic muscles of the feet is also affected. Numbness and paresthesias are initial symptoms of the sensory neuropathy; eventually the affected areas lose sensation entirely. As the disease continues to affect the nerves, symptoms move proximally. When the sensory impairment reaches the knees, similar changes may be expected in the hands, as the length of the nerve fibers to the hands approximates those to the knee. Loss of sensation and muscle wasting can then be seen in the hands as well.

A second variety of diabetic neuropathy is **diabetic mononeuritis**. In mononeuritis, individual nerve fibers are damaged, possibly as a result of impairment of the nerve's blood vessels. The nerves most commonly affected are the seventh cranial nerve (Bell's palsy), the third cranial nerve, the sixth cranial nerve, and the peroneal nerve (foot drop).

Another common diabetic neuropathy is **autonomic neuropathy** in which control of involuntary and body maintenance functions is affected.

- The most common symptom of autonomic neuropathy is constipation, caused by diminished GI tract motility.
- Diabetic gastroparesis is autonomic neuropathy involving the stomach. Patients with gastroparesis experience early satiety and vomiting after meals. As you would expect, this leads to inconsistent absorption of food and in turn may play havoc with blood sugar control. Diabetic gastroparesis does, however, respond well to treatment with cisapride, domperidone, or metoclopramide.
- In males erectile function may be disrupted as a result of autonomic neuropathy. Patients may be reluctant to discuss this problem, so you should remember to question male patients about any impotence. Erectile dysfunction may be satisfactorily treated by the use of vasoactive medications, vacuum devices, or implants.
- The urinary bladder may be damaged by diabetes. Usually urinary retention, that is incomplete emptying of the bladder, results and these patients are at risk of frequent urinary tract infections. Drugs which increase bladder wall tone or intermittent catheterization may be useful for these patients.
- Orthostatic hypotension, a dramatic drop in blood pressure when a patient stands up, can be caused by diabetic autonomic neuropathy.

Bladder damage causing urinary retention is sometimes referred to as "neurogenic bladder."

Table 16-3. Types of Diabetic Neuropathy

Type	Frequency	Key signs and symptoms/ unique features
Distal symmetric polyneuropathy	Most common	• Feet affected first • Burning pain in soles of feet, often at night • Eventually sensation lost in affected areas
Diabetic mononeuropathy	Common	• Individual nerve fibers damaged • Most commonly affected are cranial nerve VII (Bell's palsy), cranial nerves III and VI (double vision due to eye muscle paralysis), and the peroneal nerve (foot drop)
Autonomic	Common	• May cause constipation, diarrhea, gastroparesis ("paralyzed stomach"), erectile dysfunction (impotence), bladder dysfunction with urinary retention, and orthostatic hypotension
Diabetic radiculopathy	Uncommon	• Damaged nerve root at its exit from the vertebral column • Pain or numbness in area of that nerve's distribution
Diabetic amyotrophy or diabetic neuropathic cachexia	Uncommon	• Pain and muscle wasting of thighs and sometimes shoulders and trunk

An individual patient can have more than one type of neuropathy at any time.

Another form of neuropathy is **diabetic radiculopathy** in which a nerve root is damaged, and symptoms are experienced in the distribution of that root.

The least common category of diabetic neuropathy is the syndrome termed **diabetic amyotrophy** or **diabetic neuropathic cachexia**.

These patients usually have severe pain and muscle wasting especially in the thighs and also in the shoulders and trunk. Usually severe weight loss and loss of appetite occur and lead to a search for malignancy. When no malignancy is found, diabetic neuropathy can then be diagnosed. The patient's pain and loss of function may be severe, but in general the symptoms will improve or even resolve completely over 6–18 months. No single test is diagnostic of this condition, but electromyelography, nerve conduction studies, or muscle biopsy can help to establish the diagnosis.

Diabetes is a major risk factor for the development of **atherosclerosis**. Blood vessels supplying the heart, lower extremities, and brain are most often affected.

The majority of deaths in people with diabetes are caused by cardiovascular disease.

- Coronary artery disease is the most common atherosclerotic complication of diabetes.
- Peripheral vascular disease is four times more common in people with diabetes. Claudication, pain in the thigh or leg during exercise which is relieved by rest, is the main symptom. Peripheral vascular disease is a major risk factor for amputation of the lower extremities.
- Cerebrovascular disease is also increased in patients with diabetes, who have a two to four times greater incidence of stroke than people without diabetes.

Clearly, in patients with diabetes you must address all other reversible risk factors for the development of vascular disease such as hypertension, hyperlipidemia, and cigarette smoking.

HISTORY AND PHYSICAL EXAMINATION

Developing the HPI

When you see a patient with diabetes mellitus in a routine office visit, certain specific inquiries must be made.

- First, ask about symptoms of **hyperglycemia** such as polyuria, polydipsia, nocturia, weight loss, hunger, skin infections, visual changes, and sensory changes in the extremities.
- For patients on medications for their diabetes, especially insulin, you must also ask about symptoms of **hypoglycemia**. These include shakiness, tachycardia, cold sweats, feelings of deep gnawing hunger, or even sleepiness or confusion.

- Good diabetic control, for most patients, requires significant lifestyle changes. You should assess the *psychosocial and economic impact of the disease* on your patient as these effects have a great influence on the success or failure of therapy. For example, ask the patient about diet, exercise patterns, and medication adherence.
- And always ask the patient if any new symptoms have occurred which might indicate the onset of diabetic complications.

Physical Examination

Certain parts of the physical examination are of particular relevance in patients with diabetes.

- *Weight and blood pressure* are important to see whether dietary interventions and blood pressure treatments are working. In children with type 1 diabetes, maintenance of normal growth is a critical goal, so height and weight should be followed closely. Deviation from the child's usual growth pattern may indicate a deterioration of blood sugar control and a need for a change in therapy.
- *Funduscopic examination* is important in screening for retinopathy. The blurred vision commonly reported by patients when their blood sugars are unstable reflects an osmotic change in the lens. This altered shape of the lens persists until glucose levels inside and outside the lens equilibrate. Periodic examination by an ophthalmologist is recommended for *all* patients with type 2 diabetes and for those who have had type 1 diabetes for at least 5 years. Suspected proliferative retinopathy requires urgent ophthalmologic evaluation.
- *Oral examination* should be performed periodically to look for evidence of dental infection which could contribute to poor glycemic control.
- *Thyroid palpation* is relevant, especially in type 1 diabetic patients. Thyroid autoimmunity is often associated with other autoimmune endocrinopathies, and an enlarged or nodular thyroid gland in a diabetic patient will be an early clue.
- *Cardiovascular examination* is important. Check for point of maximal impulse (PMI), heaves, murmurs and gallops and evaluate the peripheral circulation for pulses and bruits.
- *Examine the hands and fingers* to look for muscle wasting due to neuropathy. Diabetics are prone to tendon tightening

(Dupuytren's contractures), caused by glycosylation of tendon proteins with resultant shortening.

- Careful *examination of the feet should be done at every visit, including neurologic and vascular exams*. Testing for sensory deficits can be performed with monofilaments, and a tuning fork (128 Hz) is useful to document vibratory sensory defects. Circulation in the feet should be assessed.

- Also look for evidence of *conditions which may secondarily cause hyperglycemia*, for example Cushing's syndrome (hypercortisolism), acromegaly (growth hormone excess), and hemochromatosis (iron overload disease).

> Patients with *both* sensory deficits and vascular compromise are at much increased risk for the development of foot complications such as ulcers, gangrene, and neuroarthropathy (Charcot foot).

Laboratory Tests

The main laboratory test for following your diabetic patients is the plasma glucose. Both fasting and random glucose determinations are valuable and one or the other will be checked at virtually every visit.

To a greater extent than with any other disease, your diabetic patients will monitor their own laboratory tests. Home glucose monitoring is a well established process which has contributed greatly to many patients' glucose control. Many patients will check their glucose a few times a week and some will do it multiple times daily and keep records to show you when they come to your office.

Patients should also be followed with periodic **glycosylated hemoglobin determinations**. This test measures the amount of glucose which has become attached to the hemoglobin molecule; the higher the average blood sugar the greater the glycosylation. Values are usually reported as **hemoglobin A1c** (with a normal range 3–6%) or **total glycosylated hemoglobin** (with a normal range 4–8%). Either value gives an assessment of the average blood sugar level over the past two to three months. The measurement of **glycosylated serum protein (fructosamine)** assesses glycemic control over the preceding 1 to 3 weeks.

Other laboratory studies needed for patients with diabetes mellitus are tests for the presence of complications.

- Check for microalbuminuria to screen for nephropathy. In patients with diagnosed nephropathy, 24-hour urine protein determinations are useful to follow the response to treatment and/or progression of the disease.

- In patients with neuropathy, other potential causes of neuropathy should be excluded. Thyroid function studies, serum vitamin B_{12}, and a serologic test for syphilis (RPR) would detect the most likely other causes.
- Other baseline studies to obtain at first diagnosis of diabetes include a lipid profile to assess for other risk factors of vascular disease, a complete blood count, and a chemistry profile including liver function tests, blood urea nitrogen (BUN), creatinine, calcium, phosphorus, albumin, and magnesium.

CASE RESOLUTION

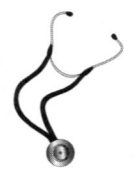

You now have sufficient information to work through the case presented at the beginning of this chapter.

A 60-year-old man came to the office because of an abnormal laboratory test found during health screening at his work place. A nonfasting blood sugar was found to be 230 mg/dl. His previous health care had been intermittent, with occasional visits to an emergency room for sore throats, bronchitis, and muscle strain. He reports to you, "I feel fine for a man my age, but the nurse at work told me I had better see a doctor right away."

You first need to complete your history.

He noted no recent weight change but did have nocturia twice nightly which he attributed to "getting old". He did not complain of thirst, but he felt that he drank more liquids during the day than previously. He also drank water when he arose at night to urinate. His vision was "not as good as it had been in the past", but did not think it had suddenly worsened. His mother had diabetes and she died of a myocardial infarction at age 55. He did not smoke cigarettes; he consumed two to three alcoholic drinks per week. Additionally, he perceived a decrease in the sensation of his toes. He has no sexual dysfunction.

Now you know that you have a patient with a high glucose and several symptoms of diabetes. He also has a positive family history. At this point you proceed with your physical examination.

Your physical examination reveals an obese male patient, 5'10" tall, weighing 230 lb. His blood pressure is 150/90. Examination of his fundi reveals small peripheral hemorrhages and exudates; no neovascular changes are found. All pulses in the lower extremities are normal. He has decreased vibratory sensation in the toes and ankles. There are no cuts or ulcers on his feet, and no tendon tightening in his hands. Another non-fasting plasma glucose done that day was 210 mg/dl.

Let's review this case: Your patient has type 2 diabetes mellitus, because two abnormal nonfasting blood sugars together with symptoms of hyperglycemia (polyuria and polydipsia) established the diagnosis. In addition, you detected abnormal findings in the eyes consistent with diabetic retinopathy and changes in his feet consistent with peripheral diabetic neuropathy. Taken together these findings suggest that his disease has been present for a long time, probably several years. Although no obvious vascular disease was detected on physical examination, the combination of type 2 diabetes, hypertension, and a family history of heart disease indicate that this patient is at significant risk for the development of vascular disease.

Next, assess his overall glycemic control and the extent of complications, and initiate treatment to improve his hyperglycemia. Now it is appropriate to educate the patient about diabetes, its complications and management, and to attempt to achieve weight reduction through dietary changes. You refer him to an ophthalmologist. To look for the presence of kidney damage, order urinalysis to see if proteinuria is present. For neuropathy, rule out other causes. Do an electrocardiogram and a fasting lipid profile to evaluate his overall cardiac risk. Finally you order a hemoglobin A1c to assess his overall glycemic control. In addition to education about diabetes and diet, the patient is taught home glucose monitoring and instructed to check blood sugars twice daily (fasting and before supper) for the next 2 weeks until he returns to see you again.

Once these tests are done, you will have an appropriate database to control and assess the complications of diabetes. You may expect to be following this patient for many years to come to help him maintain control of his diabetes.

Recommended targets for treatment include fasting plasma glucose <120 mg/dl and hemoglobin A1c <7%.

If dietary management and weight loss do not control the hyperglycemia, drug therapy will be necessary. Oral medications for diabetes include sulfonylureas, metformin, acarbose, and troglitazone. Sulfonylureas act mainly by increasing insulin secretion from the beta cells in the pancreas. Metformin and troglitazone act by reducing insulin resistance, and metformin reduces hepatic glucose production. Acarbose inhibits the breakdown of carbohydrate in the intestine. Besides oral agents, insulin is also an option for treatment. Finally, treatment is planned for the patient's hypertension and hyperlipidemia, if these problems remain after attempts at dietary modification and weight loss. Adjustments to therapy will be ongoing depending on responses to treatment of blood sugar and hemoglobin A1c.

SUMMARY

Diabetes mellitus is an *extremely* common disorder, and every office practice will include a number of diabetic patients. Treatment requires a lifelong commitment by the patient and the doctor, and your relationships with your diabetic patients can be enormously rewarding.

STUDY QUESTIONS*

1. Type 1 diabetes is associated with:
   A. Insulin resistance
   B. Ketoacidosis
   C. Cushing's syndrome
   D. Iron overload.

2. Screening for retinopathy in patients with type 2 diabetes usually begins at diagnosis, whereas it begins 5 years after diagnosis for patients with type 1 diabetes. The reason for this difference is:
   A. Blood sugars are higher in patients with type 2 diabetes.
   B. Patients with type 2 diabetes are more susceptible to complications.
   C. Patients with type 2 diabetes are more likely to have other eye diseases.
   D. The actual date of onset of type 2 diabetes is unclear in most patients.

3. Most often the earliest indicator of nephropathy in patients with type 2 diabetes is:
   A. Glycosuria
   B. Hypertriglyceridemia
   C. Microalbuminuria
   D. Urinary tract infections.

4. The Diabetes Control and Complications Trial demonstrated that improved glycemic control reduces:
   A. Retinopathy, nephropathy, and neuropathy
   B. Myocardial infarction
   C. Only retinopathy
   D. Foot amputation.

5. Mortality in patients with type 2 diabetes is most frequently related to:
   A. Renal failure
   B. Proliferative retinopathy
   C. Cardiovascular disease
   D. Peripheral vascular disease.

*For answers, see page 347.

A Patient with HIV $\boxed{17}$ or AIDS

Thomas C. Rushton

INTRODUCTION

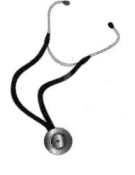

CASE PRESENTATION

J.B., a 25-year-old white man (MSM, males who have sex with males) was tested for HIV recently. He returns for a follow-up visit. He is very concerned about his HIV test results and he called the office in advance of his visit today. The office staff appropriately told him that *his test results would not be provided over the phone.* He was given an appointment for today. He sits nervously in the examination room. Before you walk into the room, you review the chart and note that the ELISA test is positive, but a confirmatory test has not been done. The patient asks you "Am I HIV positive?"

When patients infected with the human immunodeficiency virus (HIV) develop complications because of low CD4 lymphocyte counts, they have the acquired immune deficiency syndrome (AIDS). Working with these patients can be professionally rewarding. Nonetheless, the care and management of AIDS patients is complicated by the difficulty in securing the diagnosis, the variety of possible opportunistic infections and other serious complications, and the changing recommendations for therapy as new drugs become available. These factors challenge the physician caring for patients with AIDS.

Only within the last year or two has optimism developed among those caring for these patients, because *aggressive retroviral therapy with three drugs shows a marked decrease in mortality.* Recent data from the Centers for Disease Control and Prevention (CDC) indicates a 19% decline in mortality for AIDS in the US, and similar decreases are being reported elsewhere. Nonetheless, the number of cases worldwide continues to

climb. This chapter will provide a foundation for approaching the patient with HIV and AIDS.

DEFINITIONS

Anergy: the condition of being unable to respond to skin tests because of an immunologic deficiency

Branched-chain DNA assay:

method of quantitating HIV RNA in human plasma by hybridizing nucleic acids on the surface of microtiter wells (a signal amplification technique)

Cytopenia: abnormally low quantity of a given cell type in the peripheral blood (for example, a decreased number of granulocytes is known as granulocytopenia)

Dysentery: a clinical syndrome characterized by diarrhea (often bloody), abdominal pain, and dehydration

ELISA: Enzyme-linked immunosorbent assay (or enzyme immunoassay) a serologic test used for initial screening for HIV

Kaposi's sarcoma: a neoplastic condition which occurs with increased frequency in AIDS—characterized by multiple blue to reddish-purple plaques and nodules usually on the hands, feet and legs. Histologically, the lesions consist of bands of spindle-shaped neoplastic cells and fragile vascular channels; these tumors are more aggressive in AIDS patients than in idiopathic cases. It is caused by human herpes virus 8.

Opportunistic infection: disease caused by organisms which would not invade human tissue except for an "opportunity" because the host has an immunodeficiency or is otherwise debilitated.

Oral hairy leukoplakia: white, "corrugated-appearing" thickening of the sides of the tongue caused by Epstein–Barr virus infection.

Polymerase chain reaction: a laboratory method of substrate amplification applied to the determination of HIV viral load.

Retroviruses: viruses which translate genetic information from RNA to DNA via an enzyme called reverse transcriptase.

Statistical terms:
- *Sensitivity* the frequency a test is positive when the disease is present
- *Specificity* the frequency a test to determine a disease is negative when the disease is absent
- *Predictive value* the frequency diseased patients are detected among all patients with positive tests; or the frequency normal patients are detected among all patients with negative tests. Predictive values of tests are dependent upon the prevalence of the disease in the test population.

Thrush: *Candida* (yeast) infection in the oral cavity, characterized by white plaques or patches on the tongue or mucosa.

DIAGNOSING HIV INFECTION AND AIDS

Prior to 1985, no reliable test existed for determining whether an individual was infected with HIV. After 1985, an enzyme-linked immunosorbent assay (ELISA) was developed. Although it has excellent sensitivity and specificity (>99%), its predictive value depends upon the population being tested. In a geographic area or a population group of relatively low AIDS prevalence, the ELISA will have a high negative predictive value, but a low positive predictive value. This means that *a negative value in general represents a true negative result; however, a positive value may be falsely positive*.

If the ELISA test is interpreted as indeterminate or positive, the test is repeated. If the result is abnormal again, then the confirmatory test, Western blot (WB) assay, is performed. If the WB assay shows specific bands of GP120/160, P24, and GP41, the WB is positive. With these results, you can inform your patient that they tested positive for HIV; nonetheless you may consider repeating HIV testing and/or obtaining a

Throughout the testing process, and in treating HIV positive patients, it is mandatory to maintain patient confidentiality. Explain to your patient how records and conversations are protected.

viral load test for additional confirmation. *You must not tell a patient or put into the record that they tested positive or negative for HIV until the confirmatory WB assay result is available.*

Who should be tested?

- Test anyone who has a *history of sexually transmitted disease(s)* (STDs) or who falls into a **high risk category**. Persons at high risk include users of intravenous drugs, males having sex with males (MSM), and persons who have sexual contact with persons in high risk categories.
- Test *prostitutes* and *persons who received blood transfusions between 1978 and 1985;* they are at increased risk compared to the general population, though at lower risk than persons in the high risk category as defined above.
- Test women of child-bearing age.
- Test anyone who requests a test.
- Test patients in whom you find generalized lymphadenopathy, thrush, oral hairy leukoplakia, unexplained cytopenias, or active tuberculosis.
- Test *selected patients* with unexplained dementia, diarrhea, fever or weight loss.
- Test anyone who sustains blood and/or body fluid exposure(s).

Once you determine that the patient is HIV positive by both ELISA and WB assay, certain other tests are needed:

- A viral load determination: this assay measures the number of copies of virus in blood; it can be done either by polymerase chain reaction (PCR) or the branched chain DNA assay.
- A CD4 count: This count provides a guide for estimating the patient's risk for opportunistic infections.

CLINICAL COURSE AND PROGNOSIS

The HIV/AIDS patient's prognosis depends upon both the severity of illness and prior or existing complications. The highest risk for debilitating sickness and death comes from opportunistic infections. Usual human pathogens cause disease in otherwise healthy persons, but opportunistic infections (OI) involve only those persons whose immune systems are compromised. The most common OI is *Pneumocystis carinii*. Importantly, this infection was identified in much higher than expected

Opportunistic infections are characteristic of patients with compromised immune systems.

Pneumocystis carinii is probably a fungus. It is found in the environment and causes life-threatening pneumonia.

numbers among young MSMs in San Francisco in 1981, providing the first indication that HIV is an epidemic new disease. Other OIs include *Mycobacterium avium* complex (MAC), cytomegalovirus (CMV), Herpes simplex, *Mycobacterium tuberculosis*, toxoplasmosis, and candidiasis. Cryptococcus and histoplasma also cause systemic infections. Developing a serious infection with any of these OIs suggests impaired cellular immunity.

Persons with AIDS are at higher than average risk of developing neoplastic disease. Several forms of lymphoma are more common in AIDS, especially primary central nervous system (CNS) lymphoma. Kaposi's sarcoma is another neoplasm which is far more common in AIDS than in the general population.

Persons with AIDS may develop severe clinical problems associated with their medications. With several billion virus particles produced every day in an infected individual, the risk of developing resistance to the drugs used to treat HIV is a significant problem. When resistance does develop, that drug becomes ineffective. Side effects of the drugs often prove too difficult to tolerate and other drugs must be substituted. Additionally, drug–drug interactions are likely because nearly all AIDS patients take multiple drugs.

CLINICAL EVALUATION

The exceptionally detailed History and Physical Examination section described in this chapter reflects the unique needs of HIV/AIDS patients. You must pay careful attention to the subtle changes these patients experience which may be only of minor interest in other patients.

Prior treatment for syphilis may not be adequate in an HIV positive patient.

Attention to these details may mean the difference between success with the therapeutic regimen and poor adherence possibly leading to early demise.

Developing the HPI

Your HPI of the HIV/AIDS patient will resemble the Review of Systems (ROS) of other patients. A number of systemic symptoms are very important and because opportunistic infections can affect many organ systems, the HPI must be quite inclusive. Ask *especially*, at every visit, about:

- Weight loss
- Fatigue/malaise
- Appetite
- Rashes or other skin lesions

- New lymph nodes or other masses
- Medication side effects.

It is not unusual for a patient with AIDS to take a dozen or more medicines, amounting to several hundred tablets a month. Drug interactions are likely and adverse drug reactions (allergies or severe side effects) occur frequently. Document drug allergies as they occur. Reactions to sulfa drugs are very common. Your patient's medication list should include not only those medicines prescribed by a physician, but *all* over-the-counter products, including herbal and alternate therapies. The patient should not be made to feel ashamed for using alternate therapies, but it is important to know all medicines the patient takes in order to anticipate any difficulties which may occur. Liver toxicity is not uncommon with certain herbal preparations.

Relevant Other History

Past medical history

- Note prior hospitalizations and surgeries.
- Inquire about previous tuberculosis testing, exposure, or infection.
- Ask about previous sexually transmitted diseases (STDs), especially syphilis.
- Reproductive history is important, as it is necessary to test for HIV infection in all children of HIV positive mothers.
- Finally, thoroughly review vaccination status including measles, mumps, rubella, polio, pneumococcal, *Haemophilius influenzae* Type B, and tetanus vaccines.

Social history

The social history is critical because the patient has now learned of a devastating diagnosis, one for which there is no cure, that they will need to deal with every day of their life.

- Who are his/her friends?
- From where does he/she receive support?
- What funding is available for his/her medications and laboratory tests?
- Does he/she have a job?

Use of substances is important.

- Does he/she smoke?
- Does he/she drink alcohol?
- Does he/she use intravenous drugs?
- Does he/she smoke crack?

You must know the patient's sexual preferences in order to tailor instructions for preventing new infections. The patient may not share the same sexual orientation as you, but you must be nonjudgmental in obtaining the data and in instructing the patient.

- Discuss contraceptive use.
- Determine the patient's use of barrier methods such as condoms, the female condom, and dental dams. A latex dental dam creates a barrier in oral sexual intercourse.

Inquire into the patient's preferred leisure-time activities and exposures to the environment.

- What activities does the patient enjoy?
- Does he/she own any pets? In general, it is safe for AIDS patients to have cats and dogs if the animals receive routine veterinary care. Flea infestations are dangerous, as fleas may be the vector of *Bartonella* infections. Reptiles have been associated with *Salmonella* infections.
- Gardening exposes the patients to soil and its potential pathogens such as histoplasmosis.

As many of these patients are still reasonably healthy, they may travel out of their home area. You will need to advise them of potential exposures to endemic infections.

- Where have they been?
- Where are they planning to go?

Antiretroviral therapy will severely strain a patient's financial resources. Insurance companies may provide coverage only up to a predetermined limit or may provide no medication benefits at all.

- Periodically review financial status so that the patient does not suddenly find himself without the means to continue anti-HIV therapy.
- Compassionate supplies of medication are available, from pharmaceutical companies or charitable sources. Procurement of drugs by this means, however, may be a slow process.

Those who use crack are at increased risk of tuberculosis.

Consult with a social worker when one is available to you, for assistance with many issues in caring for HIV/AIDS patients.

Finally, discussion regarding end of life issues must be approached early in your care of HIV/AIDS patients. Handle this discussion in a gentle and sensitive manner. These patients are too young and healthy to readily accept that they have a terminal illness; it is presumptuous to suggest a no-code status. The patient will almost certainly want anti-retroviral therapy early in their illness. When they become progressively debilitated, they may begin to question the utility of continued aggressive therapy. Thus, assessing a patient's knowledge and wishes regarding end of life issues becomes important.

When possible, ascertain whom the patient wants as a surrogate when he or she becomes unable to make medical decisions. Ideally, patients should appoint a relative or friend as a legal medical power of attorney, but if the patient fails to do this while they have clear decision-making capacity, a physician is allowed, in most states, to assign a surrogate decision maker. With this illness, it is not unusual for the patient to be estranged from their family and to want his or her significant other to fulfill this role. Most states will allow this action as long as the choice is justifiable. Patients should be encouraged to create or revise their wills.

Family history

Next, obtain the family history. HIV/AIDS patients are as likely as other patients to develop familial illnesses, especially as patients with HIV live longer. It is common for HIV-positive patients to have diabetes mellitus or other chronic medical illnesses. Thus, a patient with a family history of diabetes mellitus who develops new onset of fatigue, polyuria, polydipsia, and weight loss is probably developing diabetes mellitus, not just showing another manifestation of AIDS.

Physical Examination

Vital signs

Patients will usually have normal vital signs. Any fever must be *thoroughly* evaluated.

Head and neck

- Inspect the skin and scalp visually and palpate any lesions. Pay particular attention to purplish lesions, suggesting Kaposi's sarcoma, and to any rashes. One type of rash, eosinophilic folliculitis, produces very severe pruritus. The scalp may have fungal lesions; hair may show the nits (eggs) of the human head louse.

Nodes that are plentiful and less than 1 cm, are described as "shotty" to reflect their shotgun-ammunition-like size.

- Do a thorough ophthalmoscopic examination with special attention to the detection of retinal lesions. Hemorrhages are ominous signs, suggesting CMV or herpes zoster infections. Zoster produces a progressive outer retinal necrosis (PORN).
- Look for nasal discharge which may be due to sinusitis, allergic or viral rhinitis, or fungal infection.
- Examine the mouth for the condition of the teeth and gums. Gingivitis is common; thrush, leukoplakia (white plaques), aphthous ulcers, herpetic lesions, and Kaposi's sarcoma can occur in the mouth.
- Examine the neck for cervical adenopathy. Small nonfixed "shotty" nodes are frequently present in HIV infection. Larger lymph nodes that are fixed to the surrounding tissues suggest mycobacterial infection, lymphoma, Kaposi's sarcoma, and other pathology. A node greater than fingertip size in diameter, or enlarging, should be biopsied.

Cardiovascular examination

- Examine the heart for murmurs and for evidence of congestive heart failure, including presence of jugular venous distention or extra heart sounds.
- The lung examination is especially important in the HIV/AIDS patient due to frequent occurrence of pulmonary infections such as *Pneumocystis carinii* pneumonia. Listen for signs of consolidation and pneumothorax.

Abdominal examination

Examine the abdomen for hepatosplenomegaly, for presence of normal bowel sounds, and for tenderness. Tenderness, especially when acute, suggests lymphoma, CMV colitis, or dysentery caused by enteric pathogens. Remember that an HIV patient with abdominal discomfort may have ordinary appendicitis and not an HIV-associated opportunistic infection.

Rectal and genital examinations

Sensitivity and communication skills are important to explain to the patient the necessity for a rectal or genital examination. A chaperon should be present regardless of the gender of the examiner and the patient.

- Look for lesions caused by sexually transmitted diseases such as syphilis, chlamydia and herpes.
- Women with HIV may show signs of vaginal candidiasis.
- Do Pap smears every 6 months in female HIV patients. If the Pap smear is abnormal, refer the patient to a gynecologist as further diagnostic testing may be needed.
- Prostate examination should be performed at the initial visit for baseline information and again when there is unexplained fever or a complaint related to urination or defecation. *Cryptococcus* may cause isolated prostatitis in HIV patients.

Neurologic examination

A neurologic examination is important to evaluate for signs of dementia or for focal deficits. HIV infections alone, CNS lymphoma, and opportunistic CNS infections can all cause abnormalities in the neurologic examination. Important CNS infections in AIDS patients include: cryptococcus, progressive multifocal leukoencephalopathy (caused by a virus), and atypical mycobacteria. Toxoplasmosis also causes seizures and focal deficits in patients with AIDS.

Laboratory evaluation

With advances in monitoring the progression of HIV infection, laboratory evaluation plays an important role in management of patients with AIDS (Table 17.1). Earlier, physicians relied primarily on surrogate markers which reflected damage done by the infection, but did not directly measure the extent of the infection. The CD4 count, a measurement of T lymphocytes with the CD4 receptor, remains the most important surrogate marker. Its value is reported both as an absolute number and as a percentage; in general, the absolute number is used as one of the criteria for starting treatment and adding medicine for prophylaxis of OIs. Natural CD4 variability remains an important factor. If the test is drawn in the afternoon, the results will be higher than if drawn earlier in the day: exercise also elevates the level. Be aware that interlaboratory variability is significant.

> In general, the CD4 count and viral load (as either PCR or branched chain assays) should be determined every 3–4 months if the patient is stable, or more frequently if therapy is changing or the patient is doing less well than predicted.

The polymerase chain reaction (PCR) test is an important test for assessing progression of the disease as well as effectiveness of antiretroviral therapy. It measures the viral load in the patient's blood. The PCR takes a small amount of nucleotide, in this case RNA, and amplifies it. The test can measure up to 750 000 copies of the virus per ml of blood, but cannot detect under 40 copies. Newer assays promise greater resolution. The branched chain DNA assay, unlike the PCR in which substrate is amplified, relies on a signal being amplified. This should

Table 17-1. Laboratory Tests for Following HIV/AIDS

Test	Purpose	Suggested frequency of testing
HIV ELISA	Screening for possible presence of HIV infection	Once for screening. Repeat if equivocal, or for confirmation
Western blot (WB)	Confirmatory test when ELISA is positive	Once, to confirm a positive HIV ELISA
CD4 count	Surrogate marker reflecting damage to immune system	Every 3–4 months, or more often if patient is unstable
Polymerase chain reaction (PCR)	Measurement of viral load by substrate amplification	Every 3–4 months, or more often if patient is unstable.
Branched chain DNA	Measurement of viral load by signal amplification	Do *either* this test *or* PCR every 3–4 months

reduce the possibility of cross-contamination as a small contaminant would not produce a very large signal.

A new assay, not yet widely available, determines the presence of viral mutations which confer resistance to antiretroviral therapy. With this information, treatment can be adjusted to treat the majority of the viral load with the drug to which it is most susceptible.

Other routine evaluation should include a test for syphilis, such as an RPR (Table 17-2). Also obtain hepatitis B and C serologies. If the patient is not immune to hepatitis B virus, then vaccination is indicated. CMV immunoglobulin G (IgG) and toxoplasma IgG tests are useful as these illnesses may reactivate when the patient progresses to AIDS. Screening for tuberculosis includes the routine Mantoux skin test using purified protein derivative (PPD) and chest X-ray. Anergy testing is no longer recommended, as a negative result in a patient with HIV is of questionable significance.

CARE/TREATMENT ISSUES

Care of HIV/AIDS patients includes many ongoing issues which are approached differently or followed more intensely than in patients with other diseases. These are preventive medicine issues, prophylactic treatments, and active drug therapy.

Table 17-2. Screening Tests for Secondary Infection in HIV/ AIDS

Test	Purpose	Clinician's response to test results
RPR	Test for syphilis	Ensure that sufficient treatment has been given
Hepatitis B and C screening	Test for evidence of previous infection and/or immunity	Hepatitis B immunization if patient not immune
Cytomegalovirus IgG, *Toxoplasma* IgG	Test for evidence for previous infection and/or immunity	Observe for potential reactivation
PPD skin test and chest X-ray	Screening for exposure to or infection with *Mycobacterium tuberculosis.*	If +PPD and no *active* disease, give 12 months prophylactic treatment with INH. If active disease present, multiple drugs

In recording test results, "+" is a common abbreviation for "positive," and "−" for "negative."

Preventive Medicine Issues (Table 17-3)

As soon as possible, while the CD4 count is relatively high (preferably >300), complete a standard **immunization** regimen.

- Pneumococcal, hepatitis B and influenza vaccinations are given routinely.
- *Hemophilus influenzae* type B vaccine should be considered in adults and should be routine in children.
- *Live vaccines should not be administered except for the measles, mumps, rubella vaccine given to children.* (This will preclude the use of some travel-related immunizations such as yellow fever.)
- Tetanus (Td) should be administered every 10 years.

For those patients who continue to engage in sexual activity, instruction for **safer sex** is necessary. Advise patients in condom use and other barrier protection such as dental dams and the female condom.

Other elements of preventive medicine include **common health issues** such as alcohol and smoking. Smoking will predispose a patient to infections. Cessation should be encouraged and assisted. Alcohol increases the amount of viremia and also reduces the effectiveness of CD8-containing cells which are important in suppressing HIV.

Table 17-3. Care and Treatment of HIV/AIDS Patients: General Preventive Medicine

Preventive medicine concern	Action
Immunizations	Pneumococcal vaccine every seven years
	Influenza vaccine yearly
	Hepatitis B vaccine if not already immune
	H. influenzae type B (HiB) vaccine if not previously immunized
	Tetanus (Td) every 10 years
	No live vaccines except MMR for children
Safer sex practices	Barriers
Smoking	Predisposes to infection; encourage and assist patient to stop
Alcohol use	Increases viremia and decreases protective CD8 cells; encourage and assist patient to stop
Nutritional status	Evaluate weight, albumin, prealbumin, total lymphocyte count
	Try appetite stimulants if necessary
	May occasionally need parenteral nutrition
Female reproductive health	Pregnancy test, STD screens when clinically indicated
	Pap smears every 6 months
	Birth control—advise long-acting injectable progesterone
	Zidovudine therapy during pregnancy
HIV transmission to household contacts	Do not share items which may be blood contaminated (razors, etc.)
	Clean body fluid-exposed items or surfaces with chlorine bleach and use latex gloves
	Generally, casual contact is not a risk for transmission

An accurate **nutritional assessment** should be made early on. Patients with HIV require increased energy intake, but often the patient experiences a degree of anorexia. Agents such as megestrol and dronabinol are useful; adjunctive therapy such as peripheral parenteral nutrition and certain growth hormones may be more therapeutic, as they increase lean body mass and not body fat.

Reproductive health maintenance is very important in women with HIV/AIDS. Do a pregnancy test whenever clinically indicated. Testing for sexually transmitted diseases should be performed also. Regular Pap smears are important as papillomavirus infections progress more rapidly and lead to earlier cervical cancer in these patients.

Birth control and family planning need to be emphasized. Some women may decide not to become pregnant for fear of transmitting the virus; others will give it consideration. Discuss with your patient her fears and desires about pregnancy, and her feelings about the possibility of terminating a pregnancy in the event it would need to be considered. Without zidovudine therapy approximately 33% of infants born to HIV positive mothers will be infected. With zidovudine, this number can be reduced by 60%. For those who choose not to risk pregnancy, birth control using long-acting injectible progesterone is preferable.

Men are at increased **risk of anal carcinoma**. Appropriate screening is still controversial; Pap smears and anoscopy have been recommended. Certainly, when any abnormality is detected, referral to a surgeon for biopsy and definitive treatment is recommended.

Patients have concerns about **transmission of HIV to household contacts**. In general, personal hygiene instruments (such as razors) or jewelry (such as earrings) where small amounts of blood may be present should not be shared among family members. Furthermore, latex gloves and bleach should be used for cleaning where exposures to bodily fluids may occur. Otherwise, casual household contact does not transmit infection.

Infection Prophylaxis (Table 17-4)

You should provide information about and prophylactic treatments for opportunistic infections.

- Include an agent such as trimethoprim/sulfamethoxisole for the prevention of *Pneumocystis carinii* pneumonia. This regimen also prevents central nervous system toxoplasmosis. PCP prophylaxis should be started with any AIDS-defining illness, or a CD4 count <200.

Table 17-4. Care and Treatment of HIV/AIDS Patients: Infection Prophylaxis

Potential infection	Available prophylactic treatment
Pneumocystis carinii	Trimethoprim/sulfamethoxasole
CNS toxoplasmosis	Trimethoprim/sulfamethoxasole
Tuberculosis exposure without active disease	INH
Mycobacterium avium complex (MAC)	Rifabutin, clarithromycin, azithromycin • Consider with CD4 count <100 • Definitely give with CD4 count <50
Cytomegalovirus retinitis	Ganciclovir

- If a Mantoux test with PPD is positive, and the patient does not have *active* tuberculosis, then isoniazid (INH) prophylaxis should be administered for 12 months.
- As a patient's CD4 count declines even further, *Mycobacterium avium* complex (MAC) infection may develop. When the CD4 count is <100, MAC prophylaxis may be considered, and definitely given once the CD4 count is at 50 or below. Choices include rifabutin, clarithromycin, or azithromycin.
- CMV retinitis is another devastating process in patients with a low CD4 count (<100 cells). Oral ganciclovir for prophylaxis is available. Recommendations frequently change; refer to guidelines from CDC or IDSA (see Suggested Reading).

Antiretroviral Therapy (Table 17-5)

Antiretroviral therapy has become much more complicated and expensive, and has a much greater incidence of side effects. Adherence to the therapeutic regimen by the patient is of utmost importance to minimize development of resistance. You must determine how much understanding the patient has and engage in educational dialogue to promote both understanding and adherence. Some patients have insufficient social support networks, and a few have psychological dysfunctions which preclude meaningful retroviral therapy adherence.

Table 17-5. Care and Treatment of HIV/AIDS Patients: Antiretroviral Therapy

Therapeutic class	Available agents
Nucleoside reverse transcriptase inhibitors	Zidovudine (AZT)
	Didanosine (ddI)
	Zalcitabine (ddC)
	Stavudine (d4T)
	Lamidavine (3TC)
Nonnucleoside reverse transcriptase inhibitors	Nevirapine
Protease inhibitors	Saquinavir
	Retonavir
	Indiravir
	Nelfinavir

Treatment with only a single antiretroviral drug rapidly leads to resistance and ineffectiveness. The only exception to this is in pregnancy where monotherapy is useful. In general, a **triple combination regimen** is recommended. With the introduction of protease inhibitors and other agents, stabilization as well as reversal of the infection can be achieved. However, this is not a cure.

Reverse transcriptase inhibitors were the first successful drugs for treating HIV. When zidovudine (AZT) was introduced in 1987, it revolutionized therapy for HIV. Originally, it was used in very high doses which caused bone marrow suppression. Today, the usual dose is much lower and it is used in combination regimens. Didanosine (ddI), zalcitabine (ddC), stavudine (d4T) and lamivadine (3TC) are other reverse transcriptase inhibitors. Newer agents called "nonnucleoside reverse transcriptase inhibitors" are available including nevirapine. If all three agents chosen for triple therapy are reverse transcriptase inhibitors, this is called concordant therapy; such therapy has been shown to reduce the viral load by 10–90%.

Proteases are necessary for viruses replicated in human cells to become independently functional, therefore, protease inhibitors have been developed as therapeutic agents.

Protease inhibitors are the newest antiretroviral drugs. While very effective, they have proved to be problematic in terms of drug interactions and side effects. You must carefully instruct your patients to avoid concomitant use of other medications. Saquinavir and retonavir are among the drugs in this class.

Other sites of HIV production are being examined for potential therapeutic drug development. For example, an integration inhibitor

would block the intercalation of the copy DNA into host DNA. It can be anticipated that over the next several months and years the choices of therapy will change dramatically.

CASE RESOLUTION

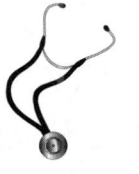

J.B., a 25-year-old white man (MSM, males who have sex with males) was tested for HIV recently. He returns for a follow-up visit. He is very concerned about his HIV test results and he called the office in advance of his visit today. The office staff appropriately told him that his *test results would not be provided over the phone.* He was given an appointment for today. He sits nervously in the examination room. Before you walk into the room, you review the chart and note that the ELISA test is positive, but a confirmatory test has not been done. The patient asks you "Am I HIV positive?"

You are unable to answer his question today, but you arrange for the necessary confirmatory tests.

J.B. returns a week later and learns that his WB assay is positive. Repeat ELISA/WB assays are performed and are positive.

You confirm to the patient that these tests are positive and he is indeed HIV positive. He is willing to continue with a full history and physical examination today.

While you have examined him in the past, he has never needed a comprehensive examination. Now you take a detailed history and perform a physical examination.
Your findings include:

- He currently feels fairly well and has not lost weight. He does notice easy fatiguability and his appetite has decreased this week because his mouth is "sore." He does not have skin rashes or enlarged nodes.
- J.B. had previously been healthy and has no known allergies. He has had no STDs and has received all routine immunizations.
- He has been in a monogamous homosexual relationship for the past 2½ years and had no previous sexual partners. His partner had been in several relationships previously and had found out 6 months ago that he was HIV positive.
- J.B. is currently employed in a clerical position and has medical insurance. He has no pets and hasn't traveled recently. He is estranged from some family members, but is still close to his sister. Since his partner is also ill, he asked his sister to be his power of attorney.

At this point you conclude that while J.B. may have serious problems to face ahead, he currently has a fairly straightforward presentation and

relatively few social complications. You proceed with his physical examination.

J.B.'s physical examination is entirely normal except for his mouth examination which shows several white patches with some surrounding erythema. The white material can be scraped off with a tongue blade. On examination it is found to be *Candida*.

Your patient's examination is normal except for "thrush" (oral candidiasis). You discuss this with him and proceed to further laboratory tests.

You order a viral load assay and a CD4 count. He has a viral load of 250 000 viruses/ml and a CD count of 275. You order a PPD which is negative and a chest X-ray which is clear.

You advise J.B. that he needs treatment for his oral candidiasis, PCP prophylaxis, and triple drug antiretroviral therapy. He agrees and starts his medications. You will see him back in for follow-up in about 2 weeks.

SUMMARY

Worldwide, deaths related to HIV and AIDS continue to decline, but even in the United States the number of *new cases* of HIV is increasing. While therapy is effective in slowing the progression of HIV infection and preventing some deaths, these are not yet considered cures. The information base in HIV pathology, clinical features, and treatment is expanding rapidly. Review recent update articles to keep informed and to learn the newest data regarding therapeutic intervention.

STUDY QUESTIONS[*]

1. A 30-year-old woman comes to your office requesting an "AIDS test." She has discovered that her current partner is a bisexual male who admits to having had a previous encounter with a man who is now known to be HIV positive. Your best advice to her would be:
    A. She is at low risk of having the virus and shouldn't worry about being tested
    B. She is at low-to-moderate risk of disease but if she insists she might have the test in the future
    C. She is at moderately high risk and should be screened with an HIV ELISA test
    D. She is at very high risk of disease and should have HIV ELISA, Western blot, and PCR tests now.

[*]For answers, see page 347.

2. Opportunistic infections which are fairly common in AIDS patients include all of the following except:

    A. *Mycobacterium avium* complex (MAC)
    B. *Pneumocystis carinii* pneumonia
    C. Cytomegalovirus retinitis
    D. *Escherichia coli* urinary tract infection

3. Which of the following findings on the HEENT examination is more common in AIDS patients than in the general population?

    A. A 1 cm tender anterior cervical node associated with pharyngitis and a positive strep screen
    B. A white corrugated appearing thickening of the sides of the tongue
    C. A subconjunctival hemorrhage
    D. A 1 cm nodule in the left lobe of the thyroid gland

4. In female patients being evaluated for possible HIV all of the following are important questions about sexually transmitted diseases (STDs) except:

    A. Have you had sexual partners whose STD history is unknown to you?
    B. If you have had syphilis in the past, how was it treated?
    C. Have you ever had hepatitis B?
    D. Have you ever had vaginal bleeding between your periods?

5. Medical advice to your patients who have been diagnosed with AIDS should include all the following except:

    A. All commercially available vaccinations should be administered as soon as the diagnosis is made, especially if the patient plans to travel.
    B. Safer sex measures, including barriers, are still important.
    C. *Pneumocystis carinii* risk can be decreased with prophylactic treatment.
    D. Antiretroviral drug therapy should generally consist of a three drug regimen.

Suggested Reading

Boswell, S. Screening for HIV Infection and Approach to the Patient with HIV Infection in Primary Care Medicine: Office Evaluation and Management of Adult Patients, 3rd edn, pp. 29–32, 58–68. J.B. Lippincott Co., Philadelphia, 1994.

DeVita, V., S. Hellman, and S. Rosenberg (eds) AIDS: Etiology, Diagnosis, Treatment, and Prevention. 4th edn. Lippincott-Raven, Philadelphia, 1997.

1997 USPHS/IDSA Guidelines for the Prevention of Opportunistic Infections in Persons Infected with a Human Immunodeficiency Virus. Annals of Internal Medicine 127: 922–946; 1997.

A Patient with  18 Altered Mental Status

Shirley M. Neitch

INTRODUCTION

CASE PRESENTATION

A 67-year-old man is brought to the office by his wife. She gives the reason for the visit as "He seems sort of confused. We just couldn't overlook his poor memory anymore." As you develop your history she tells you the following story. "John retired a little sooner than planned, about 4 years ago, because he was having trouble keeping up with everything at work. At that time we thought it was just because of all the job changes and new computers. But it wasn't much better after he quit working; he began having trouble keeping up with his volunteer work and then he couldn't seem to play cards with his friends anymore. My daughter finally made this appointment because he actually got lost driving home from the grocery store last week! You know he's really never been sick before except for his bronchitis and a little arthritis, so this is so hard to understand. I think a few times he's actually not recognized his neighbors, and I've seen him talk to the television like he believes there are real people on it."

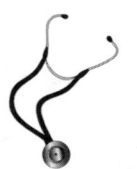

Patients with "altered mental status" come to their doctors because of a variety of complaints. Often, the patient offers *no* complaints, but rather concerned family members bring the patient to the doctor. They describe the patient's actions as "confused," "forgetful," or "not acting like himself." They may overstate or minimize the situation depending upon their own interpretations or motives. Your main goal is to promptly and aggressively evaluate the patient, identify correctable problems, and treat quickly to prevent permanent damage to the brain.

Three broad categories of disease states must be differentiated among patients with altered mental status, namely **dementia**, **delirium**, and

psychiatric disorders. Although each category presents challenges in evaluation and treatment, the primary care physician should certainly be able to make a tentative diagnosis and treat most of these patients. In selected instances, the primary care physician may need to refer the patient to an appropriate specialist.

Coma, the state of complete unconsciousness, may be caused by several of the disorders mentioned in this chapter. However, comatose patients are rarely brought for initial evaluation to an ambulatory care setting, and therefore coma will not be specifically discussed.

DEFINITIONS

Cortical functions:	complex brain functions such as language, which can only be accomplished with an intact cortex ("gray matter"), as opposed to more basic brain functions which are coordinated by subcortical ("white matter") centers.
Delirium:	acute confusional state characterized by clouded consciousness, inattention to the environment, and usually agitation and incoherence (for example, severe alcohol intoxication).
Dementia:	chronic defect in cognitive function involving impaired memory and intellect, and emotional or behavioral abnormalities (for example, Alzheimer's disease).
Depression:	mood disorder characterized by sadness and inability to experience pleasure.
Encephalopathy:	any disease of the brain; usually refers to central nervous system (CNS) disturbances caused by diseases outside the CNS; often characterized by alterations in consciousness and sometimes by headache or seizures.
Focal signs:	localized motor or sensory abnormalities found on neurological examination representing damage to specific controlling areas of the brain (for example, arm weakness after a stroke).

Intoxication:	conditions caused by intake of an excess of a drug or a poisonous substance (for example, alcohol or an opiate).
Lethargy:	decreased alertness and excessive drowsiness; a lethargic person will be easily arousable, but if unstimulated will become drowsy again.
Meningitis/encephalitis:	infection or inflammation of the meninges or brain tissue.
Metabolic disorder:	abnormalities related to disorders of metabolic processes including thyroid or pancreatic dysfunction or imbalances in water, acid/base, or electrolyte stability (for example, diabetes, abnormal thyroid, dehydration).
Pseudodementia:	a condition with clinical symptoms of dementia but not due to organic disease and without permanent cognitive sequelae; usually refers to depression-related symptoms.
Schizophrenia:	a psychiatric disease characterized by disordered thinking, hallucinations and delusions.
Sepsis:	a syndrome associated with bloodstream infection.
Space-occupying lesions:	abnormal structures which cause symptoms and signs because they impinge upon normal brain tissues; usually refers to tumors, abnormal collection of blood or fluid, or circumscribed infections within the skull.

CAUSES OF ALTERED MENTAL STATUS

Dementia

Indolent changes in mental functioning are the hallmark of dementing illnesses. Early in the course of most dementias, these changes may be quite subtle, sometimes unnoticeable to all but the most astute observer. Eventually, however, the demented person will have clearly abnormal mental function.

Unlike delirium, dementia does not cloud the consciousness. The patient may be quite alert and interactive with the environment, sometimes even pretending to recognize people and situations when they do not. The "social intactness" of early dementia may contribute to delay in diagnosis as, at this same time, the patient's spouse and others will be deftly attempting to cover memory and word-finding deficits.

Inexorably, the dementing process will rob the patient of a variety of higher cortical functions (such as calculation, recall, language, and the ability to follow commands) to the extent that activities of daily living (ADLs) become impossible. The ability to perform complex ADLs, such as keeping a checkbook or maintaining a busy schedule, is lost first, and ultimately even basic activities such as bathing, toileting, and dressing are affected. Whether the functional collapse is gradual or occurs in abrupt declining steps depends upon the cause of the dementia (see Figure 18-1).

For the most part, dementias are problems of the elderly. While anyone who has attained normal mental capacity may lose it (i.e., become demented), the processes which usually cause this are far more common in the elderly. Those who never reach a normal intellectual capacity due to congenital disorders or early life brain injury, are considered developmentally delayed or challenged, not demented.

A wide variety of disorders cause dementia. They may be classified into three broad divisions (Table 18-1).

- Primary degenerative neurologic disorders
- Vascular dementias
- Dementia related to systemic disease.

Primary degenerative neurologic disorders

Alzheimer's disease (dementia of the Alzheimer's type, DAT, senile dementia) This devastating disease is the most common of the primary dementias, affecting 3–5% of all persons over 65 years old. Most victims are in the "old-old" age group, over 85 years old; indeed the incidence in this age group is thought to be greater than 40%. The disease follows an extremely variable time course, from about 3 to as long as 15 years, and the degree of mental deterioration depends upon the stage of the disease. Typically patients have demonstrable deficits in memory, word-finding, and calculations; many show agitation or signs of depression also. The vast majority of Alzheimer's patients do not come in themselves for evaluation, but are brought in by concerned family members to whom the deficits have become apparent. *Patients have a variable awareness of the deficits*, and the depression which sometimes accompanies the

Alzheimer's disease is extremely common, but not an inevitable part of aging.

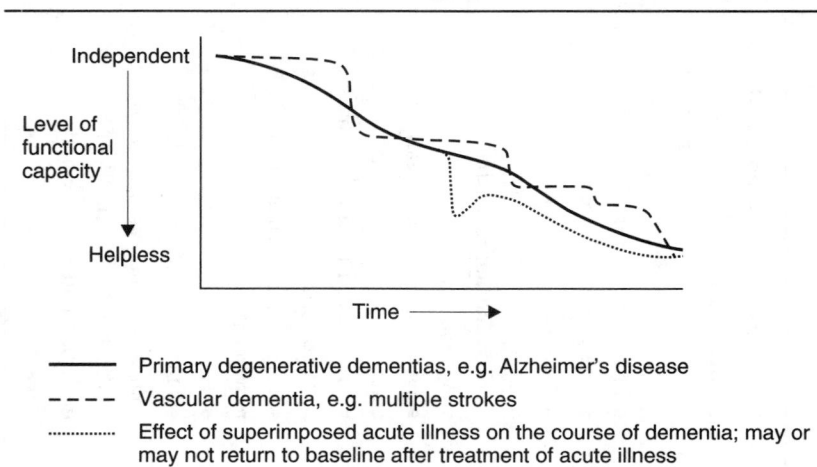

Figure 18-1. The expected clinical course of common dementias.

dementia seems closely related to the patient's perception of intellectual decline.

Pick's disease Very similar in clinical appearance to Alzheimer's disease but much more rare, Pick's disease involves more localized damage in the frontal and anterior temporal lobes of the brain. This leads to more pronounced personality changes than in Alzheimer's.

Creutzfeldt–Jakob disease Patients who have symptoms similar to DAT, but with an extremely rapid progression often prove to have Creutzfeldt–Jakob disease (CJD). Unlike other dementias, *CJD is transmissible, and body fluids and tissues must be handled extremely carefully.* The transmissible agent (a "prion" or infectious nucleic acid) is similar to, but not identical to, the agent causing bovine spongiform encephalitis or "mad cow disease."

Dementias with other CNS diseases

Several other degenerative disorders of the central nervous system may be associated with dementia. Most of them are diagnosed prior to the onset of any intellectual loss because of their characteristic *motor dysfunctions*. These include: Parkinson's disease, Huntington's chorea, progressive supranuclear palsy, and Wilson's disease. They are *not* invariably associated with dementia; for example, in Parkinson's disease approximately 1/3 of patients will become demented after many years of tremor, paucity of movement, and muscle rigidity.

Researchers are currently attempting to sort out the relationship of Parkinson's-related dementia to a clinically similar entity called Lewy Body Disease.

Table 18-1. Differentiating the Dementias

Disease	Usual age of onset	Usual duration	Relative incidence	Key signs or symptoms, and unique features
Alzheimer's disease	Rare <50 yrs Occasional 50–75 yrs Common >75 yrs	3 to 15 years	**Most common dementia**	• Primarily a deficit of memory • Predictable decline in function, almost a reversal of normal developmental sequence; however, time course and rapidity of change variable and unpredictable • Agitation common • Depression common early in the course
Pick's disease	Same as AD	3–10 years	Very rare	• Pronounced personality changes
Creutzfeldt–Jakob disease	Variable	Few months	Very rare	• "Myoclonus" is common (jerky, seizure-like involuntary limb movements) • Transmissible
Parkinson's dementia complex	Usually >65 years	Years	Uncommon	• Onset of dementia *very late* in course of some Parkinson's patients • May be closely related to a newly described entity "Lewy-body disease"

Table 18-1. Continued

Disease	Usual age of onset	Usual duration	Relative incidence	Key signs or symptoms, and unique features
Multi-infarct dementia	Usually >65 years	Years	Common	• Caused by multiple small infarctions of cortical tissue • Decline is usually in abrupt steps rather than gradual downslope as in Alzheimer's (See Figure 18-1)
Binswanger's syndrome	Usually >65 years	Years	Rare	• Caused by longstanding hypertension • Patients demonstrate nonspecific slow mentation and movement
Dementias due to systemic diseases	Variable	Variable	Uncommon	• Features of the specific illness will be present on physical examination or laboratory tests • Causes include hypothyroidism, B_{12} deficiency, neurosyphilis, AIDS

Normal pressure hydrocephalus is relatively uncommon but it is potentially partially correctable so it must be searched for aggressively. It is characterized by the clinical triad of **dementia, urinary incontinence,** and **ataxic gait**. It is caused by an enlargement of the cerebral ventricles and increased volume of cerebrospinal fluid without any blockade in the cerebrospinal fluid (CSF) circulation or increased CSF pressure.

Vascular dementias

Multi-infarct dementia Patients who suffer multiple small strokes may develop mental status changes which are *clinically* similar to the degenerative dementias. Impairments in memory, recall, attention, and calculations occur, the severity of which will be dependent upon the stage of the disease. Unlike Alzheimer's dementia, the changes in multi-infarct dementia tend to occur in abrupt declining steps. Each new stroke causes further damage, and thus further decline in function. The accumulated damage from multiple events leads to dementia. (Single large strokes may cause confusion, especially acutely, but do not lead to global decline in intellectual function.)

Binswanger's syndrome Longstanding poorly controlled hypertension sometimes leads to a condition known as Binswanger's syndrome. Binswanger's occurs when the brain tissue just below the cortex is damaged by small brain infarctions called lacunes. There are no diagnostic clinical features, although patients with this *subcortical* dementia show overall slowness of movement early in their disease and demonstrate unusual difficulty in *planning* tasks. Patients with DAT and other cortical dementias manifest disorders of memory, language, and other cortical functions earlier, and motor dysfunction only late if at all.

Cerebral hemorrhages Most patients who survive an **intracerebral** or **subarachnoid hemorrhage** will *not* have residual dementia. However, a few patients suffer sufficient damage to show intellectual deficits. Undiagnosed **subdural hematomas**, especially bilateral ones, may cause permanent cortical damage and dementia.

Dementias related to systemic diseases

Because some non-CNS systemic diseases cause symptoms of dementia, it is critical to identify and treat such diseases to minimize brain damage. While proper treatment is absolutely *necessary*, it may not be *sufficient* to

reverse all the symptoms of dementia, especially if they have existed for more than 6 months. It is preferable to designate these disorders as "partially treatable" dementias rather than using the more common designation "reversible dementia."

Some of the important causes of these "partially treatable" dementias include:

* Hypothyroidism
* Vitamin B$_{12}$ deficiency
* Neurosyphilis
* AIDS
* Depression (This tends to be a true "pseudodementia," more likely to disappear completely with adequate treatment.)

> In these disorders, some improvement in intellectual function *may* be achieved when the underlying disease is treated, but complete recovery is rare.

Delirium

Delirium is an abrupt change in mental functioning occurring over hours to days. This rather nonspecific term denotes a state of confusion, often with agitation and incoherence, with the important feature of "clouded consciousness". This means that the patient doesn't appear to recognize his or her environment and does not pay attention to events and people. This feature differentiates **delirious** persons from **demented** patients who, while confused, remain alert to their immediate surroundings.

Delirium is caused by a multitude of medical conditions. Because most causes of delirium can be reversed with early treatment, it is critical that the causative condition be diagnosed quickly. Permanent brain damage will result if the causes of delirium are treated too little or too late. Patients of any age and with any previous state of health may become delirious.

Major causes of delirium can be roughly grouped into five categories:

* Metabolic disturbances
* Intoxications/poisonings
* Infections
* Alterations in blood supply to the brain
* Miscellaneous.

> Delirium is abrupt in onset, and usually includes incoherence and agitation.

Metabolic disorders (Table 18-2)

Hypoglycemia An abnormally low blood glucose level is one of the most critical, and fortunately, an easy to diagnose cause of altered mental status. It causes mental status changes varying from agitated confusion to

Table 18-2. Metabolic Causes of Delirium

Diagnosis	Patients commonly affected	Key signs and symptoms or unique features
Hypoglycemia	• Diabetics who do not eat regularly or who exercise too heavily without eating • Other less common clinical situations listed in text	• Cold sweats, gnawing hunger, and shakiness occur early • Confusion progressing to coma *may* occur • May mimic stroke
Hyperglycemia	• Diabetics who do not take their insulin or who develop infections	• Signs of dehydration such as dry mouth and low blood pressure • Acetone-like odor on breath
Fluid and electrolyte imbalances	• Elderly • Critically ill • Patients with malignancies • Patients taking diuretics ("fluid pills")	• Signs of dehydration *or* of fluid overload (latter would include swelling, fluid in the lungs causing shortness of breath)
Thyroid diseases	• Rare today, as thyroid disease seldom goes undiagnosed long enough to cause delirium	• Other signs dependent upon specific disorder • Multiple organ systems involved and clinical manifestations vary
Hepatic encephalopathy	• End stage liver disease patients	• Usually in late stages of liver failure, after patient has shown jaundice, abdominal swelling and other signs • "Asterixis" common
Uremic encephalopathy	• End state renal failure patients, but rarely seen unless patient is not receiving dialysis	• Occurs in late stages of kidney failure

symptoms mimicking stroke to frank coma. *The blood glucose level must be determined promptly in every delirious patient and glucose administered intravenously even before the level is reported.* The degree of permanent brain damage from this condition depends upon how low the level falls and how long it stays below normal.

Causes of low blood sugar (hypoglycemia) include:

- Common:
  - ▸ Excess insulin
  - ▸ Excess oral diabetic medication
  - ▸ Normal insulin or oral medication with insufficient food intake or excessively heavy exercise.
- Uncommon:
  - ▸ Alcohol ingestion in a poorly nourished person
  - ▸ Insulin-producing tumors
  - ▸ Liver failure
  - ▸ Congenital liver enzyme deficiencies.
- Very rare:
  - ▸ Glycogen deficiency
  - ▸ Addison's disease
  - ▸ Extremely large soft tissue tumors.

> When the blood sugar either rises too high or falls too low, delirium may result.

Hyperglycemia Extreme elevations of blood glucose may also lead to altered mental status. The blood glucose may go high enough to cause mental changes in either type 1 or type 2 diabetes mellitus. In type 1 diabetes the condition is called diabetic ketoacidosis (DKA), and in type 2 diabetes it is called nonketotic hyperglycemia. By the time mental status changes occur in these conditions they are life-threatening medical emergencies requiring intense treatment and monitoring.

Fluid and electrolyte imbalances *Any severe or rapidly progressive disturbance of electrolyte stability may be associated with delirium.* Severe dehydration, extremely high or low sodium or potassium, and certain other electrolyte changes cause mental alteration. Disordered calcium metabolism, particularly hypercalcemia, is an important diagnostic consideration in delirium, especially in patients with malignancies, thyroid or parathyroid disease, or renal dysfunction.

> Remember, consider hypercalcemia as a cause of delirium in patients with malignancy, thyroid, parathyroid or renal dysfunction.

Thyroid disease Severe **hyperthyroidism** (thyrotoxicosis) may present with agitation, and in its severest form, "thyroid storm," a patient may exhibit a near psychotic state. **Hypothyroidism** may be manifested by slowness in mentation, lethargy, and forgetfulness; untreated it can

Table 18-3. Intoxications and Poisoning Causing Delirium

Causative agents	Common examples	Key signs or symptoms, or unique features
Acute alcohol intoxication	• Legal alcoholic beverages (ethanol; EtOH)	• Usually apparent from history but *never presume* a delirious patient to be EtOH intoxicated without proof
	• Rubbing alcohol, shaving lotion, cough syrups	• Ethanol substitutes used occasionally by alcoholics
	• Wood alcohol	• Wood alcohol (methanol) causes blindness
	• Wernicke's encephalopathy	• Wernicke's is caused by thiamine deficiency and is characterized by eye muscle paralysis
Chronic alcohol use	• Delirium tremens	• DTs may be fatal in as many as 15% of victims

eventually lead to a stuporous state which may be fatal (myxedema coma).

Liver failure Fulminant acute, or far advanced chronic, liver disease can lead to various mental status changes known by the general term **hepatic encephalopathy**. Multiple metabolic defects are present in patients with this disorder and no individual factor is specifically responsible for the central nervous system effects. "Asterixis" or "liver flap", a characteristic physical finding in hepatic encephalopathy, is seldom seen in other delirious states.

Renal failure Severe failure of kidney function may lead also to delirium from metabolic encephalopathy, known in this case as "uremic encephalopathy". Occasionally asterixis will be seen in this disorder.

> Asterixis is an inability to voluntarily maintain the position of an extremity. When a patient showing asterixis is asked to hold out their arm with wrist extended, they will drop the wrist in a non-rhythmic, jerky way.

Intoxication/poisonings (Table 18-3)

Alcohol Acute alcohol intoxication is a common cause of altered mental status, and is usually reversible. However, brain damage from *chronic* excessive alcohol consumption may produce delirium in two specific neurologic syndromes—Wernicke's disease and delirium tremens—and these may or may not reverse with treatment.

Wernicke's disease is caused by the thiamine deficiency which may accompany chronic alcoholism. It is characterized by abnormal eye movements, gait disturbances and confusion. The eye muscle abnormalities may become so severe as to completely paralyze the eye (ophthalmoplegia). In about 5% of alcoholics, delirium tremens results from the abrupt discontinuation of alcohol ingestion. It is the most serious alcohol withdrawal syndrome and sometimes occurs without any preceding milder symptoms. Up to 15% of persons who develop "DTs" will die of this disorder, which is characterized by fever, severe agitation and evidence of autonomic nervous system hyperactivity.

Drugs Illicit drug use, as well as accidental or deliberate overdosage of therapeutic drugs, must always be considered in the differential diagnosis of delirium. In certain patient populations, especially the elderly, even therapeutic doses of some common drugs can cause changes in mental status. This is especially likely when the patient takes multiple drugs, thereby risking drug interactions as well as primary drug effects.

> Potential intoxicants include correctly and incorrectly used medicines, as well as illegal drugs.

Plant and chemical toxins Numerous plants and household and industrial chemicals produce delirium when ingested accidentally (or deliberately, in suicide or homicide attempts). Poisonous mushrooms, jimson weed, a few household plants, and marijuana, are plants known to cause delirium syndromes. Among the many chemical compounds which produce delirium are several heavy metals (especially lead in children), insecticides (organophosphate and various chlorinated agents), atropine and related belladonna alkaloids, and carbon monoxide.

Infection

Meningitis/encephalitis Not surprisingly, acute or chronic infection of the brain causes delirium in many cases. As rapid diagnosis and treatment are critical, one's "index of suspicion" must be high. That is, if a patient has symptoms and signs suggesting the possibility of brain infection, you must recognize them quickly and do the appropriate diagnostic tests. History suggesting CNS infection includes exposure to an infected person, living in or visiting an area infested with insects carrying encephalitis viruses, or a diagnosis of immunosuppression caused by AIDS or chemotherapy.

Nearly *any* infection can lead to delirium in debilitated patients, especially the elderly.

Other infections It is less intuitively obvious, but equally important to know that severe infections *outside* the nervous system can cause delirium. This is especially true in debilitated elderly patients, in whom even an uncomplicated urinary bladder infection may provoke altered mental status. In younger patients and in healthy older persons *serious* non-CNS infections can result in mental changes occasionally, especially severe pneumonias (when the related hypoxemia may contribute) and sepsis.

Altered blood supply to the brain

Ischemia/hypoxia A number of conditions causing suboptimal blood flow or diminished oxygen delivery to the brain may cause delirium (see Table 18-4).

Subarachnoid hemorrhage More often a cause of coma, subarachnoid hemorrhage can sometimes cause delirium in its early stages.

Miscellaneous

Tumors and other space-occupying lesions Rarely, brain tumors present with symptoms of delirium, even before the usual focal neuro-

logic signs and headache appear. This may occur also in subdural hematoma though not commonly.

"Sundowning" *Delirium may be superimposed on dementia.* Sometimes this happens with the onset of other medical problems such as infection or congestive heart failure, but sometimes it is related only to environmental changes which occur in the evening (such as decreased natural light, change of caregivers, etc.). This is commonly called "sundowning".

Psychiatric Disorders

The three broad categories of psychiatric disorders—neuroses, affective disorders, and psychoses—all manifest some degree of disordered thinking (Table 18-5). However they differ dramatically in clinical presentations, in the degree to which the patients' thoughts are different from "normal," and in the extent to which function is affected. Typically, psychoses begin between the ages of 15 and 45. Neuroses and affective disorders have no specific ages of onset.

Neuroses

Panic disorder, **phobias**, **obsessive–compulsive disorder**, and **hysteria** comprise the neuroses. These are least likely of the common psychiatric disorders to alter higher cognitive functions. A patient beset by a panic attack or engaged in a compulsive behavior will be impaired functionally on a temporary basis. Nonetheless they will recognize the abnormality of their actions and would achieve a normal score on mental status testing.

Mood disorders

Mood or "affective" disorders include severe **depression**, **mania**, and **bipolar disorder** (in which the two conditions alternate). They can be substantially debilitating and interfere with the patient's ability to *cooperate* with mental status testing. However, they do not fundamentally alter the cognitive function of the patient. Mood disorders are diagnosed primarily by careful observation of the patient's behaviors. Depression leads to a slowness in movement and thinking (psychomotor retardation), and to a variety of so-called vegetative signs such as sleep dis-

Table 18-4. Other Causes of Delirium

Cause	Specific diagnosis	Key signs or symptoms, or unique features
Infection	Meningitis/encephalitis	• Rapid diagnosis and treatment are critical • Always consider this diagnosis in immunosuppressed patients (such as those with AIDS or those receiving chemotherapy) • Remember to look for fever, stiff neck and rashes on your physical examination
	Other infections	• Infections outside the nervous system can also cause delirium, if the infection is very severe or if the patient is debilitated
Decreased blood supply to brain "ischemia/hypoxia"	Sudden onset (acute)	• Causes include cardiac arrest and airway obstruction
	Slow onset, fluctuating (chronic)	• Causes include congestive heart failure and severe anemia which cause insufficient oxygen delivery to the brain; and diseases of the brain's blood vessels such as blood clots, arterial inflammation and severe hypertension which directly block blood flow
Miscellaneous	Tumors, intracerebral bleeding	• Usually cause more headache and focal neurologic signs than delirium
	"Sundowning"	• A common event in demented patients, consisting of agitation and increased confusion in the evening hours

turbances, nonspecific physical complaints, and voluntary withdrawal from social activities. Mania on the other hand, is characterized by hyperactivity, insistent voluminous speech, and interactions with other persons which often are intrusive and of an unwelcomed personal nature.

Psychoses

This group of serious psychiatric disorders includes those patients who present with the most obviously altered mental status. The two categories of psychotic disorders—the **schizophrenic syndromes** and the **schizoaffective disorders**—are closely related to each other.

Schizophrenia Diagnostic hallmarks of schizophrenia are signs and symptoms which show that the patient is misinterpreting reality. They include a variety of clinical findings such as the following:

- **Hallucinations** occur commonly and typically are *auditory*. They tend to be complex, involving external voices commenting upon the patient's actions or giving instructions.
- **Delusions** are fixed beliefs which are in conflict with reality, such as when a patient believes he is a public or historical figure.
- **Loose associations** are characterized by thoughts or speech veering off in unexpected directions due to the patient's making connections among words or events which ordinarily are not connected. This aspect of schizophrenia is manifested by flight of ideas, pressured speech and tangential speech.
- **Flat affect**, the presence of facial and behavioral expressions inappropriate to a given situation, typically occur in schizophrenia (for example, a patient remaining emotionless while describing a frightening auditory hallucination).

Schizoaffective disorders The schizoaffective disorders are closely related to both schizophrenia and the mood disorders. Typically the diagnosis applies to a delusional or hallucinating patient whose demeanor is either obviously depressed or overly excited. Distinguishing the patient with a pure mood disorder (depression, mania, or bipolar) in a very severe phase of illness from a schizoaffective patient presents a difficult problem requiring the expert assistance of a psychiatric consultant.

Table 18-5. Psychiatric Disorders Causing Altered Mental Status

Category	Specific diagnosis	Key signs or symptoms, or unique features
Neuroses	• Panic disorder • Phobia • Obsessive–compulsive disorder • Hysteria	• All four disorders are usually episodic rather than continuous • Mental status testing usually normal in neuroses
Mood (affective) disorders	• Depression	• Slowness in movement and thinking • Patient usually looks sad or makes the examiner feel overwhelmed
	• Mania	• Patient is hyperactive and intrusive • May go long periods with little or no sleep • Episodes of depression and mania alternate
	• Bipolar disorder	• Often responds to lithium treatment • A variety of subtypes occur but all consist of a break with reality;
Psychoses	• Schizophrenia	• A variety of subtypes occur but all consist of a break with reality; hallucinations common
	• Schizoaffective disorder	• Schizophrenic symptoms in patients with signs of depression or mania

HISTORY AND PHYSICAL EXAMINATION OF THE PATIENT WITH ALTERED MENTAL STATUS

Developing the HPI

A hallmark of clinical medicine is that an accurate history yields a wealth of information needed for diagnosis. In the case of altered mental status, it will usually not be the patient who relates the history and this creates some potential problems. For example, a sense of the patient's coping with the symptoms will be lacking, or information about environmental exposures may be missing. When you must obtain a history from someone other than the patient, attempt to talk to at least *two* persons, to develop a more accurate picture. Patients with altered mental status are potentially vulnerable to exploitation by unscrupulous persons. Seeking confirmation of the history can ensure that you don't get a skewed view of the patient and help prevent such exploitation.

Given these limitations, you must determine:

- Exactly how is the patient's current behavior, appearance, or feeling different from his/her usual pattern? *(Is he/she agitated, lethargic, hallucinating, forgetful, talking strangely, being aggressive, demonstrating disinhibition such as unaccustomed cursing or sexual behavior, or getting lost in familiar surroundings?)*
- How long have such abnormal behaviors or complaints been occurring?
- How rapidly did the abnormal symptoms appear?
- Does the patient have any additional new symptoms, such as fever, headache, nausea, or change in food intake?
- Is there knowledge of or suspicion of ingestion of poisons, toxins, or drugs?
- Did any physical changes occur at the same time that the mental status changed, e.g., weakness or numbness of the face or an extremity?
- Do the changes wax and wane, and if so, is there a predictable time when the changes occur?
- Does the patient appear to have very bizarre thoughts, or is there a simple deficiency in thought content and memory?
- What is the patient's current functional level regarding activities of daily living?

Additional History

All of the patient's history may be important but most relevant to your evaluation of altered mental status will be past history of hypertension, diabetes, neurologic disease, thyroid disease or syphilis. As part of the social history, it is especially important to learn whether the patient has a history of substance abuse, and to gather information about their usual home situation.

Physical Examination

This portion of your evaluation is especially difficult to conduct in the patient with altered mental status. Through no fault of their own, these patients are often uncooperative and, not infrequently, overtly combative. Your examination must be tailored toward *obtaining the critical items of information without further agitating the patient*. On rare occasions, it may be necessary to restrain a patient, but only when critical information cannot be otherwise obtained, or when the patient's actions are of immediate potential danger to the patient or staff. Sedative drugs must be avoided assiduously, until a diagnosis is made, as you certainly don't wish to risk altering the patient's mental status further.

Given the limitations imposed by a particular patient's behavior, you must do as comprehensive a physical examination as possible because the causes of altered mental status are so broad ranging. The portions of the physical examination which are especially important include:

Vital signs

Presence of fever, tachycardia or bradycardia, hypertension, and abnormal breathing patterns are very critical clues. *Elderly patients may present atypically*, for example having serious infections without fever, so *even if an older patient has normal vital signs there may still be a serious disease*.

Head and neck

Look for eye movement abnormalities, pupillary responses, and papilledema. Evaluate the tympanic membranes, and if possible, the pharynx. Examine cranial nerves as thoroughly as possible. Evaluate the neck for stiffness and thyromegaly.

Abdominal examination

You may need to do *serial* abdominal examinations looking for masses, enlarged liver, tenderness or rigidity, and presence or absence of bowel sounds. Be mindful that in some patients, especially the very young and very old, mental status may be altered by the disease process before complaints or classic physical signs appear. The patient may not complain and yet be experiencing catastrophic abdominal disease such as a ruptured organ or infarcted bowel.

Neurologic examination

This will be difficult to accomplish but important in the patient with altered mental status. As extensively as possible, examine the cranial nerves, the patient's movement, gait and strength, and, if possible, the sensory and cerebellar function. Most important of all is a formal assessment of mental status, including the following elements.

- *Level of consciousness* Is the patient alert, lethargic, somnolent/stuporous, obtunded, or comatose?
- *Screening for cortical functions* Once you have determined the patient's level of consciousness, you must screen other cortical functions by a simple test called the Folstein Mini-Mental Status Exam (MMSE) (Table 18-6). This brief test evaluates the patient's orientation, attention and calculation, short-term memory, language, and constructional ability. The total possible score is 30, and normal people will usually score no less than 28 points. Only patients with dementia or severe states of delirium or psychiatric illness will score below 20. Between 21 and 27, the scores are a bit "gray"; the patient's previous functional and educational level will influence your interpretation.

Evaluation of thought content

The notion of "evaluating the thought content" of another person may seem presumptuous or judgmental. However, once you have encountered a patient very ill with psychiatric disease it will be obvious that their thought processes are not simply eccentric, odd, or illogical. Rather they are bizarre and disconnected, and not in any way conducive to the patient functioning in the real world. Examples of abnormal thought content are delusions, hallucinations, use of "neologisms" (words made up by the patient) and inability to think abstractly. The latter is sometimes called "concrete thinking", and can be demonstrated by proverb interpretation, for example, explaining "A rolling stone gathers no moss", as "Moss won't grow on rocks that are moving."

Table 18-6. The Folstein Mini-Mental State Exam

Max. Score	Pt. Score	Questions
		Orientation
5	_____	1. What is the (year) (season) (date) (day) (month)?
5	_____	2. Where are we (state) (county) (city) (hospital) (floor)?
		Registration
3	_____	3. Name 3 objects (e.g., "ball,", "flag," "tree") and have the patient repeat them to you and score one point for each repeated correctly. Repeat until all are learned. (# trials ___)
		Attention and Calculation
5	_____	4. Begin with 100 and subtract 7. Then subtract 7 from that answer and continue through 5 answers. Alternatively, spell "world" backwards with one point for each letter in the right position (D,L,R,O,W).
		Recall
3	_____	5. Ask the patient to repeat the 3 objects named in question #3.
		Language
2	_____	6. Show a pencil and a watch and ask the patient to name them.
1	_____	7. Ask the patient to repeat "No ifs, ands, or buts."
3	_____	8. Ask the patient to follow this three-stage command "Take a paper in your right hand, fold it in half and put it on the floor."
1	_____	9. Instruct the patient to read and obey the following (_write this out for the patient in large letters_): CLOSE YOUR EYES.
1	_____	10. Instruct the patient to write a sentence.
1	_____	11. Instruct the patient to copy this design. (_Show the patient a larger copy, and give one point credit for any two intersecting 5-sided figures._)
	30	Total possible score

Source: Adapted from M.F. Folstein, S. Folstein, and P.R. McHugh, Mini-Mental State: A Practical Method for Grading the Cognitive State of Patients for the Clinician, Journal of Psychiatric Research 12: 189–198; 1975.

Neuropsychological testing

More sophisticated evaluation of cognitive functions may be necessary, especially in the dementias. These batteries of tests of intellectual function are generally done by psychologists rather than physicians.

APPROPRIATE ANCILLARY TESTS IN EVALUATION OF ALTERED MENTAL STATUS

As in all clinical situations, further testing with laboratory studies, X-rays, or other special studies will follow directly from the preliminary diagnosis suggested by your history and physical. For example, if you are reasonably sure that a patient's altered mental status is caused by purely psychiatric disease, you may need relatively few laboratory tests. On the other hand, if you assess that there is a high probability of delirium, extensive testing will likely be initiated as you search for the cause and possible treatment.

Laboratory Tests

- *CBC (complete blood count)* This test will show evidence of infection, and will demonstrate anemia, a finding common to a number of the diseases which cause altered mental status.
- *Chemistry profile* Each laboratory offers a slightly different set of tests in their standard profile, but virtually all screen electrolytes, renal function, and liver function.
- *Thyroid function tests* The levels of thyroid stimulating hormone and circulating free thyroid hormones are important diagnostic clues in cases of altered mental status, whether you suspect delirium, dementia, or psychiatric disease.
- *Vitamin B_{12} and folate levels* These are particularly important in evaluation of dementia.
- *Drug and toxin screens* These tests are critical in cases of delirium and psychiatric disorder.
- *Urinalysis* This will show evidence of infection which may contribute to delirium.
- *Lumbar puncture* A LP will be necessary if meningitis or encephalitis is suspected.

Imaging Studies

Patients with altered mental status will not often need extensive X-rays or other imaging studies. A few which *may* be necessary are:

- *CXR (chest X-ray)* These will be useful if lung infection is suspected or if there is significant heart disease.
- *CT (computerized tomography) scans of the head* Many patients with altered mental status will need a head CT. These are useful to evaluate space-occupying lesions, normal pressure hydrocephalus, and stroke. Dementia cannot be diagnosed with CT.
- *MRI (magnetic resonance imaging)* MRIs are helpful in evaluating the same potential diagnoses as noted for CT scans. They give more specific images of smaller lesions.
- *PET scans (positron emission tomography)* PET scans are capable of demonstrating metabolic patterns in the brain tissue. However, they are not widely available except in tertiary care research centers and not of use currently in early evaluation of mental status changes.

PUTTING IT ALL TOGETHER

Medical decision making represents an extraordinarily complex task, involving probabilities that certain diseases exist, the depth and breadth of the physician's knowledge, reliability of medical diagnostic tests, availability of treatment options, and the patient's own preferences and responsibilities. Early in your medical education your goal is to perfect your knowledge of disease processes, their prevalences and incidences in the patient population, and their clinical presentations. This background knowledge then comprises one aspect of the decision-making process, and quickly you discover in your clinical years that treatment options and patient preferences complicate this process dramatically. However, you may remain optimistic that the pieces will fall into place in this medical decision-making puzzle relatively easily if you approach the process systematically.

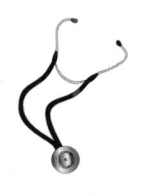

CASE RESOLUTION

The following discussion demonstrates resolution of the case presented earlier by using the steps we have outlined in this chapter:

knowledge of diseases + *history and physical examination*
+ *ancillary testing*
→ *synthesis of the problem* → *treatment*

A 67-year-old man is brought to the office by his wife. She gives the reason for the visit as "We just couldn't overlook his poor memory anymore." As you develop your history you get the following story. "John retired a little sooner than planned, about 4 years ago, because he was having trouble keeping up with everything at work. At that time we thought it was just because of all the job changes with new computers and things. But it wasn't much better after he quit working; he began having trouble keeping up with his volunteer work and then he couldn't seem to play cards with his friends anymore. My daughter finally made this appointment because he actually got lost driving home from the grocery store last week! You know he's really never been sick before except a little arthritis, so this is so hard to understand. I think a few times he's actually not recognized his neighbors, and I've seen him talk to the television like he believes there are real people on it."

Pause at this point and organize your historical information. Your patient is a 67-year-old, previously healthy man with about a 4-year history of increasing memory problems. There are some delusions but the main problem seems to be with his memory.

You complete the patient's past history, review of systems, and family and social histories. They are generally negative except that he had two grandparents and two uncles who were "senile," and he formerly drank a moderate amount of alcohol in social situations, though none for 7 or 8 years. The patient's physical examination is normal except for his mental status. His Folstein MMSE score is 18.

Again, pause here to organize. Now we know that your patient shows deficits in his mental function and has had family members with similar problems. His symptoms are progressing gradually and his history and physical do not indicate any obvious diseases. At this point you may tell the patient's family that he appears to have a dementia and you will need to order some additional tests to determine whether any disease is present which might be at least partially treatable.

You order a CBC, chemistry profile, thyroid function tests, a test for neurosyphilis, and a vitamin B_{12} level. You also obtain a CT scan of the patient's head. All tests are within normal limits.

Now you may inform the family that the patient's dementia does not appear to have a reversible component and that it may be Alzheimer's disease. You will educate the patient, if possible, and the family, as to

what they may expect if he does have Alzheimer's disease, and follow him periodically to confirm your diagnosis as his clinical course progresses.

One year later you see the patient in your office. Now his MMSE score is 14 and he is reported to have "mixed up his nights and days." He sleeps off and on all day and stays up wandering around all night. He is often belligerent with his wife and once or twice has been incontinent of urine.

The patient is showing progressive decline, as expected in Alzheimer's disease. His family is now interested in trying one of the new drugs for Alzheimer's which you prescribe after educating them about possible side effects.

SUMMARY

A very large variety of diseases cause altered mental status. As you gain clinical experience you will be able to differentiate among the causes of this disorder, and rapidly and accurately treat your patients.

STUDY QUESTIONS*

1. The Folstein Mini-Mental State Exam tests all of the following except:
    A.   Language
    B.   Constructional ability
    C.   Basic activities of daily living
    D.   Registration and recall.

2. You are regularly seeing an 80-year-old patient with Alzheimer's disease. She has been stable, with a sort of pleasant confusion and gradually worsening memory loss. Her family calls to report to you that suddenly overnight, she has become agitated, refuses to eat, and seems to be hallucinating. The most likely problem is:
    A.   Her Alzheimer's disease has worsened overnight
    B.   Something has occurred to cause delirium to be superimposed on her dementia
    C.   She has become schizophrenic
    D.   She has developed a brain tumor.

---

*For answers, see page 347.

3. A 23-year-old man is brought to the emergency room by the County EMS ambulance after he was found lying on the sidewalk in front of a downtown bar. He is disheveled appearing, incoherent, and agitated. He is uncooperative with staff and does not pay attention to you when you try to examine him. At this point you may proceed with a preliminary diagnosis of:
   A. Alcohol intoxication
   B. Schizophrenia
   C. Delirium
   D. Myxedema

4. The ER nurses finally get the patient described in question 3 undressed and they find a Medic-Alert necklace which indicates that the patient is an insulin-dependent diabetic. You immediately:
   A. Send a blood sample for glucose determination and give him i.v. glucose even before the results are known
   B. Check his thyroid gland for enlargement
   C. Ask for help from your psychiatry consultant
   D. Restrain the patient's arms and legs so you can do his neurologic exam.

5. The patient receives a sufficient amount of intravenous glucose, and he wakes up suddenly and is completely alert and normal. He apologizes for his behavior and explains that he took his insulin that morning but didn't get to eat because his 26-year-old cousin "went off the deep end" and he had been busy all day arranging to get the cousin into the hospital. "You probably saw him here in the ER, Doc. What do you suppose is wrong with him? He said he heard voices telling him that aliens were coming to make him King of England, and when he became King he would be able to fly."

   You explain to the patient that you can't really discuss another patient's case, but privately you wonder if the cousin was the patient you admitted to the hospital an hour ago with:
   A. Alzheimer's disease
   B. Diabetic ketoacidosis
   C. Binswanger's syndrome
   D. Acute schizophrenia

Isselbacher, K.J., *et al.* (eds). Harrison's Principles of Internal Medicine, 13th edn. McGraw-Hill, NY, 1994.

Moore, D.P. and J.W. Jefferson. Handbook of Medical Psychiatry, Mosby-Year Book, St. Louis. 1996.

Strub, R.L. and F.W. Black. The Mental Status Examination in Neurology, 2nd edn. F.A. Davis Co., Philadelphia, 1985.

When You Suspect  19
Alcohol Abuse

Marie C. Veitia and Shirley M. Neitch

INTRODUCTION

CASE PRESENTATION

Mr. J.H., a 39-year-old man, comes to the office at his wife's insistence complaining of "stomach pain". You have followed this patient for several years for mild hypertension, but you notice that he has missed several appointments recently. You also notice that, while you've enjoyed a pleasant relationship with him in the past, he seems irritable and somewhat evasive today.

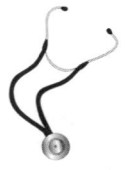

By your routine questioning, you have determined that his problem may be gastritis. As you ask about certain exacerbating factors of his pain, he brusquely replies, "Look, Doc, I don't know why what I eat or drink is any of your business! If you can't give me something for my stomach, I'll go back to the Emergency Room. I've already been there twice for this in the last 6 months."

Abuse of alcohol and other substances is a common but under-recognized problem; a frequently cited obstacle to recognition is the subtlety of the clinical picture presented by the substance abuser. In this chapter we introduce you to the knowledge, attitudes and skills necessary to recognize patients who may abuse alcohol. As alcohol is the number one mood-altering drug in use in the United States, it will be our major focus. However, many of the criteria for recognizing alcohol abuse are the same for other illicit substances.

Demographics

FAS usually includes facial deformities, abnormally slow growth, and a variety of neurologic problems.

Alcoholism is the third leading cause of death in the United States today, accounting for as many as 200 000 deaths annually. It is a major contributing factor to motor vehicle accidents, homicide, suicide, domestic violence, child abuse and neglect, homelessness, and criminal behavior. Fetal alcohol syndrome (FAS), a constellation of congenital defects caused by excess alcohol intake during pregnancy, is a leading *preventable* cause of mental retardation. The monetary costs to society in increased health related expenditures, lost productivity, and premature death are estimated in the many billions of dollars.

Substance abusers utilize medical services proportionally more than non-abusers. *Estimates are that one in five outpatients meet the criteria for alcoholism and that 25–60% of all hospital admissions may be linked to alcohol consumption.* Primary care physicians are in the ideal position to recognize the early manifestations of alcoholism. However, they fail to do so in 50–90% of cases.

Abuse of alcohol (or other substances) is not confined to any one demographic group. Male and female, young and old, substance abuse victimizes all gender, socioeconomic and ethnic groups. A few high risk profiles do exist, and you must learn to recognize them. Moreover, you *must* be alert to the potential for this problem in virtually any patient.

High Risks

More men than women abuse alcohol; about two-thirds of alcohol abusers are male. When alcoholism occurs in women, the prevalence is greatest in women ages 35–49. Contrary to popular belief, women with multiple roles (e.g., wife, mother, worker) have *lower* rates of alcoholism than women who do not have multiple roles. Married women appear to be at less risk than single, divorced, or separated women.

The physiological effects of alcohol also differ among men and women, with chronic alcohol abuse exacting a greater toll on women. Women alcoholics have a 50–100% higher case fatality than male alcoholics and a greater percentage of deaths from suicides, alcohol-related accidents, circulatory disorders, and cirrhosis of the liver. Alcohol abuse *may* increase the risk of breast cancer in women.

The usual age of onset of alcoholism is in the late teens to early twenties. The elderly are often not seen as potential alcoholics, but this stereotype is incorrect. The prevalence of alcoholism may be as high as

8–10% in persons over 65, and as many as one-third of them will not have started their excess alcohol use until they were over 65.

Alcoholism and the Family

A great deal has been written about the impact of alcoholism on the family. Because the causes and consequences of alcoholism extend well beyond the individual, physicians should recognize and treat alcoholism as a *family disease*. Families of alcoholics are at risk for financial, emotional, medical, and marital problems. Dysfunctional patterns of interaction develop as a result of denial, anger, family isolation, and secrecy. Family members may engage in *enabling* behaviors which protect the drinker from the natural consequences of his or her behavior. Physicians can be most helpful to alcoholic families by identifying the presence of the problem and developing a treatment plan that includes the family.

> Enabling behaviors tolerate, support, or even encourage the progression of the disease.

RECOGNIZING ALCOHOLISM

Definition

One reason for alcoholism being missed in the medical work up is the nebulous nature of the diagnosis itself. It is naturally harder to recognize a problem when we are uncertain of the criteria for its diagnosis. Of the many **clinical indicators suggested as diagnostic signs of alcoholism** (Table 19-1), the four most frequently cited are: quantity and frequency of intake, development of tolerance or physical dependency, severity of social consequences, and behavior surrounding the substance.

> Dependence = presence of withdrawal symptoms when use of the substance stops.

- The *quantity of alcohol consumed* is thought to be the *least sensitive diagnostic indicator*.
- Establishing physical dependence and tolerance can be useful in distinguishing use from abuse, though there are no universally accepted diagnostic criteria.
- Judging *severity of social consequences* is a bit difficult because abusers are adept at explaining away problems created by alcohol abuse. However, the AMA definition of alcoholism emphasizes social consequences stating that alcoholism is *a chronic, progressive disease that exists when the patients' compulsive and repetitive drinking results in*

> Tolerance = requiring greater and greater amounts to produce the desired effect.

Table 19-1. Diagnostic Indicators of Alcoholism

- Quantity and frequency of alcohol intake
- Physical dependence upon and tolerance of alcohol
- Severity of the social consequences of excess alcohol intake
- Behavior surrounding obtaining and using alcohol

---

impairment of some essential aspect of the patients' life (e.g., health, home, work or school and interpersonal relationships).
- Perhaps the best indicator of a diagnosis of alcoholism is the *behavior surrounding the acquisition of alcohol*. As the individual progresses from normal consumption to abuse and dependence, more and more time and energy is devoted to the pursuit of the substance and the state of consciousness it provides.

The essence of alcoholism, then, can be characterized by the three Cs: (1) **compulsive** use of alcohol, (2) loss of **control** of alcohol consumption, and (3) **continued** use despite adverse consequences.

Screening Patients for Alcohol Abuse

A number of screening instruments have been developed to facilitate physicians' recognizing alcoholism. The most extensively studied and widely used instrument is the "CAGE questionnaire" (see Table 19-2). An affirmative answer to any one of the four questions should arouse suspicion about alcoholism. Two affirmative answers are highly suggestive, and three affirmative answers confirm the diagnosis with 95% certainty. The CAGE questionnaire has not been validated in special populations such as women, adolescents, and the elderly. Although it may be less sensitive in these populations, specificity is probably not affected and answers should not be ignored.

CLINICAL MANIFESTATIONS

Several alcohol abuse syndromes are easily identified. The acutely intoxicated person, the patient with end-stage alcoholic cirrhosis, or the patient suffering delirium tremens may be recognized even by laymen, and certainly will be diagnosed by the physician. But, how will you know when your patient is *becoming* a problem drinker, or that he or she has

Table 19-2. The CAGE Questions

1. Have you ever felt that you should **C**ut down on your drinking?
2. Have people **A**nnoyed you by criticizing your drinking?
3. Have you ever felt **G**uilty about your drinking?
4. Have you ever had a drink first thing in the morning (an **E**ye-opener) to steady your nerves or get rid of a hangover?

© American Medical Association, 1984.

become alcohol addicted before such obvious changes occur? Several clues are seen in persons using alcohol to excess, but an important clinical point is that *most manifestations of alcohol use are nonspecific signs and symptoms which occur in many medical conditions*. You must not be judgmental in dealing with patients you suspect of alcoholism. Do not be too quick to assume that your findings are caused by alcohol.

Behavioral Signs

Undiagnosed alcoholics may significantly change their social patterns. They may develop new contacts and withdraw from previous friends and activities. Evasiveness about their habits is nearly universal. They may or may not exhibit signs of depression. Job attendance and performance may decline, though many "binge" drinkers successfully avoid alcohol during times when they may need to be at work.

Physical Signs

Patients may withdraw from contact with their personal physicians or alternatively, may seek more than usual medical attention because of the multitude of symptoms associated with excess alcohol use. Particularly common are GI tract disorders, cardiovascular problems, and signs of the effects of alcohol on the bone marrow (Table 19-3). Central nervous system effects of long-term alcohol use are discussed in Chapter 18.

Laboratory Tests

In evaluating patients, you will have many occasions to do specific blood tests or panels of laboratory studies. A few clues to otherwise unknown alcohol abuse may be encountered in routine laboratory studies.

Table 19-3. Common Medical Syndromes Associated with Alcohol Intake

Affected system	Specific diagnosis	Signs and symptoms/unique features
Gastrointestinal system	"Hangover"	Morning nausea and sometimes vomiting; due to the mild alcohol withdrawal syndrome experienced "the morning after" heavy alcohol consumption.
	Gastritis	Abdominal pain, nausea, vomiting and sometimes hematemesis due to irritation of stomach lining.
	Peptic ulcer	Symptoms like gastritis but more severe and persistent. Deeper ulceration of stomach lining. May bleed seriously.
	Upper GI bleeding	May occur with ulcers, as noted, or also with torn esophageal lining (Mallory–Weiss tear caused by repeated retching) or with ruptured esophageal varices (engorged esophageal veins caused by liver disease).
	Alcoholic hepatitis	Patients have abdominal pain and elevated liver function tests. May be jaundiced. Due to direct toxic damage to liver cells.
	Fatty liver	Infiltration of liver cells with fat; partially nutrition related. Enlarged liver. May be asymptomatic.
	Cirrhosis	End stage of chronic liver damage; normal cells replaced by scar tissue. The liver's synthetic function is prominently affected (i.e., it cannot make albumin, clotting factors, etc. as usual).
	Pancreatitis	May cause *severe* abdominal pain and vomiting. Often recurrent with continued alcohol use.

Table 19-3. Continued

Affected system	Specific diagnosis	Signs and symptoms/unique features
Cardiovascular system	Hypertension	Frequent problem with long-term alcohol use.
	"Holiday heart"	Atrial fibrillation caused by high intake of alcohol over short period of time (name comes from frequent occurrence of this disorder after persons increase their alcohol intake over a holiday).
	Cardiomyopathy	Cardiac muscle disease caused by alcohol (and by many other disorders as well). Multiple clinical manifestations including arrhythmias and congestive failure.
Hematologic system	Anemia	Caused by alcohol abuse through several mechanisms: • GI blood loss • Nutritional deficiency, especially folic acid • Direct bone marrow depression
	Thrombocytopenia	Platelets are especially sensitive to marrow toxicity of alcohol

- The most sensitive test of alcohol ingestion is one of the liver function tests, the gamma-glutamyl transpeptidase (GGTP). But while elevated GGTP is a very sensitive indicator, it is *nonspecific*. (Alcohol intake predictably increases the GGTP, but so do many other agents.)
- Thrombocytopenia (low platelet count) occurs frequently.
- An increase in red cell size (macrocytosis) with or without anemia, may be a clue.
- A lower than normal BUN (blood urea nitrogen) is common in alcoholics who have deficient diets.

Alcohol abuse causes numerous other laboratory test abnormalities, but these four are the most likely to be discovered coincidentally during your investigation of unrelated problems.

TREATMENT

Once identified, alcohol abuse *can* be treated, providing the patient agrees to commit him or herself to attaining and maintaining sobriety. This is a challenging goal, for patient and health care provider alike. Most estimates are that only 20% of alcoholics will be fully rehabilitated and remain alcohol-free, while 20% never attempt to stop drinking, and the remaining 60% have lifelong recurring courses of withdrawing from alcohol and then relapsing.

Treatment consists of detoxification, withdrawal from alcohol, and finally rehabilitation.

Detoxification refers to supportive treatment for the patient until the liver metabolizes the alcohol. In the most severe cases ("alcohol poisoning"), this supportive treatment may need to be as extreme as hemodialysis. Usually only respiratory support and prevention of aspiration is necessary. Patients must always be given i.v. thiamine to prevent Wernicke's encephalopathy, and many need magnesium supplementation.

Mild **withdrawal** symptoms (tremulousness and perhaps hallucinosis) may be treated with mild sedatives. Moderate withdrawal symptoms, ranging from moderate agitation to seizures, require i.v. sedatives and/or anti-convulsants. The most severe withdrawal state, delirium tremens (DTs), includes confusion, vivid hallucinations, increased autonomic activity (such as fever, tachycardia, and profuse sweating), and sometimes seizures and coma. These patients need intensive observation and supportive care.

Rehabilitation is the final step in treatment. Patients are usually hospitalized for a period of weeks. Most treatment approaches emphasize education, family involvement, complete abstinence, and individual and/or group therapy. Alcoholics Anonymous, for example, emphasizes the *admission of a loss of control* over alcohol, then rebuilding through fellowship and mutual support.

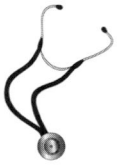

CASE RESOLUTION

Mr. J.H., a 39-year-old man, comes to the office at his wife's insistence complaining of "stomach pain". You have followed this patient for several years for mild hypertension, but you notice that he has missed several appointments recently. You also notice that, while you've enjoyed a pleasant relationship with him in the past, he seems irritable and somewhat evasive today.

By your routine questioning, you have determined that his problem may be gastritis. As you ask about certain exacerbating factors of his pain, he brusquely replies, "Look, Doc, I don't know why what I eat or drink is any of your business! If you can't give me something for my stomach, I'll go back to the Emergency Room. I've already been there twice for this in the last six months."

While you will likely be taken aback by this exchange, it is certainly still possible to salvage this encounter to the patient's benefit.

"I'm sorry these questions have upset you, Mr. H. These are just routine issues we must discuss. It sounds like you may have a significant problem if you had to go to the ER because of it, so let's see if we can go ahead and work this out."

You do not need to be confrontational at this time, even though you may suspect that the patient is using alcohol to excess. Clues which raise this suspicion include the nature of the patient's complaint, his behavioral changes, and his decision to go to the "anonymous" ER facility for his previous treatment, rather than coming to your office.

After an appropriate evaluation, you determine that the patient does have gastritis and you begin treatment. With sufficient support from you, he finally acknowledges his excessive alcohol use and you refer him to a rehabilitation facility.

SUMMARY

The primary care physician can play a key role in early recognition and treatment of alcoholism. Medical students can become familiar with the subtle clinical picture presented by the alcoholic patient and develop skills in history taking as well as knowledge of pertinent physical and laboratory findings that characterize this progressive disease. Physicians should maintain a high level of suspicion of substance abuse in their patients and expect denial of the disease by the patient and his or her family. Alcoholism can have a profound impact on families, so it is useful

for physicians to view alcoholism as a family disease and include family members in the evaluation and treatment process.

STUDY QUESTIONS*

1. Which is the most accurate statement regarding recognition of alcohol abuse?
    A. Primary care physicians usually don't miss early signs of alcohol abuse in patients.
    B. You do not need to consider alcohol abuse as a potential problem in patients over 65 years old.
    C. Alcoholics seldom seek medical attention, so it's difficult to diagnose the problem.
    D. Dysfunctional family behaviors may be a clue of possible alcohol abuse.

2. Treatment of alcoholism includes all the following steps except:
    A. Detoxification
    B. Plasmapheresis
    C. Withdrawal treatments
    D. Rehabilitation

3. Which of the following indicators is most sensitive in distinguishing alcohol use from alcohol abuse?
    A. Severity of the social consequences of alcohol use
    B. Quantity of alcohol consumed
    C. Development of physical tolerance
    D. Behaviors surrounding acquisition of alcohol

Suggested Reading

Ewing, J.A. Detecting alcoholism: The CAGE questionnaire. JAMA 252: 1905–1907; 1984.

Graham, A.V., N. Berolzheimer and S. Burge. Alcohol abuse: A family disease. Primary Care, 20 (1): 121–130; 1993.

Maly, R.C. Early recognition of chemical dependence. Primary Care, 29 (1): 33–50; 1993.

*For answers, see page 347.

When You Suspect 20
Depression

Gretchen E. Oley

INTRODUCTION

CASE PRESENTATIONS
CASE 1

Mrs. D, a 54-year-old woman, comes to the office complaining of headache, fatigue and intermittent abdominal discomfort. Eight months ago, her physical examination and blood tests were normal. At this visit, there is nothing particularly alarming about her individual complaints and her physical examination is unchanged. You prescribe over-the-counter analgesics, and advice for an exercise program and extra fiber in her diet. Three weeks later she returns complaining of similar symptoms. Blood tests are normal again, and a barium enema is normal.

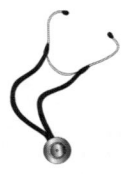

CASE 2

Mr. M. is a 66-year-old man who comes in for a regular appointment for follow-up of essential hypertension, gout, and diet-controlled diabetes. The patient has always seemed reasonably happy and well-adjusted. Before this appointment, his wife called your nurse and reported that her husband has been acting very strangely lately. He is withdrawn, has resigned from his golf league, and stays up all hours of the night. She is concerned that his diabetes may be worse or he may have had a "small stroke" and wants the doctor to "check him over good." On physical examination, the patient has no new or worrisome findings. His blood sugar, blood cholesterol, and blood pressure are stable. However, his weight has decreased by 15 lb. You observe a blunt, sad affect when sitting with the patient. Eye contact is poor and occasionally the patient gets tears in his eyes.

CASE 3

Miss B. is a 26-year-old woman who comes to the office for the first time. In the last year she began working at a firm whose health care plan for employees is obtained through a Health Maintenance Organization (HMO). She considers herself healthy but describes herself as "being depressed" for a long time, with a low energy level, barely dragging herself through her work-day. She has gained 25 lb over the last several years. She has difficulty making long-range plans or thinking in positive terms about her future. She has felt this way off and on since her college years and has rarely felt totally free of these unwanted feelings. Both her mother and older sister have been treated with antidepressants and have had counseling at various points in their lives.

Depession is an extremely common medical disorder.

Patients like the three described in these vignettes are seen very frequently in doctors' offices. All three suffer from depression. If their physicians correctly identify and treat them, their symptoms will improve.

An estimated 5–10% of patients treated in a family practice or general internal medicine practice suffer from a major depressive illness, and another 25% suffer from less severe depressive disorders. Indeed, depression is the second most common emotional disorder in this country, after anxiety disorders, which occur slightly more often. At least 75% of patients who receive treatment for depression are treated in primary care settings. *Unfortunately, only 30–50% of patients who need treatment for depression are accurately identified, diagnosed, and treated within this same setting.*

Patients report that depression is one of the most distressing and painful conditions they have ever experienced; depression causes inestimable suffering and disability among the general population. As all humans feel sad at one time or another, it is difficult for physicians, particularly those not trained in psychiatric medicine, to fully grasp the idea that depression can be a very real, persistent, and debilitating disease. Depression results from the interplay of a multitude of factors, including fixed genetic and biochemical determinants, and variable behavioral and social influences. Clearly, it is important for you to begin early in your career to understand the epidemiology, pathophysiology, diagnostic techniques, and basic therapy of this disease.

TYPES OF DEPRESSIVE DISORDERS

The term **mood disorder** is used by the American Psychiatric Association (APA) to encompass all the disturbances physicians usually call "depression." The APA publishes guidelines for defining these illnesses; their latest Diagnostic and Statistical Manual, (DSM-IV), classifies depression into eight major categories: major depression, adjustment disorder with depression, dysthymic disorder, seasonal affective disorder, bipolar disorder, cyclothymic disorder, postpartum depression, and premenstrual dysphoric disorder. The major clinical features of these depressive disorders are outlined in Table 20-1.

As your medical career progresses, you will discover that patients' depressive disorders cannot always be easily classified. The term "Depressive Disorder, Not Otherwise Specified," is a useful and meaningful classification for patients who suffer from depression, but fail to meet all criteria for any specific disorder. Though depression should not be a wastebasket diagnosis, employed to label all troubled patients, you will find certain patients who do not readily fit any depressive category but still respond positively to our interventions.

> The diagnosis of depression has a high degree of precision that is frequently not appreciated.

EPIDEMIOLOGY

Gender

Major depressive disorder occurs two to three times more frequently in women than in men, with a lifetime prevalence of 10–20% in women and 5–10% in men. Women also predominate in the categories of seasonal affective disorder and the cyclic disorders, and by definition, only women suffer from postpartum depression and premenstrual syndromes.

Age

Mood disorders occur in all age groups and should be considered in patients of any age. The highest rates of major depression occur between the ages of 25 and 34 years. Previously, it was commonly held that depression occurred at a higher rate in the elderly but recent epidemiologic data suggests that, in fact, there is a slightly lower prevalence rate in the older population.

> Mood disorders have some very well-defined characteristics statistically in the US population.

Table 20-1. Classification of Depressive Disorders

Diagnosis	Features required for diagnosis
Major depressive disorder	• Two or more consecutive weeks of depressed mood or major loss of interest in life *and* any four of the following: ▶ Weight loss or gain ▶ Psychomotor agitation or retardation* ▶ Insomnia or hypersomnia ▶ Feelings of worthlessness or inappropriate guilt ▶ Decreased ability to concentrate ▶ Recurrent thoughts of death or suicide
Adjustment disorder with depressed mood	• Mood drop, but less serious than major depression • Identifiable stressor in the environment within 3 months of onset of mood change, and not persisting more than 6 months past the stressful event.
Dysthymic disorder	• Chronically depressed personalities • Symptoms for at least 2 years, never free of symptoms more than 2 months • At least two of the following: ▶ Appetite change ▶ Sleep disturbance ▶ Fatigue ▶ Poor self-esteem ▶ Poor concentration ▶ Feelings of hopelessness
Seasonal affective disorder	• Onset of depressive symptoms in fall or winter with definite improvement in spring • Pattern present for at least 2 years *with no nonseasonal depression*
Bipolar disorder	• Patients cycle between depressive illness and manic behaviors • Severe functional impairment in family and occupation
Cyclothymic disorder	• Milder form of bipolar disorder with at least two years of shifting moods • Less functional impairment than bipolar disorder
Postpartum depression	• Onset after giving birth (immediate or up to 6 months later) • May occur in 10–20% of women • Severe, true psychosis is rare, no more than 1 in 1000 cases, but can be very dangerous to mother and baby
Premenstrual dysphoric disorder	• Sometimes called premenstrual syndrome (PMS) • Slightly more vague diagnostic criteria than other depressions • May not occur at same level of severity every month

*"Psychomotor agitation and retardation" refers to moving and talking either rapidly and aimlessly, or inappropriately slowly.

Table 20-2. Epidemiologic Features of Depression

Feature	Statistic for US population
Gender	• 2–3 times higher frequency in women • Lifetime prevalence 5–10% in men, 10–20% in women
Age	• Highest rate of onset between ages 25–34, but can occur in all age groups
Length of episode	• First episode usually lasts 6–12 months • Subsequent episodes usually become gradually longer

Suicide risk	• A rare complication of depression, *but* prevalence of depression is so high that:
	  ▶ Suicide among top 10 causes of death in all age groups
	  ▶ Among top three causes of death in adolescents and young adults
	  ▶ Highest rate of *successful* suicide attempts—elderly white males

Temporal Patterns

Though mood disorders are frequently chronic in nature, remitting and exacerbating over time, any one patient's pattern is difficult to predict. First episodes tend to last 6–12 months with subsequent bouts of depression gradually lasting longer.

Susceptibility to Depression

There is a familial or biological susceptibility to depression, though the exact mechanism has yet to be defined. Persons without familial susceptibility tend to have their first depressive illness later in life, are less likely to have repeated episodes, and are more likely to experience it in association with a severe loss or stressor. The strongest predictive factors for any one individual to experience major depression are:

- recent stressful life event
- a prior episode of depression
- a family history of mood disorder
- the presence of another psychiatric problem.

Suicide Risk

The most dramatic and life-threatening result of serious depression is attempted or successful suicide. Suicide ranks among the 10 leading causes of deaths in all age categories, and always among the top three causes of death in adolescents and young adults. While suicidal ideation is a rare result of depression, depression is such a common problem that suicidal attempts become a major problem. Depressed, elderly white males have the highest rates of *successful* suicide; other risk factors for successful attempts include alcoholism or other drug dependency, chronic physical illness, and lack of social support. Patients who exhibit more severe, psychotic features accompanying a mood disorder also have a somewhat higher risk of suicide.

Resource Utilization

Patients with mood disorders are very major users of nonpsychiatric medical services, including emergency room visits. Reasons for this include the high incidence of mood disorders, the lack of public and professional awareness of the scope of the problem, and the rather diffuse or nonspecific presentation of symptoms. Depressed patients' frequent use of medical resources has begun to increase awareness of depression as a significant public health issue.

PATHOPHYSIOLOGY

The specific cause(s) of mood disorders remains to be elucidated. It is unclear whether a single or many factors contribute to the etiology. Most researchers and clinicians operate with a construct known as the "Biopsychosocial Model of Depression," acknowledging that both environmental and biologic factors play a role in depression.

Biologic Factors

- Central nervous system chemoreceptor systems appear very important in depression. These systems involve serotonin, norepinephrine, dopamine and endorphin neurotransmitters in mood regulation.
- Estrogen and progesterone physiology may play a role in depression in women.

- The hypothalamic–pituitary–adrenal axis, including thyroglobulin-releasing hormone, prolactin, growth hormone, and cortisol are involved.
- Sleep physiology holds an important key to depressive disorders, as alterations in rapid eye movement (REM) sleep patterns occur in clinically depressed patients.
- Positron emission tomography demonstrates different patterns of regional brain metabolism in depressed patients.

> Depression clearly has a biological basis which may be multifactorial and is being widely investigated.

At this point, the conservative conclusion is that *biochemical "markers" are present in depressed patients*, but whether they play a causative role or whether they can be specifically tied to individual cases remains unclear.

Genetic and Environmental Factors

- There is *no* Mendelian pattern of inheritance in depressive disorders.
- Social factors such as poverty, domestic abuse and caretaking burdens may be highly operational in certain subsets of depressed patients and may explain why more women are affected by mood disturbances than men.
- Predisposing personality factors may be present.
- Environmental factors such as cultural and ethnic expectations and uncontrollable personal stressors clearly enter the picture.
- Iatrogenic causes of mood disturbances (e.g., prescribed medicines) have been identified.

MAKING THE DIAGNOSIS

How do primary care physicians discover whether their patients are depressed? Uninformed physicians frequently fall into the trap of assuming (as their patients might, as well) that depression is not a medical problem or illness at all. If it is viewed as personal failure, lack of moral fortitude, or as a shameful, weak response to life's stressors, it is unlikely that either the physician or the patient will make or accept the diagnosis.

Doctors often avoid opening the infamous "Pandora's Box" when evaluating patients with possible depression because they think it will take an inordinate amount of time to diagnose and treat. However, this is a self-fulfilling prophecy supported by very little objective evidence.

With important ramifications for public health, all clinicians must recognize that depression is an important and well defined medical entity.

Rarely do patients walk into their physicians' offices and say, "I think I have significant depression, can you treat me?" In the hospital patients may be identified by suicide attempts or gestures. Sometimes families will pressure patients to seek out psychiatrists, or finally legally commit loved ones who are obviously depressed. However, in the primary care office setting, the symptoms and signs are more subtle and your skill in evaluating the sometimes elusive clues to depression is critical in making the diagnosis.

Interviewing skills are paramount in helping establish a diagnosis of depression.

You may surmise that a patient has emotional problems through answers to the questions of the Review of Systems. More likely, you will become aware of the situation by *nonverbal clues* such as tearfulness, slow speech, or downcast eyes. Many patients expressly deny depression; however, with patience and probing questions you eventually can identify the problem. A fully accurate assessment frequently can't be made during one visit; it is necessary to schedule frequent follow-up visits for these patients until the clinical situation is defined.

Patients may deny depression because of the stigma of psychiatric disease, the patient's lack of awareness about their own emotional state, or because the patient is focused on their physical symptoms and complaints.

Because patients self-select symptoms to report, you may easily miss asking important questions. Some specific questions to define a patient's emotional state, not often included in the interviewing section of your standard text book, include:

1. Tell me about your sleeping habits.
   Have you lost or gained weight for no clear reason?
2. What do you like to do for relaxation or a good time?
   Are you still doing these things?
3. Has there been a recent tragedy or very stressful event in your life?
4. Do you feel helpless or hopeless about certain things in your life? Do you feel you are pessimistic about things in general? Do you feel inadequate or not up to coping with certain situations? Are you feeling more guilty or worrying more than you used to?
5. Are things okay with work, your family, your sex life?
6. Have you or others noted that you are more irritable or inappropriately angry lately?
7. Are you more tired than usual? Can you complete or finish your usual daily activities?
8. Do you have difficulty making decisions, starting or finishing tasks?
9. How much of your life have you felt like this?

10. Have you ever been diagnosed with depression or another "nervous disorder" before?
11. Is there a fluctuation or seasonality to your feelings?
12. Have you given birth in the last year?
13. Do you use/abuse alcohol or other drugs?
14. Are there periods of time when you have unusual amounts of energy. Have you had times where you couldn't sleep, went on spending sprees, felt hypersexual?
15. Do you live alone? Do you have help and support from friends or family?
16. Have you ever felt that it didn't matter if you lived or died? Have you ever considered killing yourself? Have you ever made a plan for killing yourself or actually tried to harm yourself? How does the future look to you?

Several patient self-report questionnaires have been developed to screen for depression efficiently and accurately. Primary care practitioners can use these questionnaires to supplement their personal screening of patients. These questionnaires have been validated as sensitive to detect depressive symptoms, i.e., patients with feelings or emotions that relate to depression *can* be identified. *However, answers to these questions do not make a diagnosis of depression*. Only the physician can make that important decision based on clear-cut clinical criteria.

> There are practical short-hand techniques that may help screen groups of patients for depression.

The four self-report scales often used in ambulatory care are the General Health Questionnaire (GHQ), the Center for Epidemiological Studies-Depression Scale (CES-D), the Beck Depression Inventory (BDI), and the Zung Self-Rating Depression Scale. More recently, the Short Depression Screen was developed and used in the Medical Outcomes Study. It is an eight-question instrument that accurately identifies patients with major depression. A high score on one of these instruments is a fairly *sensitive* measurement to identify *potentially* depressed patients, but is not very *specific*. (These instruments have low positive predictive values.) Despite these drawbacks, self-report screening tools are under-utilized, and you should learn how to use at least one of them. (See the suggested readings for details of these instruments.)

DIFFERENTIAL DIAGNOSES

Depression is not a diagnosis of exclusion, though many well-meaning physicians stubbornly cling to this idea. After all the appropriate history is collected, you must do a physical examination and problem analysis.

Unreasonable searches for diseases not at all suggested by the history, symptoms, or findings should be avoided.

Symptoms or findings that *reasonably* suggest a physical reason for the patients' difficulties should be investigated (see Table 20-3).

You will often find it worthwhile to *quiz the patient as to exactly what they feel is wrong*. Sometimes, strange or inappropriate concerns (for example, about fatal diseases) can be a large part of the problem, easily rectified by physician reassurance.

The most common diseases which resemble depression (i.e., the differential diagnoses) are listed in Table 20-4. Some of these diseases, such as multiple sclerosis, are subtle and may have classic findings only late in their course. Fibromyalgia and chronic fatigue syndrome are nonspecific and poorly defined diseases which have some characteristics of depression but not enough to clearly fulfill all criteria. Personality disorders, particularly drug or alcohol dependency or a somatization disorder may mimic depression. Uncomplicated bereavement can look like depression, but only becomes a clinical problem if patients are still clearly dysfunctional for more than 6 months after their loss.

Medications may contribute to a patient's symptoms. Depression can be seen with a variety of drugs including antihypertensives, anticonvulsants, hormones, steroids, digitalis, antiparkinsonian drugs, antineoplastic drugs, and antibiotics. A high level of suspicion and knowledge of basic pharmacology assist in identifying medication-related depression. Symptoms may be fully treated by simply eliminating the offending drug(s).

TREATMENT

Treatment of depression frequently involves drug therapy.

The good news is that the treatment of depression is effective in over 90% of patients. Psychotherapy (usually short-term, interpersonal, cognitive and supportive) and medications are the main therapeutic approaches. Psychotherapy alone is as helpful as medication in *mild* depressive disorders, but not effective alone in more severe forms. Most patients need 6–9 months of drug therapy after full remission. Whether medication is used once, recurrently, or chronically/prophylactically is determined by the patient's response.

Several drugs with differing mechanisms of action are available. Some of the newer agents have fewer side effects than the earlier prototype medications. Drug treatment of depression in the elderly is more challenging in that these patients frequently are frail, have more comorbid illnesses and metabolize drugs differently.

Table 20-3. Physical Examination and Laboratory Tests in Evaluation of Major Depression

1. Vital signs including height, weight
2. Complete neurological examination
3. Examination of any system in which there are clinical symptoms
4. Relevant laboratory tests including complete blood count, electrolytes, liver function tests and thyroid functions
5. Radiological studies appropriate to history and physical examination findings

Table 20-4. Differential Diagnoses of Depression

Thyroid disease
Occult malignancies
Collagen vascular or rheumatoid disease
Infectious diseases
    (e.g., hepatitis, mononucleosis, Lyme disease and AIDS)
Degenerative neurologic disorders
    (e.g., Parkinson's and dementias)
Chronic fatigue syndrome and fibromyalgia
Bereavement
Substance abuse and personality disorders
Side effects of drugs
Hematologic disorders with anemia

When to Refer

Patients should be referred for specialty psychiatric care under certain circumstances.

- If the patient does not respond to usual drugs or combination of drugs after several trials of therapy, referral is indicated.
- If the patient is suicidal or psychotic or the diagnosis is ever in question, the patient should be referred.
- More specialized techniques of therapy such as certain drugs, electroconvulsive therapy, and intense psychotherapy invariably require the skills and expertise of a specialist in psychiatric or behavioral medicine.

- Developing reliable and efficient referral patterns helps the primary care practitioner get the best treatment available for their patients.

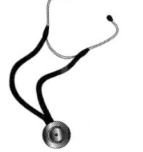

CASE RESOLUTION

So what do you think were the diagnoses of the three patients presented at the beginning of the chapter? Using the knowledge obtained in this section, the diagnoses should become clear.

CASE 1

Mrs. D, a 54-year-old woman, comes to the office complaining of headache, fatigue and intermittent abdominal discomfort. Eight months ago, her physical examination and blood tests were normal. At this visit, there is nothing particularly alarming about her individual complaints and her physical examination is unchanged. You prescribe over-the-counter analgesics, and advice for an exercise program and extra fiber in her diet. Three weeks later she returns complaining of similar symptoms. Blood tests are normal again, and a barium enema is normal.

You take some extra time with the patient and reassure her that all her tests are normal. She concludes that she is "just getting old" and will have to learn to adjust.

She returns again in 1 month complaining of intermittent dizziness, muscle aches, new abdominal symptoms, and an inability to concentrate or remember things clearly at work.

Before you see the patient this time, your nurse tells you that she has heard at church that within the past 6 months, Mrs. D's father has died and her mother has been diagnosed with cancer. Also, there are rumors that her son has had legal problems with his business.

This time you only briefly examine Mrs. D, then you sit and talk with her about her emotional state. She opens up to you quickly and confirms the problems noted by your nurse. She then says, "I believe that is really what has been wrong with me. I just worry too much."

This patient suffers from an adjustment disorder with depressed mood. As you now identify, she had some of the symptoms of depression but not enough to meet the criteria for a major depression. She had an identifiable stressor within 6 months of the onset of her symptoms and no clear physical illness.

CASE 2

Mr. M. is a 66-year-old man who comes in for a regular appointment for follow-up of essential hypertension, gout, and diet-controlled diabetes. The patient has always seemed reasonably happy and well adjusted. Before this appointment, his wife called your nurse and reported that her husband has been acting very strangely lately. He is withdrawn, has resigned from his golf league and stays up all hours of the night. She is concerned that his diabetes may be worse or he may have had a "small stroke" and wants the doctor to "check him over good." On physical examination, the patient has no new or worrisome findings. His blood sugar, blood cholesterol, and blood pressure are stable. However, his weight has decreased by 15 lb. You observe a blunt, sad affect when sitting with the patient. Eye contact is poor and occasionally the patient gets tears in his eyes.

So far you do not identify a specific diagnosis for Mr. M. Therefore you take additional history.

The patient admits to a profound sense of sadness and despair that he can't explain. He's had "the blues" before but they have always left within weeks or at least several months. He's tired but can't sleep at night. He quit golfing because it became too much of an effort to get his "clubs ready and go face his friends." On some days he has felt so worthless that he had thought it better if he simply "didn't wake up in the morning," though he has never made a plan to actively harm himself.

The second patient had a major depressive disorder. He clearly met many criteria for a major depressive disorder:

- He has a major loss of interest in life
- He has lost weight
- He has developed insomnia
- He feels worthless
- His activity and energy level are much decreased.

Though he had some chronic diseases, none was severely debilitating, and the doctor has found no new findings to otherwise explain the symptoms.

CASE 3

Miss B. is a 26-year-old woman who comes to the office for the first time. In the last year she began working at a firm whose health care plan for employees is obtained through a Health Maintenance Organization (HMO). She considers herself healthy, but describes herself as "being depressed" for a long time, with a low energy level, barely dragging herself through her work day. She has gained 25 lb over the last several years. She has difficulty

making long-range plans or thinking in positive terms about her future. She has felt this way off and on since her college years and has rarely felt totally free of these unwanted feelings. Both her mother and older sister have been treated with antidepressants and have had counseling at various points in their lives.

Miss B. has a dysthymic disorder. She has much milder symptoms than Mr. M., not meeting criteria for major depression. But she clearly does have symptoms which interfere with her functioning, especially fatigue and appetite changes.

All three patients were quickly and appropriately diagnosed and successfully treated. Over the next year, all required a combination of counseling and support from you and your staff as well as antidepressant medication, though doses and lengths of therapy varied.

SUMMARY

As your medical career progresses, you will need to continue to develop and appropriately apply the skills that this chapter covers. They will help you adequately understand and support your patients who suffer from depression.

STUDY QUESTIONS[*]

1. All the following features are necessary for a diagnosis of major depression *except*:
    A. Two or more consecutive weeks of depressed mood or major loss of interest in life
    B. Feelings of worthlessness
    C. Recurrent thoughts of death or suicide
    D. Paranoid-type delusions

2. Depression in the primary care setting is:
    A. The rarest emotional disorder
    B. Common but often not diagnosed
    C. Common and usually diagnosed
    D. Present to some extent in every patient

---

[*]For answers, see page 347.

3. Which of the following is *not* a category of depression recognized by the APA?
   A. Seasonal affective disorder
   B. Postpartum depression
   C. Disappointment reaction
   D. Bipolar disorder

4. Predictive factors for experiencing depression include all the following except:
   A. A family history of mood disorder
   B. A prior episode of depression
   C. A family history of schizophrenia
   D. A stressful life event

5. Which of the following is *not* true of suicide?
   A. Elderly white females have the highest rate of successful suicide attempts.
   B. Suicide is among the top three causes of death among adolescents.
   C. Serious depression is a risk factor for suicide.
   D. Patients with more severe psychotic features of depression are at higher risk of suicide attempts.

Suggested Reading

Depression in Primary Care: Volume 1. Detection and Diagnosis. Clinical Practice Guideline, Number 5. Rockville, MD, U.S. Department of Health and Human Services. Public Health Service, Agency for Health Care Policy and Research. AHCPR Publication No. 93-0550, 1993.

Depression in Primary Care: Volume 2. Treatment of Major Depression. Clinical Practice Guideline, Number 5. Rockville, MD, U.S. Department of Health and Human Services. Public Health Service, Agency for Health Care Policy and Research, AHCPR Publication No. 93-0551, 1993.

Brody, David S., *et al.* The role of primary care physicians in managing depression. Journal of General Internal Medicine. 7 (March/April): 243–247; 1992.

Coulehan, J.L. Managing Depression in Primary Care. Internal Medicine. Vol. 15, No. 12: 34–49. Medical Economics Publishing. Montvale, NJ.

Goroll, A.H., May, L.A. & Mulley A.G. Jr. Primary Care Medicine. Office Evaluation and Management of the Adult Patient, 3rd edn, pp. 1033–1043. J.B. Lippincott Company, Philadelphia, PA, 1995.

Isselbacher, K.J., Braunwald, E., Wilson, Martin, Fauci, A. and Kasper. Harrison's Principles of Internal Medicine, 13th edn, pp. 2400–2409. McGraw-Hill, New York, NY., 1994.

Lemcke, D.P., Pattison, J., Marshall, L.A. & Cowley, D.S. Primary Care of Women, pp. 98–107. Appleton and Lange. Norwalk, CT, 1995.

Rosenfeld, J.A. Women's Health in Primary Care, pp. 183–203. Williams and Wilkins. Baltimore, MD. 1997.

Schwenk, T.L. Screening for depression in primary care (editorial). Journal of General Internal Medicine. 11: 437–439; 1996.

Wells, K.B., Stewart, A., Hays, R.D., *et al.* The functioning and well-being of depressed patients: results from the medical outcomes study. JAMA. 262: 914–919; 1989.

Williams, J.W., Jr *et al.* Depressive disorders in primary care: prevalence, functional disability and identification. Journal of General Internal Medicine. 10: 7–11; 1995.

When You Suspect  *Domestic Violence*

Diane W. Mufson

INTRODUCTION

CASE PRESENTATIONS

The following case reports illustrate the spectrum of domestic violence. In each case, the situation is described as it initially appeared to the physician or health care professional.

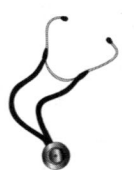

CASE 1

Ann, 28, arrives at the Emergency Room (ER) with a blackened eye, inflammation of the face, neck, and arms. She thinks her left arm is sprained or broken. Although calm, she avoids talking more than necessary and reports she fell down the basement stairs while carrying a full laundry basket. Her husband, 31, accompanies her; he is extremely concerned about her situation and answers all questions quickly and calmly.

CASE 2

Beth, 40, returns to her internist's office this year for the eighth time. All medical tests have been negative. She complains of GI problems, insomnia, and generalized anxiety. When asked about home life, she insists everything is fine.

CASE 3

Johnny, 4, is brought to his pediatrician. He appears to have broken his elbow. His mother says he is "wild" and does dangerous things. She wonders if he needs medication for ADHD (attention deficit hyperactivity disorder). The child sits quietly in the office and does not complain of pain,

as would most children with fractures. His medical record notes a broken leg at age 1 from falling down stairs; stitches required for a large gash in his head at age 2 and burns on his hands at age 3 as a result of playing with a cigarette lighter. He appears much below average in weight for size and age.

CASE 4

Mary, 5, who is visiting her aunt for the weekend, is brought to the ER. Her aunt reports that she refuses to take a bath, cries from pain when she urinates, and says Daddy "plays special games with me when Mommy is working."

CASE 5

Laura, 14, comes to a youth health center clinic and says her stepfather has been forcing her to have sex with him for the past year. Now she thinks she is pregnant. She is upset, agitated, and does not want to return home.

If one medical condition existed that resulted in over 100 000 hospital days, 40 000 ambulatory visits and 30 000 emergency room (ER) contacts per year (1), would the medical community respond? Would a program of prevention be considered? Would research be suggested? Would educational activities be designed? While the answers to these questions should be "Yes," for at least one notable problem, reality indicates otherwise. That problem is domestic violence. Notwithstanding these medical resource utilization statistics, domestic violence was not usually considered as medically important. However, in the last 25 years, the US and other similar cultures recognized the negative social, behavioral, and interactional patterns consequent to this problem that need attention because of the costs in lives and economic problems.

Domestic violence can be generally defined as aggressive, hurtful negative behavior within a group of related people who live together. Beyond this basic definition, a variety of situations, relationships, violence levels and rationalizations make domestic violence a multidimensional area.

Some medical students will become distressed when they read this material. You may recognize familiar and uncomfortable echoes of some part of your family's life. Others will recall hearing of domestic violence scenes, but not feeling closely involved. Still others of you may be sure they do not know anyone who has ever been either a victim or perpetrator of active family malevolence. Nonetheless, you can be sure that by the time you have completed medical school and a residency you will experience first hand more than one aspect of domestic violence.

The following excerpts, which represent only the tip of the iceberg, are the press clippings from one week in the fall of 1996 from a newspaper serving an area of 100 000 population:

- A 27-year-old woman told police her husband came home intoxicated late Friday and threatened her life. She stated they got into an altercation after he accused her of sleeping with other men. The woman said he hit her in the face and head with his fists, kicked her in the leg, and held a knife to her throat. Reportedly she obtained a domestic violence petition against her husband.
- A local 26-year-old man was arrested on domestic battery charges after the police observed the man kick his wife in the shins. It was reported he had two other warrants on file for domestic battery in an adjacent county.
- A 38-year-old man was arrested early on Tuesday morning. He was charged with domestic battery after it was reported he spat in his girlfriend's face, pulled her hair, brandished a 12-inch butcher knife, and threatened to kill her.
- A 16-year-old boy told police he fought with a family member after the boy refused to get out of bed Wednesday morning. He stated that the family member threw a soda bottle at him and bruised his right arm. After he got out of bed he was punched in his left eye; a window was broken during the fight.
- A letter appeared in the newspaper requesting people not to vote for the reelection of magistrate John Doe (fictional name). The letter was written by the mother of a woman who had been a domestic violence victim. She noted that the magistrate would say things like "Oh, it's you again. Why don't you just move out of town?"

If this amount of news was published in one 5-day period in a local newspaper, how many domestic violence situations occurred in this community which were unreported? Berry (2) noted that up to 6 million women may suffer abuse in their own homes each year. While possibly two-thirds of domestic violence cases are reported, the National Coalition Against Domestic Violence suggests that as many as 90% of battered women never make a report.

Three main types of situations/victims characterize domestic abuse. As we discuss them, notice that they share something in common: each situation includes domination of individuals who are in a dependent, weaker, and subservient or less powerful role. This is particularly true when the person with power, strength, and control has a need to dominate, and lacks warmth, self-control or nurturance.

- *Partner abuse* Usually this is abuse of a wife by a husband. Men for the most part, are larger, possess a stronger muscular frame, weigh more than their spouses and have been accorded a dominant role by society. As same sex relationships are more openly recognized today, the incidence of violence towards same sex partners will probably increase. In recent years, a few cases of females abusing significant male partners, often with fatal results, have been reported.
- *Child abuse* Child abuse is an independent type of family violence. For years much child abuse has been camouflaged under rubric of "making men out of boys," "this is how I was raised and see how well I turned out," and "one can do whatever one wants with one's children." Child abuse can also include child sexual abuse.
- *Elder abuse* The third main type of domestic violence involves elders and those incompetent to fend for themselves. As the number of elderly, frail and dependent senior citizens increases, more of them are likely to become victims of hurtful actions.

Some progress has been made in the past 25 years in understanding and coping with domestic violence, primarily in the area of child abuse/neglect. Effective programs and laws are in place to direct health care professionals in dealing with child abuse. As yet, no cohesive program exists for spouse abuse. As Gelles (3) reported, a United States Senator was asked why the Senate was not holding hearings in wife abuse, as they did for child abuse; he is reported to have replied that eliminating wife abuse "would take all the fun out of marriage." Similar comments were reported of a district court judge following a wife's complaint about her husband's violence. The judge leaned over the bench and smiled at the husband and said, "If I were you, I would have hit her too."

Understanding elder, step and other relative abuse is just in its infancy. As a variety of kin become responsible for the health and wellness of family members, as the nuclear family shrinks, and as less support is evident for the caregiver, it is likely that domestic violence will occur more often in these situations.

DEFINITIONS

Domestic violence is an all-encompassing situation that includes physical violence, threats of violence, emotional abuse and sexual violence, among or with any legal or surrogate family member(s). The physical and emotional damage which results is beyond that which could be

accounted for by any reasonable disagreements ordinarily expressed in daily encounters. In its broadest form, domestic violence involves any treatment, action or behavior within a family/living unit that results in serious hurt, pain or loss of functional ability. Thus, child and elder abuse and neglect are included in this definition.

Spouse/significant other abuse is a behavior that seeks to control, dominate, restrict a spouse or other intimate partner or their behavior, by use of force, threats of force and/or manipulation of the environment. Battering and spouse beating are common forms. Total control of money, vehicles, social contacts and even homicide are common in spouse abuse.

Child maltreatment Children need a certain amount of nurturance to be able to grow and function in a healthy manner. Our society tends to believe that any "normal" adult will provide such basics for their children. "Real life" tells us otherwise. Child maltreatment includes:

1. *Physical abuse*: injury that results in pain, broken bones, disfigurement, head or body trauma or avoidable illness.
2. *Emotional abuse*: actions that result in fear for self or others, inability to cope appropriately for age/intelligence and lack of personal security. Children who witness violence towards a parent or loved one also fall into this domain.
3. *Neglect*: whether by intentional design or inability to function properly as a caregiver, the adult/parent(s) in charge do not provide for the safety, basic shelter, supervision and health needs of the child.
4. *Sexual abuse*: occurs when a child is involved in sexual activities for which s/he is not physically, socially or emotionally prepared and is not able to give appropriate consent. Thus, a child may appear to agree to a sexual activity with an adult family member, but in reality they can not understand the present or future consequences of this action.
5. *Munchausen by proxy syndrome*: overly aggressive medical care with negative results. Infrequently, situations occur in which a parent seeks constant or repeated emergency health care for a child, who is either not ill or only has a mild illness. In this case, the adult attempts to present him or herself in the role of a supreme caregiver to meet his/her own needs, while subjecting the child to unnecessary and often painful treatment.

Elder/incapacitated maltreatment is physical, mental, emotional and/or financial abuse or neglect that results in harm or injury to an

older individual, who is no longer able to look after their own interests competently or completely.

Sibling/child relations abuse involves behavior between minors who are related or living in the same family environment where one, usually the mentally or physically stronger child, controls the younger or less able one in a way that results in harm, injury or death.

CAUSES OF DOMESTIC VIOLENCE

If specific factors always, or even usually, signalled the occurrence of domestic violence, then with appropriate prevention and treatment modalities, domestic violence could be alleviated. However, this is not the case. Several factors may predispose some individuals to becoming both victims and perpetrators of domestic violence. By understanding these, some inroads can be made into decreasing the prevalence of domestic violence.

Childhood Experiences

We know that children incorporate their modes of functioning based upon what they learn in their formative years. The family environment provides a fertile training ground for good and bad. *The messages that are often transmitted to the child include:*

- The way our family works is how people interact; it is not wrong or right—*it is just how it is.*
- Females often learn that might makes right; that arguing with a male will result in negative consequences; and, they cannot do much about this. The concept of "learned helplessness," has been described by Walker (4) who reported that psychologist Martin Seligman first used this term for situations in which women feel powerless in controlling their own lives; it may become a training ground for victimization.
- Males often learn that by domineering, threatening, and physical force they will become "real men" and receive approval from a father figure who otherwise did not show much approval or affection in childhood.
- Other variations of abuse scenarios occur, where a victim may learn dysfunctional relating styles that escalate and perpetuate abuse. Unless they have reason to change, adults often revert to

or continue the pattern of domestic relationships they experienced while growing up. Walker further noted that battering was reported to have occurred in 81% of batterers' childhood homes, in 67% of battered women's childhood homes, but in only 24% of the nonbatterers (4).

Reaction to Frustration

Many individuals do not abuse on a regular basis. However, periodically they lose their composure and show violent or aggressive behavior.

Displaced aggression, in which an individual is upset or angry with another unrelated person to whom they cannot show their true feelings, may lead to periodic outbursts. While the aggressor may want to get even with a boss or powerful relative, he or she cannot; as a result, he or she takes out these negative feelings against a "safe" and less powerful individual.

Societal Values and Expectations

We live in a society that traditionally has identified and reinforced women as weaker, dependent and less aggressive. Men, on the other hand, have been seen as independent, strong and leaders. To further magnify the disparity between the roles of the sexes, men were identified as the wage earners, and until recent generations, this was accurate for the great majority.

It is interesting that the everyday term "rule of thumb," refers to the English Common Law which permitted a husband to beat his spouse with any stick as long as it was no thicker than his own thumb. This represented an *improvement* in the treatment of wives. In earlier times, a wife could be controlled with any reasonable means (2). The female was empowered only to make a home for her husband and care for the children, with the adult male's needs taking priority. Divorce was not an option for most women until the 1960s, and when it happened, usually it relegated the woman to serious economic deprivation. Jones (5) reported that over a century ago, two of the earlier champions of women's rights, Elizabeth Cady Staton and Susan B. Anthony, interpreted marriage as "an institution devised by men, and backed by all the authority of church and state, to give husbands absolute authority over wives."

Use of Drugs and/or Alcohol

Drugs and alcohol do not cause an individual to perpetrate or become a victim of domestic violence. What these stimulants do is to *reduce any effective judgment and social decision making skills*, so that these skills and judgments can no longer filter one's emotions and behaviors.

THE MYTHS AND THE FACTS OF DOMESTIC VIOLENCE

Domestic violence is not a "warm and fuzzy," socially acceptable subject. People do not talk about it with their work colleagues, social friends or family members. Because so little information about domestic violence is exchanged, large numbers of erroneous, or at least inaccurate, beliefs or myths flourish. Consequently,

1. These myths permit us to believe that domestic violence is an esoteric behavior occurring under only very unusual conditions; and, even more importantly,
2. They permit us to feel confident that the people *we* associate with would never do anything as despicable as those acts associated with domestic violence.

The myths and the facts that encompass domestic violence include:

MYTH   Only poor, uneducated people are involved
FACT   Domestic violence affects persons of any age, income, race, occupation, religion or any other personal quality. What we do find is that persons with high status and large incomes are much more likely to be able to camouflage or successfully deny any such involvement.

MYTH   Only mentally ill or "crazy" people are violent with their loved ones
FACT   A study by Murray Straus and colleagues (6) indicated that less than 10% of all types of family violence can be accounted for by mental illness or psychiatric disorders. Therefore, at least 90% of those inflicting harm on their loved ones are considered competent, of normal intelligence and able to understand their actions and consequences.

MYTH   Family violence is a rare and modern occurrence

FACT   Family violence has occurred throughout recorded history and probably before then (3). In examples from writings of Biblical times, Middle Ages and more recent European, Asian, African civilizations, males were (are) entitled to treat their women and children as possessions, and therefore do what they will with them. Gil (7) published a 1967 study of child abuse in the US. At that time, about 6000 cases occurred throughout the country; however, some states reported no cases. We now admit that domestic violence is not a new phenomenon. What is new is the increased frequency of its report. Gelles (3) cited Kempe and colleagues (8) concerning their publication of "the Battered Child Syndrome," as the seminal study alerting physicians to recognize and diagnose child abuse. Based largely on the work of Caffey (9), they used X-ray technology to identify physical damage to children. Once child abuse was recognized as a problem in our society, wife abuse and other forms of family violence could be understood as destructive behavior, urgently in need of attention by the medical community.

Recent statistics (2) substantiate an increasing awareness of the problem. By the end of the 1960s, *all 50 states passed laws requiring professionals (physicians, social workers, psychologists, teachers, etc.) who suspect abuse of children to report it to the proper authorities.* Protection of women and the elderly as victims has taken longer and has been less comprehensive than that of child victims.

MYTH   Without alcohol and drugs there would be no violence

FACT   The use of these substances is associated with family abuse patterns. However, experts hold diverging opinions on the degree to which these stimulants are responsible. Flanzer (10) believes that they are causal agents of violence, while Gelles (11) perceives that they are related to, but not responsible for, abuse. Although the use of these substances may cause ordinary behavioral controls to lapse, many instances of abuse occur while the abuser is completely sober. Alcohol sometimes represents a convenient scapegoat, so that its use may be blamed for the entire problem. However, individuals with severe substance abuse patterns are likely to have few if any behavioral controls and their main concerns in life may be procuring the substances they crave, rather than meeting anyone else's needs.

MYTH   Once people realize what they are doing or mature, violence will stop

FACT   This is a great idea, but the sad truth is that violence usually becomes a way of functioning, a means of handling emotions or a familiar behavior. Unless some major unpleasant event happens to the abuser, little chance exists that they will change behaviors.

MYTH   Battered wives are incompetent and uneducated; anyone with any brains or gumption would remove themselves from an ongoing violent environment

FACT   While some physical and verbal abusive behaviors may begin early on in a relationship, many violence patterns develop slowly and subtly. Often, the victim cannot believe that the person who has expressed such love for them and who has been so supportive and caring can actually be so brutal. The victim often minimizes or rationalizes the events until the pattern is well established and the victim's situation becomes so restrictive, that escape from the victimization becomes extremely difficult.

MYTH   People who are violent to family members will always display this pattern

FACT   Violence and anger outbursts tend to occur periodically. Walker (12) described a cyclic theory of violence that identifies a pattern where tension builds, the violent behavior occurs and a loving, kind stage ensues. Victims of violence report that the dual feelings of hope for the future and caring, attention and often repentance from the abuser in the present, lead them to feel that the abuse, battering and destructive patterns are over. Many victims anticipate that a period of one to three months without any violence may build their hopes for the end of this cycle. Walker (12) also noted that as the cycle of battering continued, victims recognized the tension phase as more apparent and the warmth and caring episodes from the abuser as less frequent. Additionally, people who are violent or abusive at home may not exhibit these same behaviors at work or in other social settings.

FACTS AND FIGURES

Domestic violence continues to occur in the US at an embarrassingly high rate for a "civilized" society such as ours. It is not clear whether the high number of abuse reports in recent years represents a real increase

in activity or if it is due to improved recognition and reporting. Myriad facts and figures (2) attest to the magnitude of the problem (Table 21-1). They sustain the viewpoint that medical professionals will invariably be forced to deal with domestic violence in their patients at some time in their career.

WHAT TO LOOK FOR WHEN YOU SUSPECT DOMESTIC VIOLENCE

Only a small minority of domestic violence victims will spontaneously tell you what has happened to them. The question then is, "how to decide if you are dealing with someone whose complaints should be a red flag?" You need to be aware of the signs of domestic violence. Some guidelines which can alert you to domestic violence:

- *Patients who appear with unexplained or poorly explained injuries.* Often these injuries do not match the manner in which they are reported to have occurred. Professional training, experience and sometimes common sense will tell you that two plus two is not equalling four.
- *Patients who reappear with unusual frequency for treatment of results of accidents.* While most people have occasional minor household accidents, people who appear for care with recurring reports of falling off ladders, slipping down stairs, burning themselves on frying pans, and running into doors, may indeed be signaling that they are having household disasters. It is just that their disaster object may be human rather than inanimate.
- *Patients who have the ability to explain their status, but are reluctant to say much.* They may appear evasive, embarrassed, confused or uncooperative. No matter how hard you try, you just cannot obtain clear, precise information.
- *Pregnant women with injuries to the abdomen, the genital area or breasts.* Men sometimes become jealous, worried or angry during their partner's pregnancy and may direct their hostility to the physical areas they associate with pregnancy.
- *Unexplained anxiety, nervousness, withdrawal.* People who are victims of abuse find themselves isolated. They do not know where to turn and feel they cannot tell anyone about their problems. They tend to lose trust in themselves and others. They feel that if they were not smart enough to discern that they have formed a liaison with an abuser and that others will feel they are stupid. Over time these feelings can lead to depression, suicidal thoughts or panic attacks.

Table 21-1. Facts and Figures About Domestic Violence

In 1994, the Secretary of the Department of Health and Human Services indicated there were 4 million reported domestic violence incidents.

The American Medical Association reports that 1 out of 3 women treated in an emergency room is a victim of violence.

Murder is the second leading cause of death for women between 15–24 years.

Women who divorce or separate from their abusive partners report being battered about 14 times as often as those who continue living with their partners.

Up to 75% of battered women victims are trying to leave or have left men who do not wish them to leave.

Pregnant women are at high risk for domestic abuse; 25–33% of them may be battered or abused.

Close to 75% of children in an abusive home, witness the violence. Almost all of them know what is going on even if they do not see it.

Fifty to 70% of males who abuse their female partners also abuse children in the home. The more children in the home, the better the chance that one of them will be treated harshly.

A study in 1991 showed that of men who were arrested, prosecuted, convicted, and sentenced for assaulting a female partner, less than 1% served any jail time.

Ninety-five percent of battering victims are women. Rape occurs in about 50% of violent relationships.

The estimated cost of treating domestic violence victims is $3–5 billion annually.

The estimated loss annually in wages, sick leave and absences due to the effects of domestic violence is $100 million.

Wives also assault spouses at times. However, the National Crime Victimization Survey (13) indicates that the rate of assaults by males is 13 times greater than that by females.

- *Patients who are overly sensitive or "jumpy."* These people are "on guard." They expect something bad to happen and become hyper-vigilant. They cannot relax. Their behavior is incongruent with the situation from an external view. Internally, they are expecting "the other shoe to drop."
- *Overly protective husbands/partners.* What appears as great concern and warmth for the victim, may actually be a means of controlling the

victim and impressing others. If concern for a patient is so over-powering that the patient cannot express him/herself, it may be an indication of domination rather than support.

PHYSICAL AND BEHAVIORAL INDICATIONS OF DOMESTIC VIOLENCE

Recognizing Domestic Violence

There are few foolproof ways to assess domestic violence. The clearest situation would be where two people walk in to your office together and one says "in a moment of anger I hit my spouse in the face and the resulting swollen eye and loose teeth are because of that." Perhaps they even indicate that after they take care of their medical needs, they recognize and will seek help for their emotional and behavioral difficulties. While a professional *might* encounter a scenario similar to this one, it is best not to rely upon it. Therefore, you must look for some of the possible **clues indicative of a domestic violence situation**. These may include:

Physical injuries

- Swollen or blackened eyes
- Broken bones, especially if of dubious origin
- Burns and bruises, especially on difficult to reach areas, such as soles of feet and buttocks
- Broken nose
- Cauliflower ears
- Signs of choking or pressure around the neck; damaged vocal cords
- Bruises or injury to breasts and vaginal area
- Broken fingers or hands
- Multiple bruises in various stages of healing
- Unexplained hemorrhages
- Ruptured spleen or internal organs
- Missing, chipped or loosened teeth
- Split and swollen lips.

Behavioral indices in victims

- Confusion
- Avoidance or ambiguousness in answering questions
- Looking to spouse for answers
- Difficulty making eye contact
- High degrees of agitation or anxiety
- Flattened affect or depressive presentation.

Victims often display the "Stockholm Syndrome" (5) in which traumatic psychological infantilism and pathological transference come into play. The result is that a victim aligns himself or herself with his captors/abusers and sees them as support, and those who would like to offer help, as meddlers.

SUGGESTIONS FOR HELPING DOMESTIC VIOLENCE VICTIMS

As a student physician, you need to become informed about recognition and evaluation of domestic violence victims. However, you must not act alone to treat or counsel them in a definitive way. The following points speak to the evaluation of domestic violence victims:

1. Be informed and conversant with domestic violence information. Make sure you believe that "anyone can become a victim".
2. Check medical records as much as possible.
3. If you suspect abuse, examine the patient without the person present who seems to have control over her/him and could be an abuser.
4. Maintain an equal eye-level with a person you suspect has been victimized. It is much easier for people who have been controlled by others to interact and talk openly when they perceive the helping individual is not physically towering over them.
5. Be prepared to ask concrete questions such as "Tell me precisely how you acquired these injuries." "Did anyone hurt you?" Do not put pressure on the victim to say more than they choose to say, but leave the opportunity open for them to speak up in the future.
6. Be familiar with agencies, social services and domestic violence shelters that exist within your community. If national, state or regional hotlines exist, become familiar with them. Provide such information to patients when they are not with a person who may

be an abuser. Give name(s) or phone numbers of domestic violence shelters to patients if they are at all interested.

7. Do not feel unsuccessful if a victim does not take your offer of help. *It can often be dangerous to make rapid, unplanned changes in leaving an abusive situation.* Data also suggest that women may consider several "leaving scenarios" before they actually do so.

8. Remember domestic violence is not a medical diagnosis. However, in making medical diagnoses, you will at some time see cases of family violence.

9. Clearly record your medical findings and what the patient says. You or a colleague are apt to encounter that individual again and the medical records may be needed in other medical or legal situations.

10. Seek your colleague(s) help in treating domestic violence situations, as they are usually difficult for all involved.

CASE RESOLUTION

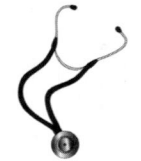

In analyzing these cases, you should consider the following:

1. There is a problem situation that cannot be ignored.
2. Medical and psychological issues are intertwined.
3. Treatment is likely to involve professionals from various disciplines.
4. The treating physician or health care professional may have personal concerns or emotional responses that may impact on patient treatment.

CASE 1

Ann, 28, arrives at the Emergency Room (ER) with a blackened eye, inflammation of the face, neck, and arms. She thinks her left arm is sprained or broken. Although calm, she avoids talking more than necessary and reports she fell down the basement stairs while carrying a full laundry basket. Her husband, 31, accompanies her; he is extremely concerned about her situation and answers all questions quickly and calmly.

Ann has been physically assaulted by her husband. He really does care about her, but loses control of his temper periodically. He has a high status job and will do anything to keep his secret. Ann comes from a family where women are supposed to take care of others and not complain.

CASE 2

Beth, 40, returns to her internists office for the eighth time this year. All medical tests have been negative. She complains of GI problems, insomnia, and generalized anxiety. When asked about home life, she insists everything is fine.

Beth has never been physically abused. However, she has been emotionally and verbally assaulted and the only way she can escape from constant demands made by her husband is to be "ill."

CASE 3

Johnny, 4, is brought to his pediatrician. He appears to have broken his elbow. His mother says he is "wild" and does dangerous things. She wonders if he needs medication for ADHD (attention deficit hyperactivity disorder). The child sits quietly in the office and does not complain of pain, as would most children with fractures. His medical record notes a broken leg at age 1 from falling down stairs, stitches required for a large gash in his head at age 2, and burns on his hands at age 3 as a result of playing with a cigarette lighter. He appears much below average in weight for size and age.

Johnny has been physically abused by both parents and his oldest two siblings; he has been neglected also. He does not have ADHD. He is the youngest of five children in a family where substance abuse and unemployment are common.

CASE 4

Mary, 5, who is visiting her aunt for the weekend, is brought to the ER. Her aunt reports that she refuses to take a bath, cries from pain when she urinates, and says Daddy "plays special games with me when Mommy is working."

Mary's physical examination indicates sexual abuse. Her laboratory report is positive for a sexually transmitted disease (STD).

CASE 5

Laura, 14, comes to a youth health center clinic and says her stepfather has been forcing her to have sex with him for the past year. Now she thinks she is pregnant. She is upset, agitated, and does not want to return home.

Laura is pregnant, but by her boyfriend. She has been miserable since her mother remarried and saw her predicament as a means to handle both problems.

SUMMARY

Domestic violence takes many forms and affects many people. Victims may be reluctant to admit to their situations and indeed may deny the problem. You must maintain a high index of suspicion to avoid missing domestic violence as a diagnostic consideration in your patients.

STUDY QUESTIONS[*]

1. Domestic violence situations may include:
    A. Threats of maltreatment and potential harm
    B. Actual physical force and battering
    C. Control of vehicles and social contacts
    D. All of the above

2. Which is not likely to be a cause of domestic violence?
    A. Childhood exposure to family domestic violence
    B. Learned helplessness in females
    C. Growing up in a heavily urban environment
    D. Messages to males to grow up to be "real men"

3. Which of the following health concerns are not likely to be associated with domestic violence?
    A. Swollen or blackened eyes
    B. Unexplained hemorrhages
    C. Frequent nonspecific anxiety or distress
    D. Rash on hands and feet

4. A Basic reason for much of the ongoing domestic abuse is:
    A. A historical pattern of dominance by more powerful individuals
    B. Poverty
    C. Mental illness among abusers
    D. Alcohol abuse among victims

5. As a medical professional, you should recognize that all of the following actions on your part may help a victim of domestic violence *except*:
    A. Sitting on the same level as the victim while talking with him/her
    B. Insisting that a victim leave the domestically violent situation immediately without any planning
    C. Accepting the idea that anyone, regardless of appearance, can be a victim of domestic violence
    D. Being prepared to consult with colleagues when domestic violence is suspected

---

[*]For answers, see page 347.

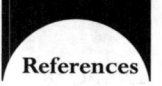

References

1. Wiebe, C. Enlisting your help in the battle against domestic violence. American College of Physicians Observer. 14 (9): 6–7; 1994.
2. Berry, D.B. The Domestic Violence Sourcebook. Contemporary Books, Chicago, 1995.
3. Gelles, R.J. Intimate Violence in Families, Sage Publications, Beverly Hills, CA, 1985.
4. Walker, L.E. The Battered Woman Syndrome. Springer Publishing Co. Inc., New York; 1984.
5. Jones, A. Next Time, She'll Be Dead: Battering and How to Stop It. Beacon Press, Boston; 1994.
6. Straus, M.A., R.J. Gelles & S.K. Steinmetz. Behind Closed Doors: Violence in the American Family. Doubleday & Co. Inc., New York; 1980.
7. Gil, D. Violence Against Children: Physical Child Abuse in the United States. Harvard University Press, Cambridge, MA, 1970.
8. Kempe, C.H., F.N. Silverman, B.F. Steele, W. Droegemueller & H.K. Silver. The battered child syndrome. JAMA 181: 107–112; 1962.
9. Caffey, J. Some traumatic lesions in growing bones other than fractures and dislocations. Br. J. Radiol. 23: 225–238; 1957.
10. Flanzer, J.P. Alcohol and other drugs are key causal agents of violence. In: Gelles, R.J. and Loseke, D.R. (eds). Current Controversies on Family Violence. Sage Publications, Newbury Park, CA, 1993.
11. Gelles, R.J. Through a sociological lens: social structure and family violence. In: Gelles, R.J. and Loseke, D.R. (eds). Current Controversies on Family Violence. Sage Publications, Newbury Park, CA, 1993.
12. Walker, L. The Battered Woman. Harper Row, New York, 1979.
13. Straus, M.A. Physical assaults by wives: a major social problem. In: Gelles, R.J. and Loseke, D.R. (eds). Current Controversies on Family Violence. Sage Publications, Newbury Park, CA, 1993.

Suggested Reading

Alpert, E.J., S. Cohen & R.D. Sege. Family violence: an overview. Academic Medicine. 72: Supplement: S3–S6; 1977.

Alpert, E., R. Sege & Y. Bradshaw. Interpersonal violence and the education of physicians. Acadenic Medicine, 72: Supplement: S41–S50; 1997.

Bronfenbrenner, U. Two Worlds of Childhood: US and USSR. Russell Sage Foundation, 1970.

Cohen, S., E. De Vos & E. Newberger. Barriers to physician identification and treatment of family violence: lessons from five communities. Academic Medicine, 72: Supplement: S19–S25, 1997.

Council on Scientific Affairs, American Medical Association. Violence against women: relevance for medical practitioners. JAMA. 267: 3184–3189; 1992.

Council on Scientific Affairs, American Medical Association. Physicians and domestic violence: ethical considerations. JAMA, 267: 3190–3193; 1992.

Flitcraft, A.H. Violence, values and gender: Editorial. JAMA, 267: 3194–3195; 1992.

Kalichman, S.C. (ed.). Children who witness violence. The Child, Youth and Family Services Quarterly, Div. 37, American Psychological Association, 17 (1); winter 1994.

Pinn, V.W. & M.T. Chunk. The diverse faces of violence: minority women and domestic abuse. Academic Medicine, 72, Supplement, S65–S71; 1997.

Sadler, A.E. (ed.). Family Violence (Current Controversies). Greenhaven Press, Incl. San Diego, CA, 1996.

Short, L.M., D. Cotton & C.S. Hodgson. Evaluation of the module on domestic violence at the UCLA School of Medicine. Academic Medicine, 72, Supplement, S75–S92; 1992.

Straus, M.A. & R.J. Gelles (eds). Physical Violence in American Families: Risk Factors and Adaptations to Violence in 8145 Families. Transaction Publishers, New Brunswick, NJ, 1990.

Sugg, N.K. & T. Inui. Primary care physicians' response to domestic violence: Opening Pandora's Box. JAMA, 267: 3157–3160; 1992.

Swisher, K.L. (ed.). Domestic Violence (Opposing Viewpoints). San Diego, CA, 1996.

Warshaw, C. Intimate partner abuse: developing a framework for change in medical education. Academic Medicine, 72: Supplement: S26–S37; 1997.

Answers to Study Questions

Chapter 5
1. B   2. C   3. True   4. A

Chapter 6
1. B   2. C   3. D   4. A   5. D

Chapter 7
1. C   2. B   3. D   4. A   5. D

Chapter 8
1. C   2. B   3. D   4. C   5. D

Chapter 9
1. B   2. D   3. A   4. D   5. A

Chapter 10
1. C   2. C   3. D   4. D

Chapter 11
1. C   2. C   3. B   4. D   5. B   6. D

Chapter 12
1. C   2. C   3. B   4. D   5. D

Chapter 13
1. A   2. B   3. B   4. B   5. D

Chapter 14
1. D   2. C   3. C   4. C   5. A

Chapter 15
1. B   2. C   3. B   4. A   5. D

Chapter 16
1. B   2. D   3. C   4. A   5. C

Chapter 17
1. C   2. D   3. B   4. D   5. A

Chapter 18
1. C   2. B   3. C   4. A   5. D

Chapter 19
1. D   2. B   3. D

Chapter 20
1. D   2. B   3. C   4. C   5. A

Chapter 21
1. D   2. C   3. B   4. D   5. B

Index

Index

ISBN 0-07-046515-0

90000

9 780070 465152